T0227245

Updates in Abdominal Core Health

Editor

DAVID M. KRPATA

SURGICAL CLINICS
OF NORTH AMERICA

www.surgical.theclinics.com

Consulting Editor
RONALD F. MARTIN

October 2023 • Volume 103 • Number 5

ELSEVIER

1600 John F. Kennedy Boulevard ● Suite 1800 ● Philadelphia, Pennsylvania, 19103-2899

http://www.surgical.theclinics.com

SURGICAL CLINICS OF NORTH AMERICA Volume 103, Number 5
October 2023 ISSN 0039–6109, ISBN-13: 978-0-443-18268-6

Editor: John Vassallo (j.vassallo@elsevier.com)
Developmental Editor: Anita Chamoli

Surgical Clinics of North America (ISSN 0039–6109) is published bimonthly by Elsevier Inc., 360 Park Avenue South, New York, NY 10010-1710. Months of publication are February, April, June, August, October, and December. Business and Editorial Offices: 1600 John F. Kennedy Blvd., Suite 1800, Philadelphia, PA 19103-2899. Periodicals postage paid at New York, NY and additional mailing offices. Subscription prices are $479.00 per year for US individuals, $1045.00 per year for US institutions, $100.00 per year for US & Canadian students and residents, $575.00 per year for Canadian individuals, $1327.00 per year for Canadian institutions, $580.00 for international individuals, $1327.00 per year for international institutions and $250.00 per year for foreign students/residents. To receive student/resident rate, orders must be accompanied by name of affiliated institution, date of term, and the *signature* of program/residency coordinator on institution letterhead. Orders will be billed at individual rate until proof of status is received. Foreign air speed delivery is included in all *Clinics* subscription prices. All prices are subject to change without notice. POSTMASTER: Send address changes to *Surgical Clinics*, Elsevier Health Sciences Division, Subscription Customer Service, 3251 Riverport Lane, Maryland Heights, MO 63043. **Customer Service (orders, claims, online, change of address): Telephone: 1-800-654-2452 (U.S. and Canada); 314-447-8871 (outside U.S. and Canada). Fax: 314-447-8029. E-mail: journalscustomerservice-usa@elsevier.com (for print support); journalsonlinesupport-usa@elsevier.com (for online support).**

Reprints. For copies of 100 or more, of articles in this publication, please contact the Commercial Reprints Department, Elsevier Inc., 360 Park Avenue South, New York, New York 10010-1710. Tel. 212-633-3874, Fax: 212-633-3820, E-mail: reprints@elsevier.com.

Surgical Clinics of North America is also published in Spanish by McGraw-Hill Interamericana Editores S.A., P.O. Box 5-237 06500 Mexico D.F. Mexico; and in Portuguese by Interlivros Edicoes Ltda., Rua Comandante Coelho 1085, CEP 21250, Rio de Janeiro, Brazil; and in Greek by Paschalidis Medical Publications, Athens Greece.

Surgical Clinics of North America is covered in *MEDLINE/PubMed (Index Medicus), EMBASE/Excerpta Medica, Current Contents/Clinical Medicine, Current Contents/Life Sciences, Science Citation Index,* and *ISI/BIOMED.*

Contributors

CONSULTING EDITOR

RONALD F. MARTIN, MD, FACS
Colonel (Retired), United States Army Reserve, Department of General Surgery, Pullman Surgical Associates, Pullman Regional Hospital and Clinic Network, Pullman, Washington

EDITOR

DAVID M. KRPATA, MD, FACS
Associate Professor of Surgery, Cleveland Clinic Lerner College of Medicine, Department of Surgery, Cleveland Clinic Foundation, Cleveland, Ohio

AUTHORS

DIVYANSH AGARWAL, MD, PhD
Department of Surgery, Massachusetts General Hospital, Harvard Medical School, Boston, Massachusetts

LUCAS BEFFA, MD, FACS
Assistant Professor of Surgery, Cleveland Clinic Lerner College of Medicine, Department of Surgery, Cleveland Clinic Foundation, Cleveland, Ohio

NOAH DEANGELO, MD
Department of Surgery, The University of North Carolina at Chapel Hill School of Medicine, Chapel Hill, North Carolina

COLSTON EDGERTON, MD
Assistant Professor of Surgery, Department of Surgery, Novant/New Hanover Regional Medical Center, Wilmington, North Carolina

RYAN ELLIS, MD
General Surgery Resident, Department of Surgery, Cleveland Clinic Lerner College of Medicine, Cleveland Clinic Center for Abdominal Core Health, Cleveland, Ohio

MATTHEW HAGER, MD
Surgical Resident, Department of Surgery, Novant/New Hanover Regional Medical Center, Wilmington, North Carolina

IVY N. HASKINS, MD, DABOM, FASMBS
Assistant Professor, Department of Surgery, University of Nebraska Medical Center, Omaha, Nebraska

ALEXANDRA HERNANDEZ, MD
Surgical Resident, Department of Surgery, Division of General Surgery, University of Washington, Seattle, Washington

RANA M. HIGGINS, MD
Associate Professor, Division of Minimally Invasive and Gastrointestinal Surgery, Medical College of Wisconsin, Milwaukee, Wisconsin

WILLIAM W. HOPE, MD
Associate Professor, Department of Surgery, Novant/New Hanover Regional Medical Center, Wilmington, North Carolina

DAVID M. KRPATA, MD, FACS
Associate Professor of Surgery, Cleveland Clinic Lerner College of Medicine, Department of Surgery, Cleveland Clinic Foundation, Cleveland, Ohio

SARA MASKAL, MD
General Surgery Resident, Department of Surgery, Cleveland Clinic Lerner College of Medicine, Cleveland Clinic Foundation, Cleveland, Ohio

MEGAN MELLAND-SMITH, MD
Department of Surgery, Cleveland Clinic Lerner College of Medicine, Cleveland Clinic Center for Abdominal Core Health, Cleveland, Ohio

NIR MESSER, MD
Department of Surgery, Cleveland Clinic Lerner College of Medicine, Cleveland Clinic Foundation, Cleveland, Ohio

BENJAMIN T. MILLER, MD
Assistant Professor, Department of Surgery, Cleveland Clinic Lerner College of Medicine, Cleveland Clinic Center for Abdominal Core Health, Cleveland, Ohio

LAUREN OTT, PA-C
Mass General Brigham, Newton-Wellesley Hospital, Boston Hernia, Tufts University School of Medicine, Boston, Massachusetts

ERIC M. PAULI, MD
David L. Nahrwold Professor of Surgery, Division of Minimally Invasive and Bariatric Surgery, Department of Surgery, Penn State Health Milton S. Hershey Medical Center, Hershey, Pennsylvania

ARIELLE J. PEREZ, MD, MPH, MS
Associate Professor of Surgery, Division of General and Acute Care Surgery, Department of Surgery, Director, UNC Health Hernia Center, The University of North Carolina at Chapel Hill School of Medicine, Chapel Hill, North Carolina

REBECCA PETERSEN, MD, MSc, FACS
Associate Professor, UW Medicine Hernia Center, Department of Surgery, Division of General Surgery, University of Washington, Seattle, Washington

CLAYTON C. PETRO, MD, FACS
Assistant Professor of Surgery, Department of Surgery, Cleveland Clinic Lerner College of Medicine, Cleveland Clinic Center for Abdominal Core Health, Cleveland, Ohio

BENJAMIN K. POULOSE, MD, MPH
Robert M. Zollinger Lecrone-Baxter Chair and Chief, General and Gastrointestinal Surgery, Department of Surgery, The Ohio State University Wexner Medical Center, Columbus, Ohio

AJITA S. PRABHU, MD, FACS
Program Director, Cleveland Clinic General Surgery Residency Program, Associate Professor of Surgery, Cleveland Clinic Lerner College of Medicine, Cleveland, Ohio

ARCHANA RAMASWAMY, MD, MBA, FACS
Chief of Surgery, Loma Linda Veterans Administration Hospital, Loma Linda, California

MICHAEL REINHORN, MD, FACS
Boston Hernia, Mass General Brigham Newton-Wellesley Hospital, Wellesley, Massachusetts; Clinical Associate Professor in Surgery, Tufts University School of Medicine, Boston, Massachusetts

VICTORIA R. RENDELL, MD
Division of Minimally Invasive and Bariatric Surgery, Department of Surgery, Penn State Health Milton S. Hershey Medical Center, Hershey, Pennsylvania

MICHAEL J. ROSEN, MD
Professor of Surgery, Cleveland Clinic Lerner College of Medicine; Director, Cleveland Clinic Center for Abdominal Core Health, Cleveland, Ohio

KATHRYN A. SCHLOSSER, MD
Associate Professor, Department of Surgery, Prisma Health, Greenville, South Carolina

ROBERT D. SINYARD III, MD, MBA
Fellow, Department of Surgery, Massachusetts General Hospital, Harvard Medical School, Boston, Massachusetts

JEREMY A. WARREN, MD
Vice Chair of Academics, Department of Surgery, Division of Minimal Access Surgery, University of South Carolina School of Medicine, Greenville, South Carolina; General Surgery, Prisma Health, Greenville, South Carolina

THOMAS Q. XU, MD
Division of Minimally Invasive and Gastrointestinal Surgery, Medical College of Wisconsin, Milwaukee, Wisconsin

Contents

Abdominal Core Health: What Is It? 827

Benjamin K. Poulose

Abdominal core health encompasses the stability and function of the abdominal core and associated quality of life. Interventions to maintain core health include surgical and non-surgical therapies that integrate the functional relatedness of the abdominal core components.

Hernia Formation: Risk Factors and Biology 835

Ivy N. Haskins

The incidence of ventral hernias in the United States is in increasing. Herein, the author details the etiology of congenital and acquired ventral hernias as well as the risk factors associated with the development of each of these types of ventral hernias.

Hernia Prevention: The Role of Technique and Prophylactic Mesh to Prevent Incisional Hernias 847

Noah DeAngelo and Arielle J. Perez

Millions of laparotomies are performed annually, carrying up to a 41% risk of developing into a hernia. Incisional hernias are associated with morbidity, mortality, and costs; an estimated $9.6 billion is spent annually on repair of ventral hernias. Although repair is possible, surgeons must prevent incisional hernias from occurring. There is substantial evidence on surgical technique to reduce the risk of incisional hernia formation. This article aims to critically summarize the use of surgical technique and prophylactic mesh augmentation during fascial closure to inform decision-making and reduce incisional hernia formation.

Primary Tissue Repair for Inguinal Hernias: The Shouldice Repair Technique and Patient Selection 859

Divyansh Agarwal, Robert D. Sinyard III, Lauren Ott, and Michael Reinhorn

It is estimated that approximately one in four men and one in 20 women will develop an inguinal hernia over the course of their lifetime. A non-mesh inguinal hernia repair via the Shouldice technique is a unique approach that necessitates dissection of the entire groin region as well as careful assessment for any secondary hernias. Subsequently, a pure tissue laminated closure allows the repair to be performed without tension. Herein, the authors describe a brief overview of inguinal hernias and discuss the relevant patient evaluation, operative steps of the Shouldice procedure, and postoperative considerations.

Inguinal hernias are one of the most common surgical pathologies faced by the general surgeon in modern medicine. The cumulative incidence of an inguinal hernia is around 25% in men and 3% in women. The majority of inguinal hernias can be repaired minimally invasively, utilizing either robotic or laparoscopic approaches.

Chronic postoperative inguinal pain, CPIP, afflicts 10% to 15% of the nearly 700,000 Americans who have inguinal hernia surgery every year. CPIP is challenging to manage because it poses many diagnostic dilemmas that can be overcome with a thorough history, examination, differential diagnosis, and imaging. The initial treatment of CPIP should explore all nonsurgical therapies including medications, physical therapy, interventional pain management and cognitive therapy. When nonoperative methods fail, surgical interventions including neurectomy and hernia mesh removal have proven to be beneficial for patients with CPIP.

Surgical repair of primary umbilical and epigastric hernias are among the most common abdominal operations in the world. The hernia defects range from small (<1 cm) to large and complex even in the absence of prior incision or repair. Mesh has generally been shown to decrease recurrence rates, and its use and location of placement should be individualized for each patient. Open, laparoscopic, and robotic approaches provide unique considerations for the technical aspects of primary repair with or without mesh augmentation.

Patients requiring abdominal wall reconstruction may have medical comorbidities and/or complex defects. Comorbidities such as smoking, diabetes, obesity, cirrhosis, and frailty have been associated with an increased risk of postoperative complications. Prehabilitation strategies are variably associated with improved outcomes. Large hernia defects and loss of domain may present challenges in achieving fascial closure, an important part of restoring abdominal wall function. Prehabilitation of the abdominal wall can be achieved with the use of botulinum toxin A, and preoperative progressive pneumoperitoneum.

to be challenging to perform and remain associated with high rates of postoperative complications and recurrences. In this article, the authors summarize the critical factors to consider when evaluating a patient for PH repair. The authors provide an overview of the current techniques for repair, including both open and minimally invasive approaches. The authors detail the mesh-based repair options and review the evidence for choice of mesh to use for repair.

Despite the heavy reliance of surgeons on mesh with which to repair hernias, less attention is paid to the technical specifications of mesh and/or regulatory processes for bringing medical devices to market during surgical training. This article summarizes some of the key controversies and points regarding mesh materials and regulatory processes related to mesh devices.

A wide array of mesh choices is available for abdominal wall reconstruction, making mesh selection confusing. Understanding mesh properties can make mesh choice simpler. Each mesh has characteristics that determine its durability, ability to clear an infection, and optimal position of placement in the abdominal wall. For clean retromuscular hernia repairs, we prefer bare, heavy weight, permanent synthetic mesh. For contaminated retromuscular abdominal wall reconstruction cases, such as parastomal hernia repairs, we typically use bare, medium weight, permanent synthetic mesh. Biologic and biosynthetic meshes also have acceptable wound event and hernia recurrence rates when used in contaminated cases.

The potential consequences of mesh infection mandate careful consideration of surgical approach, mesh selection, and preoperative patient optimization when planning for ventral hernia repair. Intraperitoneal mesh, microporous or laminar mesh, and multifilament mesh typically require explantation, whereas macroporous, monofilament mesh in an extraperitoneal position is often salvageable. Delayed presentation of mesh infection should raise the suspicion for enteroprosthetic fistula when intraperitoneal mesh is present. When mesh excision is necessary, the surgeon must carefully consider both the risk of recurrent infection as well as hernia recurrence when deciding on single-stage definitive reconstruction versus primary closure with delayed reconstruction.

SURGICAL CLINICS
OF NORTH AMERICA

FORTHCOMING ISSUES

December 2023
Emergency General Surgery
Viren Premnath Punja and
Paul J. Schenarts, *Editors*

February 2024
Liver Transplantation and Transplantation Oncology
Shimul A. Shah, *Editor*

April 2024
Trauma Across the Continuum
Marcie Feinman, *Editor*

RECENT ISSUES

August 2023
Vascular Surgery
Ravi K. Veeraswamy and
Dawn M. Coleman, *Editors*

June 2023
Burn Management
Leopoldo C. Cancio, *Editor*

April 2023
Surgical Decision Making, Evidence, and Artificial Intelligence
Jason R. Bingham, Carly M. Eckert, and
Matthew J. Eckert, *Editors*

SERIES OF RELATED INTEREST

Advances in Surgery
https://www.advancessurgery.com/
Surgical Oncology Clinics
https://www.surgonc.theclinics.com/
Thoracic Surgery Clinics
https://www.thoracic.theclinics.com/

Foreword

Abdominal Core

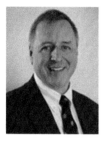

Ronald F. Martin, MD, FACS
Consulting Editor

Of all the statements one hears along the way in learning or practicing surgery, the one that by far and away is most untrue is, "hernia repairs and appendectomies are intern cases." Utter nonsense. Any surgeon who has been around for any length of time will be the first to tell you that a difficult hernia operation—or for that matter a difficult appendectomy—will try the soul of the most capable surgeon. In part, because when these cases are challenging, they are usually *very* challenging. Also, that patients and providers may expect that these cases will be "easy" further ups the emotional ante when they are not easy.

Teaching hernia operations is also an extreme challenge (at least to me) compared with helping someone learn how to do other kinds of cases. I think part of it is our general difficulty trying to explain or even draw three-dimensional structures when making our explanations. Certainly, three-dimensional computer-generated graphics are helpful in showing someone the anatomy, but even with enhanced preoperative demonstration, one still must recognize the structures as they are found in live human anatomy. Maybe virtual reality adjuncts will aid in this one day. For now, however, one must be involved in many of these cases—from whichever approach one chooses—before things actually "click" and a technical comfort level is achieved.

If I were to encourage the reader to take away one concept from the excellent issue compiled by Dr Krpata and his colleagues, it would be this: abdominal wall hernias occur in the abdominal core, and *all* the parts of the abdominal core are related in terms of structure and function. Whether it is the diaphragm, the inguinal canal, lumbar musculature, and so forth, all the parts of the core interrelate, and the forces that are found within the abdominal cavity and pelvis are distributed to the entire abdominal core. Addressing a defect or weakness in one spot will by its very nature redistribute those forces elsewhere in the core.

The contents of the abdominal and pelvic cavities are predominantly fluid in nature; even the solid organs are capable of some amount of deformity. To be sure, there are

Surg Clin N Am 103 (2023) xiii–xiv
https://doi.org/10.1016/j.suc.2023.07.007
0039-6109/23/© 2023 Published by Elsevier Inc.

surgical.theclinics.com

fluids that are compressible, noncompressible, and extremely viscous to the point of bordering on solid, yet fluid, nonetheless. The consequence of that observation is that pressure will largely distribute more or less equally to all the bounding surfaces of the abdominal/pelvic cavity. If one believes the above, then it becomes inherent that the abdominal core is an interrelated three-dimensional structure where alteration anywhere in the structure leads to alterations everywhere in the structure.

When I was first training in surgery, we predominantly focused on the various (and there were many) "this-is-the-only-way-to fix-a-hernia" operations that various staff members believed in. The focus was purely technical and limited to the concern at hand. Honestly, it worked out pretty well for most people most of the time. If we ever paid any real attention to the pathophysiology of hernia formation or recurrence, I can't recall it. We were taught that a true abdominal wall hernia was a "defect in the abdominal parieties through which passes a mesothelial lined sac and its contents." That definition is actually quite useful in that it forces one to consider variations on the theme, such as sliding hernias, that present additional challenges. If one follows the logic of the above, the solution to a hernia always becomes: return the sac and its contents to the proper cavity and obliterate the defect or return it to its proper size. What the concept does not necessarily help us with is what other forces are at play that will help you choose *how* to alter the defect.

The authors of this issue have put together a most helpful collection that will allow the reader to explore the various options of operations to reduce or reposition the sac and contents where they belong and repair the defect by any and all means available to us today. They will also guide the reader through options for prosthetic choice and reinforcement. Most importantly, the issue is all tied together with coherent explanations of three-dimensional anatomic considerations and the forces and pathology that lead to hernia formation as well as the forces that lead to higher likelihoods of postrepair success or failure.

For general surgeons, the repair and prevention of hernias are paramount to most practices. I would encourage anyone who alters the abdominal walls of humans to read this material in its entirety, as every one of these articles is relevant to your practice.

We are deeply indebted to Dr Krpata and his colleagues for assembling this excellent and complete issue for our series.

Ronald F. Martin, MD, FACS
Colonel (Retired), United States Army Reserve
Department of General Surgery
Pullman Surgical Associates
Pullman Regional Hospital and Clinic Network
825 Southeast Bishop Boulevard, Suite 130
Pullman, WA 99163, USA

E-mail address:
rfmcescna@gmail.com

Preface

Abdominal Core Health

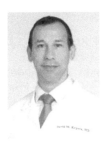

David M. Krpata, MD, FACS
Editor

The most basic definition of a hernia is a defect in the abdominal wall that allows content to go through it that should not. The historical perception of a hernia is one that fosters an inconsequential surgical problem that can often be overlooked and fall to the lap of a recent medical school grad as the "intern's case." As in most medical problems, there is an evolution in the understanding of the disease, which then leads to an advancement in its management. The disease of hernia is no different. Over the last two decades, there has been substantial growth in technique, technology, and appreciation of the abdominal core. Our increased understanding of how defects in the abdominal wall can impact our basic physiology and function has led to the concept of "Abdominal Core Health."

This issue of *Surgical Clinics* begins by introducing the reader to abdominal core health and its importance. As our understanding of how a hernia impacts the core and core physiology expands, the concept of hernia development and hernia prevention grows in importance. These are highlighted in the subsequent articles posing the question to reader: What's more important in prevention, technique or prosthetic? Following this, the reader will be exposed to changes in surgical technique for inguinal hernias that bring back the old as well as introduce the new. The art of primary tissue repair is masterfully described in the article on Shouldice technique. The antithesis is then presented with the latest technology to infiltrate inguinal hernia surgery, robotic inguinal hernia repair. What is quickly learned is that despite the presence of mesh or the presence of technology, chronic postinguinal hernia pain is a reality of inguinal hernia repair that all surgeons should respect.

The subsequent articles show the diversity of ventral hernia disease and the complexities in determining the most appropriate operation for each patient. As issues such as preoperative optimization, mesh position in the abdominal wall, advances in surgical techniques such as component separation, and new technology are discussed, the goal is for readers to understand how to tailor his or her approach to each individual

Surg Clin N Am 103 (2023) xv–xvi
https://doi.org/10.1016/j.suc.2023.04.023
0039-6109/23/© 2023 Published by Elsevier Inc.

surgical.theclinics.com

patient. Finally, the frequently misunderstood world of how medical devices make it to the surgical field is explored as it pertains to hernias. The reader can then use this as a foundation for assessing hernia mesh prosthetics and the management of their complications following abdominal core surgery.

At the end of this issue of *Surgical Clinics*, it is my hope that readers will have found some guidance and a framework to navigate what is most ideal for their patient and provide them with the best abdominal core health.

David M. Krpata, MD, FACS
Department of Surgery
Cleveland Clinic Foundation
9500 Euclid Avenue
Cleveland, OH 44195, USA

E-mail address:
krpatad@ccf.org

Abdominal Core Health
What Is It?

Benjamin K. Poulose, MD, MPH

KEYWORDS

- Abdominal core health • Hernia • Abdominal wall reconstruction

KEY POINTS

- The abdominal core musculature includes the circumferential soft tissues of the diaphragm, pelvic floor, and abdominal wall/flanks.
- Abdominal core health (ACH) describes the stability and function of the abdominal core musculature with associated quality of life.
- Maintenance of core health can include exercise, physical therapy, medical therapy, alternative medical therapies, surgical intervention, and measures to prevent disease (ie, hernia prophylaxis).
- Disease processes impacting ACH include hernia, diastasis, athletic pubalgia/core muscle injury, benign/malignant tumors, and prosthetic/intervention-associated complications.
- Emerging evidence is confirming a key principle of ACH: intervention in one component can impact another component.

HISTORY

The concept of abdominal core health (ACH) is transforming how surgeons think of hernia and abdominal wall diseases. The underlying holistic idea is that the components of the abdominal core musculature including the diaphragm, pelvic floor, and abdominal wall/flanks are functionally related. Extending this idea to include the lower back completes the functional relationships of the trunk (**Fig. 1**) that allows patients to run, jump, sit, stand, twist, work, exercise, urinate, and defecate without issue. Two ideas of physics also are important to maintain ACH. Laplace's law, as applied to the abdominal core musculature, describes that tension on the abdominal wall is directly proportional to pressure within the abdomen and to the 'radius' of the abdominal cavity and inversely proportional to the thickness of the abdominal wall. Pascal's principle describes that pressure exerted in the abdominal core is transmitted equally and undiminished to all parts of the core musculature. These two rules can only be

Center for Abdominal Core Health, Department of Surgery, The Ohio State University Wexner Medical Center, Doan Hall N729, 410 West 10th Avenue, Columbus, OH 43210, USA
E-mail address: Benjamin.poulose@osumc.edu
Twitter: @BKP_Columbus (B.K.P.)

Surg Clin N Am 103 (2023) 827–834
https://doi.org/10.1016/j.suc.2023.04.012
0039-6109/23/© 2023 Elsevier Inc. All rights reserved.

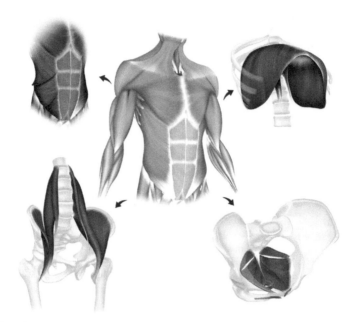

Fig. 1. The related components of the abdominal core musculature include the diaphragm superiorly, pelvic floor inferiorly, and abdominal wall and flanks anterolaterally. The lower back also plays an important role in core stability and function. These components work together to maintain ACH. An increasing body of evidence informs us that intervention on one part of the core musculature can affect other components. (*Courtesy of* the Abdominal Core Health Quality Collaborative Foundation; with permission.)

applied to the abdominal cavity/abdominal core musculature if we think of the system as an enclosed space that is functionally related. Any surgeon who has established pneumoperitoneum to perform minimally invasive surgery has proven these concepts. It is interesting to note that surgeons widely accept this law and principle, but we often fail to recognize the clinical application of the related components of the abdominal core musculature.

ACH encompasses the stability and function of the abdominal core musculature with associated quality of life (QoL). Maintenance of core health can include exercise, physical therapy, medical therapy, alternative medical therapies, surgical intervention, and measures to prevent disease (ie, hernia prophylaxis). Disease processes impacting ACH include hernia, diastasis, athletic pubalgia/core muscle injury, benign/malignant tumors, and prosthetic/intervention-related complications (**Box 1**).[1] The repair of

---

Box 1
Disease processes impacting abdominal core health

Hernia

Diastasis

Athletic pubalgia/core muscle injury

Benign and malignant tumors

Prosthetic and intervention-related complications

hernia, in most of its forms, is one of the most common interventions performed by surgeons to positively impact ACH.

Expanding the field's identity beyond hernia surgery is also important for several reasons. Many surgeons caring for abdominal wall issues address many problems beyond hernia including diastasis, core muscle injuries, and tumors. Certainly, the management of hernia makes up a large part of our practices, but is not the sole disease process the skillset is used to address. Also, there is a connotation in the lay public that hernia is a disease associated with the male sex, largely due to inguinal hernia demographics. In fact, hernia disease can significantly impact women's health.[2] Incisional hernia often affects more women than men, with worse outcomes. Post-partum diastasis remains one of the most poorly studied entities affecting ACH that negatively affects millions of women. Despite this known impact on women, the US health system largely regards surgical correction of this entity as a cosmetic procedure—precluding coverage by most insurance companies. In effect, we are penalizing women for having children. Finally, hernia surgery is the only General Surgery subspecialty that defines itself by a single disease process alone rather than by the true breadth of the field such as Transplant Surgery, Acute Care Surgery, Cardiac Surgery, Colorectal Surgery, Surgical Oncology, or Vascular Surgery.

CURRENT EVIDENCE

A clinically useful, reliable, and feasible test to assess abdominal core function or stability in the context of hernia repair has remained elusive. Generally speaking, most assessments after hernia repair have focused on QoL. This is reasonable in the long term, but misses an opportunity to increase patient engagement during the recovery period. Patients undergoing certain types of knee surgery are followed in the postoperative period with close measurements of knee extension. This important surrogate of success is incredibly motivational for both patients and providers. It would be ideal if a similar surrogate marker existed for hernia repair. Criss and colleagues measured abdominal core function using isokinetic and isometric analyses via Biodex dynamometry before and 6 months after Rives-Stoppa abdominal wall reconstruction (AWR). They found improvements in both measurements and in abdominal wall-specific QoL.[3] Chaudhari and colleagues developed a novel test to assess abdominal core stability, as opposed to core function. In this evaluation, the Quiet Unstable Sitting Test (QUeST), patients are asked to sit motionless with arms crossed and eyes closed for 60 seconds on a BOSU balance trainer which has been placed on a force plate (**Fig. 2**). The center-of-pressure excursion distance is measured and graphically evaluated. Not only was this found to be a test that can be administered in a practical clinical setting, QUeST was able to identify that patients with hernia had less core stability than control patients without hernia.[4] The results of these promising assessments for both core function and core stability deserve further investigation into practical application and patient engagement in the context of hernia repair and AWR.

To date, surgeons have a had a narrow view of the benefits of hernia repair. Our discussions with patients largely center around relieving pain at the hernia site, improving abdominal wall-related QoL, and lowering the risk of acute incarcerated and/or strangulation events. It is interesting that this limitation exists as most abdominal wall-specific QoL measures take a much more holistic approach to assess success. For example, the Hernia-Related Quality of Life Survey and Carolinas Comfort Scale collectively include questions related to activities of daily living, exercise, movement, sexual function, and psychosocial well-being.[5,6] Many of the complex activities

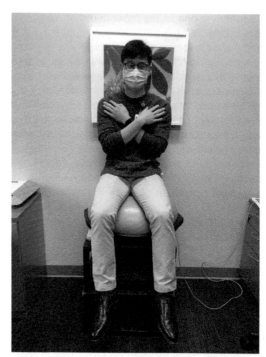

Fig. 2. The QUeST measure of core stability. A participant sits on a BOSU ball with an underlying force plate tracking center-of-pressure excursion (COPexc). The entire assembly is placed on a flat table ensuring that the patient's feet are dangling. Participants are asked to sit unmoving with eyes closed for three 60-second trials while counting backward from 60 to 0. A 1-minute rest is allowed between each of the three trials. The mean COPexc is used as a measure of postural sway representative of core stability. (*From* Chaudhari AMW, Renshaw SM, Breslin LM, et al. A Quiet Unstable Sitting Test to quantify core stability in clinical settings: Application to adults with ventral hernia. Clin Biomech (Bristol, Avon). 2022;93:105594; with permission.)

measured within these instruments are assessments of abdominal core function. That is, they assess the interconnectedness of the components of the abdominal core musculature after repair of one of the components (anterior abdominal wall/flanks).

Most experienced surgeons will relate stories of patients in whom back pain, urinary function, sexual function, and the ability to defecate have improved after hernia repair or AWR. Unfortunately, these have largely been passing observations. The experiences of these patients represent the limited knowledge we have regarding indications for hernia repair and other operations involving abdominal core musculature. An increasing body of work demonstrates that hernia repair goes well beyond simply 'fixing holes' in the abdominal wall. Haskins and colleagues showed in a small prospective cohort that Quebec Back Pain Disability Scale scores improved after AWR. Concomitant improvement was also seen in the hernia related quality of life survey (HerQLes) assessment in these patients. Interestingly, no changes were observed in the Sahrmann Core Stability Test, suggesting this particular assessment of core stability may not be appropriate for this population of patients.[7] In a remarkable body of work, Olsson and colleagues evaluated the success of linea alba plication in women with abdominal core dysfunction secondary to post-partum rectus diastasis. They prospectively evaluated 60 women up to 3 years after surgical intervention and found that both core muscle strength and stability increased. Surprisingly, measures of pelvic function including the Urogenital Distress Inventory and Incontinence Impact Questionnaire both improved after surgical intervention. Koo and colleagues described a plausible mechanism relating diaphragm dysfunction with ventral hernia. Using a 'Piston in Cylinder' model they showed that patients with large anterior abdominal wall hernias have less diaphragmatic excursion than patients with normal abdominal walls.[8] Even simple binder use was able to improve diaphragmatic excursion. Licari and colleagues[9] convincingly showed that patients undergoing ventral hernia repair had significant improvement in postoperative peak expiratory flow 3 years after surgical intervention (**Box 2**).

In addition to re-thinking the benefits of surgical intervention for known problems of the abdominal wall (eg, hernia, diastasis, abdominal wall tumors), two additional modalities of maintaining ACH are worth mentioning: hernia prophylaxis and the use of movement therapy/physical therapy in the perioperative period. First, hernia prophylaxis is gaining prominence as an accepted means preventing hernia formation. The importance of prophylaxis cannot be overstated. In patients undergoing resection for most types of abdominal malignancy, the cumulative incidence of incisional hernia formation at 2 years is 41%.[10] Schlosser and colleagues have demonstrated that a small 1% decrease in hernia formation achieved through reduction of recurrence of hernia prophylaxis can save the US health care system nearly $140 million annually in hospitalization costs alone. This can include a small bites fascial closure technique that has been shown in a randomized controlled trial to reduce incisional hernia formation rates by 38% 1 year after initial laparotomy.[11] The data for mesh use in the prevention of midline incisional hernia formation are encouraging. Jairam and colleagues[12] reported a randomized controlled trial showing a 40% reduction in hernia formation at 2 years with sublay mesh reinforcement and 57% reduction with onlay mesh. The results for prevention of parastomal hernia formation are mixed. In the most recent Cochrane systematic review including 10 randomized controlled trials with 844 total participants, a reduction in parastomal hernia formation was noted with the use of prophylactic mesh, but the heterogeneity of the methods, and large variation in long-term follow-up methods, greatly limited the overall conclusions.[13] Interestingly, the use of mesh for parastomal hernia prophylaxis is more widely accepted than for midline hernia prophylaxis largely because of the generally dismal outcomes with parastomal hernia repair. The main issue that has not been adequately assessed is the level of harm incurred with the use of prophylactic mesh. Although probably low-rate, having this information would help better advise patients, who currently do not have hernias, on the risks of mesh placement.

Probably one of the most underutilized modalities to improve outcomes in abdominal core surgery in general and hernia repair specifically involves movement/physical therapy. Similar to Orthopedic procedures, operative intervention on the abdominal

---

Box 2
Evidenced-based non-traditional symptom improvement after ventral hernia repair

Pulmonary function

Pelvic floor function

Abdominal core function

Abdominal core stability

wall involves manipulation and augmentation of one of the most dynamic areas of the body. An increasing body of evidence informs us that movement therapy can improve outcomes in patients undergoing operative intervention. Using data from the Abdominal Core Health Quality Collaborative (ACHQC), Renshaw and colleagues[14] demonstrated that ventral hernia repair patients with higher preoperative activity levels had lower odds of experiencing any complication after elective repair. Perez and colleagues[15] draw an interesting analogy between AWR and tendon repair as being collagen-based repairs that rely on movement and proscribed physical therapy for proper healing. In a small clinical trial, preoperative physical therapy was shown to have some benefit in terms of lung function after upper abdominal operations.[16] The effect of physical therapy on ventral hernia outcomes is an active area of investigation with results of ongoing prospective trials forthcoming. In a national survey of ACHQC surgeons, physical therapy was perceived to have high benefits for patients.[17] The lack of high-level empiric data to show benefit was a main barrier to the wider use of physical therapy for hernia patients.

CLINICAL RELEVANCE

The clinical relevance of ACH concepts is immediate and beneficial. Having discussions with patients about maintenance of core health over time can help motivate patients to adopt healthier lifestyles and additional therapeutic modalities in the context of undergoing hernia repair or AWR. For surgeons, re-thinking hernia from a single episode of 'fixing a hole' to a wider view of a patient's experience over time is important. Nearly every instance of long-term data have shown that recurrence rates after both ventral and inguinal hernia increase with time.[18–20] This information should inform surgeons and patients accordingly. For some patients, hernia repair may actually be a 'one and done' experience. However, with many patients, especially those with incisional hernias, having a hernia becomes a chronic disease that will need a coherent strategy over time to maintain the patient's ACH. This may involve an array of interventions performed over many years including physical therapy, movement, hernia prophylaxis, and repeat surgical interventions for recurrence (**Box 3**). Reframing conversations between patients and surgeons in this context can be very beneficial to correctly set expectations.

In addition to improving QoL with hernia repair, we can begin to think of additional benefits of stabilizing the abdominal wall in terms of improving pulmonary dysfunction, pelvic floor issues, and abdominal core function/stability. Certainly, an increasing body of evidence will need to be accrued to more definitively advise patients of specific benefits, moving away from the concept of simply 'fixing a hole.'

ACH also incorporates an area of abdominal wall practice that many specialists discover: the intersection of Surgical Oncology and abdominal wall disease

---

Box 3
Ways to maintain abdominal core health

Exercise

Physical Therapy

Medical Therapy (compression garment, binder, truss use)

Alternative Medical Therapies (acupuncture, therapeutic yoga)

Surgical Intervention

Measures to prevent disease (hernia prophylaxis)

management. With up to 41% of patients undergoing abdominal surgery for malignancy developing hernias, early surgical repair can have a positive result on cancer survivorship.[21] Many patients presenting with cancer issues involving the abdominal wall do not have hernias in the traditional sense but can require resection of the abdominal wall due to tumor invasion. The resultant defect created often requires advanced myofascial release techniques and judgment afforded by surgeons with expertise in abdominal wall management. This area of practice, which does not involve traditional hernias, is an important contribution to the maintenance of ACH for the cancer patient.

SUMMARY

The concept of ACH is already transforming how surgeons approach the management of the abdominal wall. By moving away from dwelling on a single disease process—hernia—and focusing on maintaining health, providers can embrace the true breadth of the field and its benefits to patients. A practical concept recognizes that the components of the abdominal core musculature including the diaphragm, pelvic floor, and abdominal wall/flanks function in concert with each other and the lower back to enable our daily activities.

CLINICS CARE POINTS

- Physical therapy can be an important adjunct to the routine care of the hernia patient.
- Emerging evidence informs of that stabilization of the anterior abdominal wall can have positive impacts on other areas of the abdominal core components.
- The concept of abdominal core health encompasses the breadth of the field.

DISCLOSURE

Dr B.K. Poulose receives salary support from the Abdominal Core Health Quality Collaborative and researcher grants from BD Interventional and Advanced Medical Solutions.

REFERENCES

1. Poulose BK, Adrales GL, Janis JE. Abdominal core health-a needed field in surgery. JAMA Surg 2019. https://doi.org/10.1001/jamasurg.2019.5055.
2. Cherla DV, Poulose B, Prabhu AS. Epidemiology and disparities in care. Surg Clin 2018;98:431–40.
3. Criss CN, Petro CC, Krpata DM, et al. Functional abdominal wall reconstruction improves core physiology and quality-of-life. Surgery 2014;156:176–82.
4. Chaudhari AMW, Renshaw SM, Breslin LM, et al. A Quiet Unstable Sitting Test to quantify core stability in clinical settings: application to adults with ventral hernia. Clin Biomech 2022;93:105594.
5. Heniford BT, Lincourt AE, Walters AL, et al. Carolinas comfort scale as a measure of hernia repair quality of life: a reappraisal utilizing 3788 international patients. Ann Surg 2018;267:171–6.
6. Krpata DM, Schmotzer BJ, Flocke S, et al. Design and initial implementation of HerQLes: a hernia-related quality-of-life survey to assess abdominal wall function. J Am Coll Surg 2012;215:635–42.

7. Haskins IN, Prabhu AS, Jensen KK, et al. Effect of transversus abdominis release on core stability: short-term results from a single institution. Surgery 2019;165:412–6.

8. Koo P, Gartman EJ, Sethi JM, et al. Physiology in Medicine: physiological basis of diaphragmatic dysfunction with abdominal hernias–implications for therapy. J Appl Phys 2015;118:142–7.

9. Licari L, Campanella S, Carolla C, et al. Abdominal wall incisional hernia repair improves respiratory function: results after 3 years of follow-up. Hernia 2021;25:999–1004.

10. Baucom RB, Ousley J, Beveridge GB, et al. Cancer survivorship: defining the incidence of incisional hernia after resection for intra-abdominal malignancy. Ann Surg Oncol 2016;23:764–71.

11. Deerenberg EB, Harlaar JJ, Steyerberg EW, et al. Small bites versus large bites for closure of abdominal midline incisions (STITCH): a double-blind, multicentre, randomised controlled trial. Lancet 2015;386:1254–60.

12. Jairam AP, Timmermans L, Eker HH, et al, PRIMA Trialist Group. Prevention of incisional hernia with prophylactic onlay and sublay mesh reinforcement versus primary suture only in midline laparotomies (PRIMA): 2-year follow-up of a multicentre, double-blind, randomised controlled trial. Lancet 2017;390:567–76.

13. Jones HG, Rees M, Aboumarzouk OM, et al. Prosthetic mesh placement for the prevention of parastomal herniation. Cochrane Database Syst Rev 2018. https://doi.org/10.1002/14651858.CD008905.pub3.

14. Renshaw SM, Poulose BK, Gupta A, et al. Preoperative exercise and outcomes after ventral hernia repair: Making the case for prehabilitation in ventral hernia patients. Surgery 2021;170:516–24.

15. Perez JE, Schmidt MA, Narvaez A, et al. Evolving concepts in ventral hernia repair and physical therapy: prehabilitation, rehabilitation, and analogies to tendon reconstruction. Hernia 2021;25:1–13.

16. de Toledo Piza Soares SM, Nucci LB, de Carvalho da Silva MM, et al. Pulmonary function and physical performance outcomes with preoperative physical therapy in upper abdominal surgery: a randomized controlled trial. Clin Rehabil 2013;27:616–27.

17. Renshaw S, Peterson R, Lewis R, et al. Acceptability and barriers to adopting physical therapy and rehabilitation as standard of care in hernia disease: a prospective national survey of providers and preliminary data. Hernia 2022;26:865–71.

18. Burger JWA, Luijendijk RW, Hop WCJ, et al. Long-term follow-up of a randomized controlled trial of suture versus mesh repair of incisional hernia. Ann Surg 2004;240:578–83 [discussion: 583-585].

19. Köckerling F, Koch A, Lorenz R, et al. How long do we need to follow-up our hernia patients to find the real recurrence rate? Front Surg 2015;2:24.

20. Luijendijk RW, Hop WCJ, van den Tol MP, et al. A comparison of suture repair with mesh repair for incisional hernia. N Engl J Med 2000;343:392–8.

21. Feng MP, Baucom RB, Broman KK, et al. Early repair of ventral incisional hernia may improve quality of life after surgery for abdominal malignancy: a prospective observational cohort study. Hernia 2019;23:81–90.

Hernia Formation
Risk Factors and Biology

Ivy N. Haskins, MD, DABOM

KEYWORDS

- Acquired hernia • Congenital hernia • Hernia • Incisional hernia • Risk factor

KEY POINTS

- Ventral hernias may be either congenital or acquired.
- The most common congenital ventral hernia is an umbilical hernia.
- Most congenital ventral hernias heal on their own and do not require surgical management.
- The most common acquired ventral hernia is an incisional hernia.
- Patient and surgery risk factors impact the likelihood of incisional hernia occurrence.

INTRODUCTION

A hernia is defined as a protrusion of a structure or part of a structure through the tissues that normally contain it.[1] Ventral hernias (VHs) occur when there is a defect in the fascia of the abdominal wall with a hernia sac containing peritoneum. VHs may be congenital or acquired, and their formation is often multifactorial.[1,2] Currently, more than 600,000 VH repairs (VHRs) are performed annually in the United States, with an estimated annual cost of $9.7 billion dollars.[3,4] Unfortunately, VH and VHR remain under studied. Therefore, there is a lack of awareness of the true incidence of VH and risk factors associated with their formation.[4] Herein, the author details what is currently known about the etiology and treatment of congenital abdominal wall hernias as well as the risk factors associated with acquired VH.

ETIOLOGY OF CONGENITAL UMBILICAL HERNIAS

Congenital umbilical hernias (UHs) are defined as UHs that are present at birth. The ventral body wall begins to form during the third week of gestation with differentiation of the mesoderm.[1,2,5] As the embryo begins its three-dimensional fold during the fourth week of life, the primitive umbilical cord develops at the site of the umbilical ring.[5] The

Department of Surgery, University of Nebraska Medical Center, 983280 Nebraska Medical Center, Omaha, NE 68198-3280, USA
E-mail addresses: ivhaskins@unmc.edu; ivhaskins@gmail.com
Twitter: @IvyNHaskinsMD (I.N.H.)

Surg Clin N Am 103 (2023) 835–846
https://doi.org/10.1016/j.suc.2023.04.020
0039-6109/23/© 2023 Elsevier Inc. All rights reserved.

surgical.theclinics.com

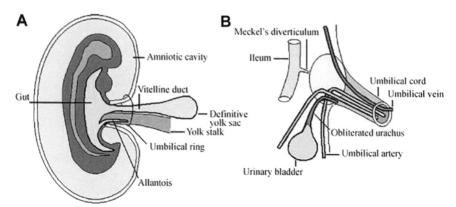

Fig. 1. (*A*) Primitive umbilical cord and (*B*) definitive umbilical cord. (*From* Hegazy, A.A. Anatomy and embryology of umbilicus in newborns: a review and clinical correlations. Front. Med. 10, 271–277 (2016); with permission.)

primitive umbilical cord contains the definitive yolk sac, which is connected to the amniotic cavity by the mesoderm-containing vitelline duct. During the sixth week of gestation, the midgut herniates through the primitive umbilical cord. The midgut then returns to the amniotic cavity during the 10th to 12th weeks of gestation. Reduction of the midgut back into the amniotic cavity leads to development of the definitive umbilical cord, which contains two veins and one artery surrounded by a collagenous mesoderm matrix known as Wharton's jelly as well as a sheath of amniotic fluid (**Fig. 1**).[6] As the embryo continues to develop, the definitive umbilical cord fuses with the linea alba and rectus abdominis musculature.[2] Fusion of the definitive umbilical cord with the linea alba and the rectus abdominis musculature facilitates formation of the umbilical cicatrix stalk and closure of the abdominal wall fascia as the umbilical veins and artery obliterate to form the falciform and umbilical ligaments (**Fig. 2**).[2] The umbilical stalk, including the area of the abdominal wall immediately adjacent to it, is the weakest part of the abdominal wall. A congenital UH is the result of abnormal development of the umbilical ring and failure of the umbilical cicatrix stalk to form.[7]

RISK FACTORS FOR CONGENITAL UMBILICAL HERNIAS

UHs are present in approximately 20% of newborns in the United States. Several risk factors have been identified to be associated with congenital UH. Genetic risk factors include a family history of congenital UH, autosomal trisomies, including trisomy 21 (Down syndrome) and trisomy 18 (Edward syndrome), metabolic disorders, including hypothyroidism and mucopolysaccharidoses (due to an associated large definitive umbilical cord), and congenital growth disorders, including Beckwith-Wiedemann syndrome and Marfan syndrome.[7,8] Black infants are more likely to have an UH compared with white infants.[8] Finally, any disorder that increases intra-abdominal pressure (IAP) in the newborn increases the risk for a congenital UH.[7] Some examples of potential risk factors for increased IAP include high gestational weight, pyloric stenosis, duodenal atresia, neonatal liver failure with associated ascites, and constipation.[7]

MANAGEMENT OF CONGENITAL UMBILICAL HERNIAS

Most congenital UHs resolve on their own without surgical repair because the umbilical ring continues to contract after birth.[9] Newborns with an underlying congenital

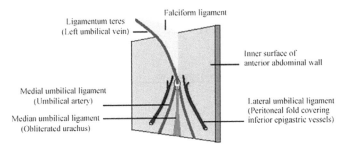

Fig. 2. Orientation of the falciform ligament and the median and medial umbilical ligaments relative to the umbilical ring. (*From* Hegazy, A.A. Anatomy and embryology of umbilicus in newborns: a review and clinical correlations. Front. Med. 10, 271–277 (2016); with permission.)

growth disorder, those with untreated increased IAP, and those with fascial defects ≥ 1.5 cm are more likely to have a persistent UH defect requiring surgical repair. Because most congenital UH close on their own, it is recommended that surgical repair be postponed until 4 to 6 years of age.[6,7,10] The only exception to this timing of repair is for fascial defects ≥ 1.5 cm as they are less likely to close spontaneously, irrespective of the age of the child and are associated with an increased risk of bowel incarceration and strangulation.[10] In the case of larger fascial defects, it is recommended that elective repair is performed once the child is 2 years of age.[7,8]

OTHER CONGENITAL ABDOMINAL WALL HERNIAS

Omphalocele and gastroschisis lead to congenital abdominal wall hernias. Omphalocele results when the midgut fails to return to the amniotic cavity during fetal development. Omphalocele can be differentiated from gastroschisis as the contents have a protective lining of Wharton's jelly and amniotic fluid because the abdominal wall defect is through the umbilical ring.[8] Gastroschisis occurs when there is an abdominal wall defect to the right of the umbilical ring through which the intestines protrude without a protective lining.[8] The cause of omphalocele and gastroschisis is unknown, and the treatment is aimed at fluid resuscitation of the newborn and gradual (omphalocele) or urgent (gastroschisis) reduction of the abdominal contents back into the abdominal cavity.[8] Subsequent abdominal wall hernia formation following the treatment of either omphalocele or gastroschisis is inherent to the small abdominal cavity and increased IAP in newborns with either of these disorders.

SUMMARY OF CONGENITAL ABDOMINAL WALL HERNIAS

Congenital abdominal wall hernias are predominately UHs. Because umbilical cicatrix stalk formation continues after birth, upward of 80% of pediatric UHs will close spontaneously.[6,7,10] Pediatric UHs with a fascial defect ≥ 1.5 cm and any baby demonstrating signs of bowel incarceration or strangulation require earlier and more urgent repair. **Table 1** further summarizes the types and management of congenital abdominal wall hernias.

ACQUIRED VENTRAL HERNIAS

For the purposes of this article, acquired VHs are defined as hernias diagnosed during adulthood. The author recognizes that this definition excludes a proportion of

Table 1
Summary of congenital abdominal wall hernias

Congenital Abdominal Wall Hernia Type	Timing of Hernia Appearance	Management
1. Umbilical Hernia	At Birth	Watchful waiting until 4–6 y of age unless fascial defect $\geq$ 1.5 cm or incarcerated
2. Omphalocele	After reduction of contents back into the abdominal cavity	Elective ventral hernia repair when older
3. Gastroschisis	After reduction of contents back into the abdominal cavity	Elective ventral hernia repair when older

congenital abdominal wall hernias that went unnoticed until adulthood and are thus misdiagnosed as acquired congenital VH. Acquired VH can be further classified as primary (or spontaneous) VH and incisional VH. Most of the VHs are acquired and the most common acquired VH is an incisional hernia (IH). The underlying etiology and risk factors that lead to the development of primary and incisional acquired VH vary to some degree and are further detailed below.

ETIOLOGY OF PRIMARY ACQUIRED VENTRAL HERNIAS

Primary acquired VHs include epigastric and UH. According to the European Hernia Society classification of primary and incisional abdominal wall hernias, an epigastric hernia is defined as an abdominal wall hernia that occurs from 3 cm below the xiphoid until 3 cm above the umbilicus, whereas an UH is an abdominal wall hernia that occurs from 3 cm above the umbilicus to 3 cm below the umbilicus.[10] Epigastric hernias account for approximately 4% of all VH, whereas UHs account for approximately 15% of all VH.[10,11]

There are two main explanations for the development of primary epigastric hernias. The most accepted explanation for the development of epigastric hernias is that proposed by Moschcowitz, which states that epigastric hernias are the result of vascular arcades perforating the linea alba.[12] At the site of vascular arcade perforation of the linea alba, a space is created between the transversalis fascia and the peritoneum of the abdominal wall, which facilitates progression of this space to a fascial defect that often contains incarcerated preperitoneal fat.[10,12] An alternative explanation for epigastric hernia formation is that proposed by Askar, which argues that epigastric hernias form due to a decreased number of decussating fascial fibers across the midline and/or due to opposite and unequal pressures occurring along vertical fibers of the abdominal wall that run from the diaphragm to a mid-point between the xiphoid and the umbilicus.[10,13]

Primary UHs are the result of weakness around the umbilical cicatrix stalk. Interestingly, the area surrounding the umbilical cicatrix stalk is weaker than the umbilical cicatrix stalk itself, resulting in most UH actually being periumbilical in location.[1] In addition to the area around the umbilical cicatrix stalk being weak, there is one additional explanation for the development of primary UH, which was proposed by Fathi and colleagues In their article published in 2012, they describe five different umbilical ring patterns based on the location and length of the falciform ligament and median and medial umbilical ligaments relative the umbilical ring. As described earlier in this article, the umbilical ring obliterates to form the umbilical cicatrix stalk as the umbilical artery and veins develop into the falciform and umbilical ligaments. More specifically, the left umbilical vein becomes the falciform ligament, the umbilical artery becomes the paired medial umbilical ligaments, and the obliterated urachus becomes the median umbilical ligament.[5] **Table 2** describes the five types of umbilical ring patterns, which are also displayed in **Fig. 3**. It is thought that the type 3 umbilical ring pattern is protective against UH formation due to coverage of the entire umbilical ring by the falciform ligament.

RISK FACTORS FOR PRIMARY ACQUIRED EPIGASTRIC AND UMBILICAL HERNIAS

Known risk factors for the development of a primary acquired epigastric hernias include extensive and repetitive coughing, such as that which occurs with uncontrolled chronic obstructive pulmonary disease (COPD), intense physical training, and in a patient who is overweight or obese.[14] The impact of these risk factors on the development of a primary acquired epigastric hernia can be explained by the previously described mechanisms for epigastric hernia formation. All three factors may lead to both increased space between the transversalis fascia and peritoneum in addition to increased strain on the vertical abdominal wall muscle fibers. Other potential risk factors for primary acquired epigastric hernia formation include older age, male sex, nicotine use, chronic steroid use, and diabetes mellitus (DM).[14]

Known risk factors for primary acquired UH include factors that lead to increased IAP and connective tissue disorders.[11] Factors that lead to increased IAP include pregnancy, especially multiparity and multiple pregnancies (twins, triplets, and so forth), ascites, obesity, chronic constipation, peritoneal dialysis, uncontrolled COPD, and intense physical activity. Connective tissue disorders associated with primary acquired UH include lathyrism, Marfan syndrome, Loeys–Dietz syndrome, and Ehlers–Danlos syndrome. Lathyrism is an acquired connective tissue disorder that inhibits collagen cross-linking when people eat a diet high in grass peas, whereas Marfan syndrome, Loeys–Dietz syndrome, and Ehlers–Danlos syndrome are all heritable connective tissue disorders.[15,16]

ETIOLOGY OF INCISIONAL VENTRAL HERNIAS

Incisional VHs occur at any location along the anterior abdominal wall through which surgery was previously performed, including both in the midline and along the lateral anterior abdominal wall. The incidence of IH ranges from less than 1% at the site of previous ports to greater than 50% at the site of an ileostomy or colostomy.[2,4,17–20] There is some variation in the cause of port site hernias, parastomal hernias, and midline and lateral abdominal wall IH. Nevertheless, a simplified explanation for the development of an IH is that it results from tissue trauma and an imbalance between tension and counter-tension created by the different forces along the anterior abdominal wall.[2]

RISK FACTORS FOR THE DEVELOPMENT OF AN INCISIONAL VENTRAL HERNIA

Risk factors for the development of an IH can be organized into several different categories. For the purposes of this article, the author divides these risk factors into patient factors and surgical factors. Patient factors include associated comorbidities, such as nicotine use, older age, male sex, obesity, COPD, DM, chronic steroid use, malnutrition, history of previous wound infection, collagen vascular disorder, chronic constipation, ascites, repetitive heavy lifting, pregnancy, and previous pelvic radiation therapy. Surgical risk factors include emergency surgery, surgical approach used (open vs minimally invasive), number and size of surgical ports used (if a minimally

Table 2 Umbilical ring pattern types	
Type	Description
1	Round UR, RL attached to top of UR, MDL, and MNL attached to the bottom of the UR
2	Slitted UR, RL, MDL, and MNL all attached to slit
3	Round UR, RL covers the UR and ends where the MNL begins at the bottom of the UR, MDL attached to bottom of UR
4	Round UR, RL bifurcates and attaches to either side of the UR, MDL and MNL attached to the bottom of the UR
5	Round UR, RL attached to the top of UR, MDL and MNL fuse before attached to the bottom of the UR

Abbreviations: MDL, medial umbilical ligament; MNL, median umbilical ligament; RL, round ligament; UR, umbilical ring.

invasive operation was performed), type and length of suture material used for abdominal wall closure, suture technique used for abdominal wall closure, location of incisions, use of mesh, presence of an ileostomy or colostomy, and surgeon volume.

PATIENT RISK FACTORS FOR INCISIONAL VENTRAL HERNIA

Under perfect conditions, tissue strength following surgery will only ever be 80% as strong as it was before surgery, with an additive decrease in strength with each subsequent operation.[21] The strength of an incision depends on the organized cascade of cell signaling, tissue growth factors, and cell migration that is responsible for wound healing and ultimately leads to type I collagen deposition and collagen cross-linking.[15] If any step of the wound healing process is impaired, the overall strength of the incision decreases and the risk for IH increases.

Postoperative wound events are associated with an increased risk for IH due to increased inflammation at the surgical site.[21,22] Inflammation impairs all phases of wound healing and increases the risk for acute wound dehiscence and evisceration as well as long-term IH formation.[15] Patient factors that have previously been found to be associated with an increased risk of postoperative wound events include nicotine use, DM, chronic steroid use, malnutrition, history of wound infection, and previous pelvic radiation therapy.

The proposed mechanism for the association of nicotine use with postoperative wound infections includes tissue hypoxia, decreased oxidative capacity of neutrophils, alterations in the ratio of type I to type III collagen, and an increase in protease degradation of connective tissue.[23] Hyperglycemia associated with DM also blunts the normal cell cycle cascade required for wound healing in addition to impairment of cell-mediated immunity.[24] Chronic steroid use and malnutrition are both associated with decreased collagen synthesis and an overall decrease in the amount of type I collagen present in wounds.[15,25] Previous wound infections have been proposed to harbor bacteria that may lead to a subsequent wound infection.[22] Finally, previous pelvic radiation therapy reduces wound angiogenesis and increases oxygen free radicals, which impair the normal cell cycle cascade for wound healing.[26]

Increased IAP is another risk factor for IH formation.[27] During periods of increased IAP, the abdominal wall must conform to compensate for the bulging of the abdominal viscera against the anterior abdominal wall. If the tension from increased IAP exceeds the failure tension of the anterior abdominal wall, a hernia results.[27] Similar to

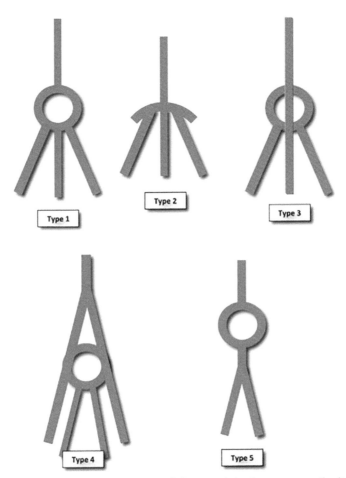

Fig. 3. Umbilical ring is the circle or spherical shape and the ligaments are the linear struc-tures. (*From* Fathi AH, Soltanian H, Saber AA. Surgical anatomy and morphologic variations of umbilical structures. Am Surg. 2012;78(5):540-544; with permission.)

postoperative wound events, increased IAP is associated with both early wound dehiscence and evisceration as well as IH formation over the long term. Patient fac-tors that lead to an increase in IAP include obesity, COPD, ascites, repetitive heavy lifting, chronic constipation, and pregnancy (especially multiparity and multiple pregnancies).

Finally, with respect to patient risk factors for hernia formation, patients with abnormal collagen deposition are at an increased risk for developing IH. These include older patients, male sex, and patients with collagen vascular disorders. Both older age and male sex are associated with decreased collagen synthesis.[27,28] This decrease in collagen synthesis in older and male patients is primarily driven by differences in sys-temic estrogen concentrations.[28,29] As mentioned above, Marfan syndrome, Loeys–Dietz syndrome, and Ehlers–Danlos syndrome are inherited collagen vascular disor-ders that impair collagen synthesis and deposition and lathyrism is an acquired collagen vascular disorder that inhibits collagen cross-linking in patients who eat high concentrations of grass peas.[15,16]

ROLE OF PATIENT COMORBIDITY OPTIMIZATION IN PREVENTING INCISIONAL HERNIA FORMATION AND RECURRENCE

In 2010, the Ventral Hernia Working Group developed a grading system for the risk of postoperative surgical site occurrences which was later modified by Rosen and colleagues (**Fig. 4**).[30,31] The purpose of these grading systems is to help identify patient comorbidities that if modified preoperatively, may lead to more durable VHR. Recently, impact of these patient comorbidities on postoperative outcomes following VHR has been found to be cumulative.[32] Although there have been other proposed VH risk calculators and recent studies that have shown that some of the previously identified patient risk factors may not actually be associated with an increased risk for postoperative wound events or IH, the author would recommend that when able to do so, the above listed patient comorbidities and risk factors be optimized before elective VHR.[22,32–35]

SURGICAL RISK FACTORS FOR INCISIONAL VENTRAL HERNIA

There are several surgery-specific risk factors associated with an increased risk of postoperative IH. First, emergency surgery is associated with an increased risk of postoperative IH due to the absence of preoperative patient optimization, increased length of the wound, increased likelihood of postoperative wound events, and the increased potential for wound ischemia (in cases of abdominal wall trauma) and inability to achieve primary fascial closure.[15,36] Open abdominal or pelvic surgery is associated with a higher risk of IH compared with minimally invasive surgery.[15] Further, bladed trocars, ports ≥ 10 mm in size, and single-incision minimally invasive surgery all have increased rates of IH due to increased tissue trauma.[17,18,37] With respect to the orientation of the incision, vertical midline incisions have the greatest risk of IH as the midline of the abdominal wall is the area of greatest tension from the wound closure and counter-tension from the lateral abdominal wall myofascial complexes and they are associated with greater disruption of the abdominal wall collagen bundles, which are oriented transversely.[2,15,37] The need for ileostomy or colostomy creation at the time of surgery is also associated with an increased risk of IH. The risk of parastomal hernia formation is higher for diverting ostomies compared with end ostomies and for colostomies compared with ileostomies. The risk of parastomal hernia formation is likely multifactorial but is related to the inherent abdominal wall defect required for ostomy creation as well as the contaminated nature of ostomy creation.[19,20]

There are also several components to closure of the abdominal wall that impact the likelihood of IH. Based on currently available literature, slowly resorbable or permanent monofilament suture is recommended over fast absorbing or multifilament suture for closure of the abdominal wall. A suture to wound length of at least 4 to 1 is recommended.[38] In addition, the "small bites technique" incorporating only fascia in a running or continuous fashion is associated with a decreased risk of IH compared with large bites that include muscle and fascia or closure of the abdominal wall using an interrupted or figure-of-eight technique.[37,38] A summary of the guidelines, which were published by the European Hernia Society, is detailed in **Table 3**. Finally, there are recent data to suggest that placement of prophylactic mesh at the time of abdominal wall closure and abdominal wall closure by higher volume surgeons may also be associated with a decreased risk of IH.[39–41]

SUMMARY OF ACQUIRED VENTRAL HERNIAS

Most of abdominal wall hernias are acquired. Acquired abdominal wall hernias may be either primary (or spontaneous) or result from previous abdominal or pelvic surgery.

A

Grade 1 *Low Risk*	Grade 2 *Co-Morbid*	Grade 3 *Potentially Contaminated*	Grade 4 *Infected*
• Low risk of complications • No history of wound infection	• Smoker • Obese • Diabetic • Immunocompromised • COPD	• Previous wound infection • Stoma present • Violation of the gastrointestinal tract	• Infected mesh • Septic Dehiscence

B

Grade 1 *Low Risk*	Grade 2 *Co-Morbid*	Grade 3 *Contaminated*
• Low risk of complications • No history of wound infection	• Smoker • Obese • Diabetic • COPD • History of Wound Infection	• Clean-contaminated • Contaminated • Dirty

Fig. 4. Evolution of the Ventral Hernia Working Group grades. (*A*) Original Ventral Hernia Working Group grades and (*B*) modified Ventral Hernia Working Group grades.

Table 3
Summary of European Hernia Society guidelines for abdominal wall closure

Recommendation	Strength of Recommendation
1. Non-midline incisions are recommended when possible.	Strong
2. Continuous suturing for closure of midline abdominal wall incisions in elective surgery is recommended.	Strong
3. The use of rapidly absorbable suture material for closure of midline abdominal wall incisions in elective surgery is not recommended.	Strong
4. Using slowly resorbable over nonabsorbable suture for continuous closure of midline abdominal wall incisions in elective surgery is suggested.	Weak
5. Monofilament suture material should be used for midline abdominal wall incisions.	Weak
6. The use of monofilament sutures impregnated with antibiotics is not advised because of insufficient data.	Weak
7. A single aponeurotic layer of closure is recommended for elective, midline abdominal wall incisions.	Weak
8. A suture to wound length of 4–1 for continuous closure is suggested.	Weak
9. The "small bites technique" for continuous closure of midline incisions is suggested.	Weak
10. No recommendation on suture material or suturing technique for use in emergency surgery can be given.	N/A
11. No recommendation on suture material or suturing technique for use in non-midline incisions can be given.	N/A

There are several patient and surgery-specific risk factors associated with acquired abdominal wall hernias. Preoperative optimization of patient comorbidities and closure of the abdominal wall as recommended by the European Hernia Society may lead to a decreased incidence of IHs over time.

DISCLOSURE

The author has nothing to disclose.

REFERENCES

1. Earle DB, McLellan JA. Repair of Umbilical and Epigastric Hernias. Surg Clin North Am 2013;93(5):1057–89.
2. Miller HJ, Novitsky YW. Chapter 52 – Ventral Hernia and Abdominal Release Procedures. In: Yeo CJ, editor. Shackelford's surgery of the alimentary tract, 2 volume Set. 8th edition. Philadelphia, PA: Elsevier; 2019. p. 571–89.
3. Gillies M, Anthony L, Al-Roubaie A, et al. Trends in Incisional and Ventral Hernia Repair: A Population Analysis from 2001 to 2021. Cureus 2023;15(3):e35744.
4. Schlosser KA, Renshaw SM, Tamer RM, et al. Ventral Hernia Repair: An Increasing Burden Affecting Abdominal Core Health. Hernia 2022. https://doi.org/10.1007/s10029-022-02707-6.
5. Hegazy AA. Anatomy and Embryology of Umbilicus in Newborns: A Review and Clinical Correlations. Front Med 2016;10(3):271–7.
6. Lassaletta L, Fonkalsrud EW, Tovar A, et al. The Management of Umbilical Hernias in Infancy and Childhood. J Pediatr Surg 1975;10(3):405–9.
7. Troullioud Lucas AG, Jaffar S, Mendez MD. Pediatric Umbilical Hernia. In: StatPearls [Internet]. Treasure Island, FL: StatPearls Publishing; 2023.
8. Abhyankar A, Lander AD. Umbilical Disorders. Surgery 2004;22(9):214–7.
9. Poenaru D. Disorders of the Umbilicus in Infants and Children: A Consensus Statement of the Canadian Association of Paediatric Surgeons. Paediatrc Child Health 2001;6(6):312–3.
10. Muysoms FE, Miserez M, Berrevoet F, et al. Classification of Primary and Incisional Abdominal Wall Hernias. Hernia 2009;13(4):407–14.
11. Coste AH, Jaafar S, Parmely JD. Umbilical Hernia. In: StatPearls [Internet]. Treasure Island, FL: StatPearls Publishing; 2023.
12. Moshcowitz AV. Epigastric Hernia without Palpable Swelling. Ann Surg 1917;66(3):300–7.
13. Askar OM. Aponeurotic Hernias. Recent Observations Upon Paraumbilical and Epigastric Hernias. Surg Clin North Am 1984;64(2):315–33.
14. Ponten JEH, Somers KYA, Nienhuijs SW. Pathogenesis of the Epigastric Hernia. Hernia 2012;16(6):627–33.
15. Franz MG. The Biology of Hernia Formation. Surg Clin North Am 2008;88(1):1, vii.
16. Meester JAN, Verstraeten A, Schepers D, et al. Differences in Manifestations of Marfan Syndrome, Ehlers-Danlos Syndrome, and Loeys-Dietz Syndrome. Ann Cardiothorac Surg 2017;6(6):582–94.
17. Bunting DM. Port-Site Hernia following Laparoscopic Cholecystectomy. J Soc Laparoendosc Surg 2010;14(4):490–7.
18. Agaba EA, Rainville H, Ikedilo O, et al. Incidence of Port-Site Incisional Hernia after Single-Incision Laparoscopic Surgery. J Soc Laparoendosc Surg 2014;18(2):204–10.

19. Temple B, Farley T, Popik K, et al. Prevalence of Parastomal Hernia and Factors Associated with its Development. J Wound Ostomy Continence Nurs 2016;43(5): 489–93.
20. Rieger N, Moore J, Hewett P, et al. Parastomal Hernia Repair. Colorectal Dis 2004; 6(3):203–5.
21. Smith J, Parmely JD. Ventral Hernia. In: StatPearls [Internet]. Treasure Island, FL: StatPearls Publishing; 2023.
22. Blatnik JA, Krpata DM, Novitsky YW, et al. Does a history of wound infection predict postoperative surgical site infection after ventral hernia repair? Am J Surg 2012;203(3):370–4.
23. Sørensen LT, Himmingsen UB, Kirkeby LT, et al. Smoking is a risk factor for incisional hernia. Arch Surg 2005;140(2):119–23.
24. Wilson RB, Farooque Y. Risk and prevention of surgical site infection after hernia mesh repair and the predictive utility of ACS-NSQIP. J Gastrointest Surg 2022; 26(4):950–64.
25. Wicke C, Halliday B, Allen D, et al. Effects of steroids and retinoids on wound healing. Arch Surg 2000;135(11):1265–70.
26. Wagh Y, Menon A, Mody B, et al. Radiation-induced wound infections in operated soft tissue sarcomas: an unbelievable challenge in a series of five cases. J Orthop Case Rep 2020;10(1):30–4.
27. Soucasse A, Jourdan A, Edin L, et al. A better understanding of daily life abdominal wall mechanical solicitation: investigation of intra-abdominal pressure variations by intragastric wireless sensor in humans. Med Eng Phys 2022. https:// doi.org/10.1016/j.medengphy.2022.103813.
28. Jorgensen LN, Sorensen LT, Kallehave F, et al. Premenopausal women deposit more collagen than men during healing of an experimental wound. Surgery 2002;131(3):338–43.
29. Lenhardt R, Hopf HW, Marker E, et al. Perioperative collagen deposition in elderly and young men and women. Arch Surg 2000;135(1):71–4.
30. Ventral Hernia Working Group, Brueing K, Butler CE, Ferozco S, et al. Incisional ventral hernias: review of the literature and recommendations regarding the grading and technique of repair. Surgery 2010;148(3):544–8.
31. Kanters AE, Krpata DM, Blatnik JA, et al. Modified hernia grading scale to stratify surgical site occurrence after open ventral hernia repairs. J Am Coll Surg 2012; 215(6):787–93.
32. Alkhatib H, Tastaldi L, Krpata DM, et al. Impact of modifiable comorbidities on 30-day wound morbidity after open incisional hernia repair. Surgery 2019;166(1): 94–101.
33. Petro CC, Haskins IN, Tastaldi L, et al. Does active smoking really matter before ventral hernia repair? an AHSQC analysis. Surgery 2019;165(32):406–11.
34. Haskins IN, Krpata DM, Prabhu AS, et al. Immunosuppression is not a risk factor for 30-day wound events or additional 30-day morbidity or mortality following open ventral hernia repair: an analysis of the americas hernia society quality collaborative. Surgery 2018;164(3):594–600.
35. Haskins IN, Olson MA, Stewart TG, et al. Development and validation of the ventral hernia repair outcomes reporting app for clinician and patient engagement (ORACLE). J Am Coll Surg 2019;229(3):259–66.
36. Kaafarani HMA, Kaufman D, Reda D, et al. Predictors of surgical site infection in laparoscopic and open ventral incisional herniorrhaphy. J Surg Res 2010;163(2): 229–34.

37. Muysoms FE, Antoniou SA, Bury K, et al. European hernia society guidelines on the closure of abdominal wall incisions. Hernia 2015;19(1):1–24.
38. Deerenberg EV, Harlaar JJ, Steyerberg EW, et al. Small bites versus large bites for closure of abdominal midline incisions (STITCH): A double-blind, multicentre, randomised controlled trial. Lancet 2015;386:1254–60, 10000.
39. Borab ZM, Shakir S, Lanni MA, et al. Does prophylactic mesh placement in elective, midline laparotomy reduce the incidence of incisional hernia? a systematic review and meta-analysis. Surgery 2017;161(4):1149–63.
40. Smith L, Coxon-Meggy A, Shinkwin M, et al. Happy to close?" the relationship between surgical experience and incisional hernia rates following abdominal wall closure in colorectal surgery. Colorect Dis 2023. https://doi.org/10.1111/codi.16537.
41. Christophersen C, Fonnes S, Baker JJ, et al. Surgeon volume and risk of reoperation after laparoscopic primary ventral hernia repair: a nationwide register-based study. J Am Coll Surg 2021;233(3):346–56.

Hernia Prevention

The Role of Technique and Prophylactic Mesh to Prevent Incisional Hernias

Noah DeAngelo, MD[a], Arielle J. Perez, MD, MPH, MS[b],*

KEYWORDS

- Hernia prevention • Mesh augmentation • Prophylaxis • Fascial closure

KEY POINTS

- Incisional hernia formation can be as high as 41% after laparotomy.
- Technical factors, within the surgeon's control, such as the location of the incision, closure technique, and materials, have been shown to reduce the risk of hernia formation.
- Non-midline incisions are associated with a reduced risk of incisional hernia formation.
- Monofilament, absorbable suture closure in a 4:1 ratio, using a running technique and ensuring to take small bites of fascia, is recommended to prevent incisional hernia formation.
- Onlay and retromuscular prophylactic mesh augmentation has been shown to decrease the risk of incisional hernia formation with minimal increase in other complications.

INTRODUCTION

Prevention has become a fundamental principle of modern medicine, with specific practices and policies aimed at preventing and optimizing risk for development of common ailments. Successfully integrated in primary care and general internal medicine, primary prevention strategies, such as vaccinations and smoking cessation, and secondary strategies, such as colonoscopies and mammograms to detect early cancer are widely accepted. However, this focus has only been used sparingly in surgery. With the expansion of outcomes-based surgical research, there has been an increased focus on identifying and optimizing high-risk patients that could benefit from early intervention and preventative strategies to reduce the risk of incisional hernia formation.

[a] Department of Surgery, University of North Carolina at Chapel Hill, 101 Manning Drive, Chapel Hill, NC 27514, USA; [b] The University of North Carolina at Chapel Hill, Department of Surgery, 160 Dental Circle, Burnett-Womack, CB #7228, Chapel Hill, NC 27599-7228, USA
* Corresponding author.
E-mail address: arielle_perez@med.unc.edu

Surg Clin N Am 103 (2023) 847–857
https://doi.org/10.1016/j.suc.2023.04.021
0039-6109/23/© 2023 Elsevier Inc. All rights reserved.

surgical.theclinics.com

Incisional hernias present a commonly encountered problem associated with high morbidity, mortality, and cost. Over the years, there has been a significant focus on discovering the most efficacious ways to repair these hernias when they occur with several different techniques and innovations revolutionizing how surgeons manage these hernias. However, incisional hernias and their associated complications remain a significant problem for patients and their providers. Ideally, surgeons must try to prevent an incisional hernia from occurring in the first place.

With that in mind, there has been substantial research to define the optimum technique for primary abdominal closure and reduce the risk of hernia formation. Despite this, the incidence of hernia formation remains high and seems to be increasing. This article aims to critically summarize the use of surgical technique and prophylactic mesh during fascial closure to improve knowledge, inform decision-making, and reduce incisional hernia formation.

BACKGROUND

Incisional hernias are a known and frequent complication of abdominal surgery. It is estimated that over 2 million laparotomies are performed annually in the United States for benign conditions alone.[1] Prior studies had estimated that at least 20% of patients who undergo a laparotomy will develop an incisional hernia.[2] However, newer data show hernia incidence can be as high as a 28% after laparotomy for benign disease and 41% for malignant disease.[3,4] With this increased incidence, it is no surprise that spending on ventral hernia repair in the United States has tripled from $3.2 billion for over 348,000 repairs in 2012 to $9.6 billion for over 610,000 repairs in 2022.[5,6]

Laparotomy and the subsequent development of incisional hernias are associated with significant morbidity, cost, and decreased quality of life.[5–8] These hernias can be associated with pain, discomfort, and negative cosmetic appearance, which significantly reduce a patient's quality of life. Most importantly, incisional hernias pose a risk for incarceration and strangulation requiring emergency surgery leading to even further associated increased morbidity and mortality.[9,10]

The development of an incisional hernia is multifactorial. Patient factors, including age, body mass index (BMI), gender, smoking status, and malnutrition, are known to increase the risk for incisional hernia development.[11–13] Perioperative factors, such as occurrence of surgical site infection, acuity of surgery (elective vs emergent), and early return to activity can impede the ability for proper wound healing and in turn increase incisional hernia formation.[3,12,14] Technical factors, at the control of the surgeon during the time of operation, such as the location of the incision, tissue handling, suturing technique, and choice of materials, have been shown to reduce the risk of hernia formation.[15,16] Although some elements are immutable, both patient and surgeon must work in concert to reduce risk factors and enhance the potential for optimal healing of the fascial closure to reduce incisional hernia formation.

SURGICAL TECHNIQUE: ABDOMINAL WALL INCISION

Abdominal incisions can be made in a midline, transverse (ie, Pfannenstiel), oblique (ie, Kocher and McBurney incisions), or paramedian manner (**Fig. 1**).[17] In a large systematic review, the risk of incisional hernia formation was found to be significantly less with non-midline incisions—transverse versus midline (relative risk [RR] = 1.77; 95% confidence interval [CI], 1.09–2.87) and paramedian versus midline (RR = 3.41; 95% CI, 1.02–11.45).[18] Although the 2005 Cochrane came to similar conclusion of the superiority of transverse over midline incisions, they tempered their

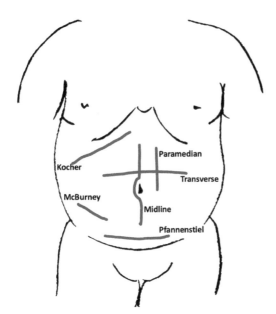

Fig. 1. Abdominal incisions.

findings due to the heterogeneity of studies and clinical situations and stated "the optimal incision for abdominal surgery still remains the preference of the surgeon."[19] Similarly, non-midline incisions made for minimally invasive specimen extraction sites have been shown in an randomized control trial (RCT) of midline versus transverse incision for colon extraction had a statistically significant lower incidence of incisional hernia formation.[20]

SURGICAL TECHNIQUE: PRIMARY FASCIAL CLOSURE

Several studies have examined the optimal suture closure technique for laparotomy incisions. These often include type of suture (absorbable vs nonabsorbable, slowly vs rapidly absorbable, monofilament vs multifilament), closure method (individual anatomic layers vs en masse closure), and closure technique (continuous vs interrupted, small bite vs large bite).

Previous meta-analyses have supported the use of slowly absorbable or nonabsorbable sutures in a continuous running technique when compared with rapidly absorbing sutures in an interrupted fashion.[21] However, a 2017 Cochrane review found suture absorption (absorbable vs nonabsorbable, slow vs fast absorbable), closure method (mass vs layered), and closure technique (continuous vs interrupted) showed no difference in the risk of incisional hernia formation, infection, and wound dehiscence.[22] The only variable which demonstrated a lower risk of incisional hernia formation was the use of a monofilament suture when compared with multifilament suture (RR 0.76, 95% CI 0.59–0.98).[23] As well, absorbable sutures had lower risk of developing chronic draining sinuses compared with permanent sutures.[23] Owing to speed, ability to distribute tension along the incision and reduced foreign body material in the wound, the most recent 2022 guidelines for abdominal wall incisional closure supported by the European and American Hernia Societies recommend continuous suturing.[17]

Several prior studies have suggested that a suture length to wound length ratio of at least 4:1 during laparotomy closure reduces incisional hernia formation.[23,24] This can be achieved by taking large bites which are father apart but incorporate more tissue or small tissue bites closer together. Two large RCTs have demonstrated a statistically significant reduction in incisional hernia rates at 1 year when using a small bite technique.[25,26] The small bite technique in both trials used a 2 to 0 slowly absorbable suture on a small 20 to 31 mm needle, "biting" 5 to 8 mm from the wound edge and including only fascia while avoiding muscle and fat with each bite (**Fig. 2**).

Despite the heterogeneity in studies, there seems to be good evidence and clinical application to support incisional closure using a monofilament absorbable suture closure using a running technique. A minimum of a 4:1 suture length to incision length ratio should be achieved with the suture by take small fascial bites while avoiding fat and muscle entrapment.

SURGICAL TECHNIQUE: PROPHYLACTIC MESH AUGMENTATION

The data supporting mesh use during hernia repair have been quite compelling, decreasing the incidence of hernia recurrence from 63% to 32%.[27,28] For this reason, mesh use has been extrapolated to laparotomy incision closure as an additional strategy to reinforce the abdominal wall and reduce incisional hernia formation. For prophylactic mesh augmentation (PMA), mesh can be placed in three defined locations: (1) underlay, (2) sublay, and (3) onlay (**Fig. 3**).

Onlay mesh involves the placement of mesh above the muscles, anterior to the fascia. Reminiscent of the hernia repair technique described by Chevrel, the midline

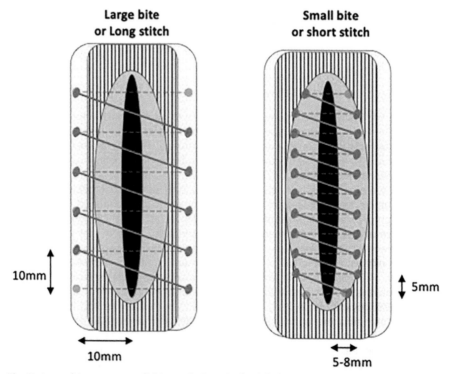

Fig. 2. Large bite versus small bite technique in fascial closure.

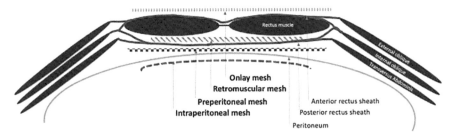

Fig. 3. Mesh placement for prophylactic mesh augmentation.

fascia is first closed then the anterior rectus sheath cleared by creating lipocutaneous flaps on both sides, often requiring the division of periumbilical perforator vessels.[29] Unlike, Chevrel's technique where flaps of the anterior rectus sheath are mobilized and flipped medially to strengthen the midline closure, onlay PMA is much simpler and leaves the anterior sheath intact. Mesh is then either tacked or glued to the anterior sheath.

Sublay mesh for PMA is most commonly placed in the retrorectus plane, posterior to the rectus muscle but anterior to the posterior sheath. Reminiscent of the hernia repair techniques described by Rives and Stoppa, the rectus sheath is opened and the retrorectus space cleared, taking care to avoid injury to the epigastric vessels and lateral neurovascular bundles.[30] To exclude the viscera, the posterior rectus sheath is first closed using an absorbable suture. Mesh is then placed in the retrorectus space and the anterior sheath closed in the manner of a primary fascial closure as above. Sublay mesh for PMA can also be placed in the preperitoneal plane—sandwiched between the posterior rectus sheath and peritoneum. This less commonly performed technique can often be quite difficult if the patient does not have a robust peritoneum.

The underlay position involves the fixation of mesh in the intraperitoneal abdominal plane. Similar to the sublay placement, underlay mesh for PMA provides the theoretic advantage of distributing tension of intra-abdominal pressures across the abdominal wall. However, intraperitoneal mesh against the viscera increases the risk of complications such as fistulization.

OUTCOMES OF PROPHYLACTIC MESH AUGMENTATION

The first published study evaluating PMA was a 1998 RCT where a Polyglactin quickly absorbable synthetic mesh was placed in the intraperitoneal space in obese patients after open gastroplasty—this showed no difference in incisional hernia formation.[31] Since then, however, there have been multiple RCT studies as well as meta-analyses demonstrating the effectiveness of PMA. Much like the real world, these studies have been performed in heterogeneous patient populations with varying closure techniques. Multiple RCTs have included clean-contaminated and contaminated cases, including bariatric and colorectal cases.[31–35] PMA RCTs have used various meshes—biologic, resorbable synthetic, polyester, and the most commonly studied, polypropylene; have used various mesh locations—preperitoneal, retrorectus, onlay, intraperitoneal; and are combined with various methods of primary fascial closure—fast absorbing, permanent and slowly absorbable sutures, and interrupted and running sutures.

With the heterogeneity of studies, multiple systematic reviews and meta-analysis using varying inclusion and exclusion criteria have been performed using up to 20

RCTs on PMA. A 2020 meta-analysis by Jairam and colleagues of 12 RCTs comparing PMA for midline laparotomy to primary fascial closure in 1815 patients demonstrated significantly reduced risk of incisional hernia formation using an onlay (RR 0.26, 0.11–0.67; P = .005) and retromuscular (RR 0.28, 0.10–0.82; P = 0·02) mesh location compared with primary suture alone.[36] No difference in surgical site infections was noted, but a higher seroma risk rate was present for onlay PMA (RR 2.23, 1.10–4.52; P = .03).[36] Similar advantages of retromuscular and onlay PMA as well as increased risk of seroma with onlay PMA have been consistently described in two other separate meta-analyses which evaluated intraperitoneal and preperitoneal PMA mesh placement and primary fascial closure alone.[37,38]

Potential negative consequences of mesh placement on surgical outcomes and complications, including surgical site infection, seroma formation, and chronic pain, must be considered when adopting a new technique such as PMA. In a 2020 meta-analysis by Ahmed and colleagues of 26 studies comparing PMA to primary fascial closure, redemonstrated the reduced the risk of incisional hernia formation and increased risk of seroma formation, but also found an increased risk of chronic wound pain.[39] With subgroup analysis, however, neither seroma nor chronic wound pain showed significant difference. No statistically increased risk of surgical site infection or hematoma was noted in this analysis and others.[38,39]

Reoperation for mesh-related complications after PMA has been described for various reasons such as mesh infection after permanent intraperitoneal composite PMA and partial mesh excision for poor mesh incorporation in the setting of mesh and fascial exposure after onlay polypropylene PMA during emergency laparotomy.[40,41] More alarming was the early termination of an RCT evaluating intraperitoneal biologic PMA during emergency laparotomy due to increased incidence of mesh-related complications requiring surgical reoperation.[42] In current studies describing only 1 to 3 year follow-up after PMA, it can be surmised that similar to Kokotovic's description of an increased incidence of mesh-related complications over time after hernia repair, so too can be mesh-related complications after PMA.[43]

The use of prophylactic mesh for abdominal wall closure has been shown to reduce the risk of incisional hernia at any position. However, the ideal position for PMA remains in question. To date, there has only been one randomized control trial that has compared onlay with retromuscular PMA.[44,45] A total of 480 patients were randomized to receive either primary suture, onlay mesh, or retromuscular mesh closure. The use of mesh for both locations significantly reduced incisional hernia formation when compared with primary closure. However, there was no significant difference between onlay versus retromuscular mesh location. Similar to other studies, onlay PMA was associated with an increased risk of seroma.

When considering PMA, the surgical setting and risks of complications should be evaluated. The RCT comparing retromuscular versus onlay mesh placement showed the risk of seroma formation was significantly greater for patients who had received onlay mesh. However, this was not found to translate into an increased risk for surgical site infection, readmission, or need for reoperation.[45,46] The potential risk of mesh infection is of critical importance considering its associated morbidity and may deter the widespread implementation of prophylactic mesh in elective and otherwise benign abdominal cases. This fear, however, seems to be inconsequential based on multiple RCT and meta-analyses.

MESH SELECTION

There are limited data comparing different types of mesh for PMA. To date, there have been no RCTs comparing different meshes for PMA. Numerous RCTs compare one mesh type (permanent synthetic, biologic, absorbable synthetic) to primary fascial closure. For now, surgeons may need to extrapolate mesh data from hernia repair when comparing mesh.

Trials comparing permanent synthetic mesh to primary fascial closure all found a significant reduction in incisional hernia rates in the synthetic arm, regardless of mesh placement. Costlier biologic and absorbable synthetic mesh has more mixed data. One RCT comparing intraperitoneal biologic PMA to primary suture closure following open Roux-en-Y showed no significant difference in incisional hernia rates after 2-year[35] However, a smaller RCT comparing onlay biologic PMA to primary suture closure after elective AAA repair showed significant reduction in incisional hernia formation after 3-year follow-up.[46] Although the 1998 polyglactin study showed no difference, an RCT of patients undergoing clean-contaminated and contaminated laparotomy had a significant reduction in incisional hernia formation after 2-year follow-up with resorbable Bio-A sublay PMA compared with double-layer midline fascial closure.[47]

ECONOMIC IMPLICATIONS

In addition to the morbidity and mortality of incisional hernias, there is a significant financial burden associated. Incisional hernias have an estimated annual cost approaching $9.7 billion in the United States for nonfederal institutions alone.[6] Although PMA does incur an additional cost for the material itself and increased operating room time associated with mesh placement, there are data to suggest the long-term impact of reducing incisional hernia formation may be overall more cost-effective. A 2015 cost-utility analysis considering the probability of possible scenarios (outcomes, complications, and management) of PMA versus primary fascial closure found PMA to be more cost-effective when considering both direct medical care costs of dealing with the multiple iterations of possible outcomes and indirect patient (ie, lost wages) and societal (ie, productivity loss due to employee absence) costs.[48]

SUMMARY

Incisional hernias are frequently encountered complications of abdominal surgeries and are associated with significant morbidity and cost. There are clear data showing adoption of certain techniques can reduce the risk of incisional hernia formation. Abdominal incisions off the midline can reduce the risk of hernia formation. Primary fascial closure with a monofilament, absorbable suture closure in a 4:1 ratio, using a running technique, and ensuring to take small bites of fascia can reduce the risk of hernia formation.

PMA offers an additional strategy aimed at reducing hernia development and its associated complications. There is convincing evidence to support the use of PMA following midline laparotomy. Research has demonstrated mesh to be effective when placed in the onlay and retromuscular positions when compared with primary suture closure. Even when accounting for increased operating time and placement of a foreign body which can increase the risk for infection, an increased risk for postoperative complications has not been observed with mesh placement. The reduction in postoperative incisional hernia development following mesh placement is cost-effective for both patients and the medical system.

Despite the overwhelming evidence of the efficacy of small bite technique and PMA, implementation remains limited. Application ultimately depends on the surgeon performing the index operation. Barriers can include the lack of knowledge of the most up to date data, additional operative time required, patient and/or surgeon worry about subsequent mesh complications, and surgeon skill to develop the appropriate tissue planes. Although the use of mesh for ventral and incisional hernia repair is becoming common, not all surgeons have a familiarity with mesh placement. Surgeons who do not perform hernia repairs routinely may require additional training and education on these techniques.

CLINICS CARE POINTS

- Incisional hernia formation can be as high as 41% after laparotomy.
- Technical factors, within the surgeon's control, such as the location of the incision, closure technique, and materials have been shown to reduce the risk hernia formation.
- Non-midline incisions are associated with a reduced risk of incisional hernia formation.
- The use of a running, monofilament, absorbable suture during fascial closure in a 4:1 suture length to incision length ratio and ensuring to take small bites of fascia is recommended to reduce incisional hernia formation.
- Onlay and retromuscular prophylactic mesh augmentation has been shown to decrease the risk of incisional hernia formation when compared with primary fascial closure alone and intraperitoneal and preperitoneal prophylactic mesh augmentation.
- Onlay and retromuscular prophylactic mesh augmentation does not increase the risk of surgical site infection, readmission, or need for reoperation.
- Onlay prophylactic mesh augmentation is associated with an increased risk of seroma formation.
- There are limited data to support the use of costlier biologic and absorbable synthetic meshes for prophylactic mesh augmentation.

DISCLOSURE

The authors have nothing to disclose.

REFERENCES

1. DeFrances CJ, Hall MJ. Advance data from vital and health statistics, no.342. 2002 National Hospital Discharge Survey, Vol. 2004. CDC hospital discharge diagnoses from 2002. Hyattsville (MD): National Center for Health Statistics; 2004.
2. Mudge M, Hughes LE. Incisional hernia: a 10 year prospective study of incidence and attitudes. Br J Surg 1985 Jan;72(1):70–1.
3. Hoer J, Lawong G, Klinge U, et al. Factors influencing the development of incisional hernia. A retrospective study of 2983 laparotomy patients over a period of 10 years. Chirurg 2002;73:474–80.
4. Baucom RB, Ousley J, Beveridge GB, et al. Cancer survivorship: defining the incidence of incisional hernia after resection for intra-abdominal malignancy. Ann Surg Oncol 2016;23:764–71.
5. Poulose BK, Shelton J, Phillips S, et al. Epidemiology and cost of ventral hernia repair: making the case for hernia research. Hernia 2012 Apr;16(2):179–83.

6. Schlosser KA, Renshaw SM, Tamer RM, et al. Ventral hernia repair: an increasing burden affecting abdominal core health. Hernia 2022 Dec 26. https://doi.org/10.1007/s10029-022-02707-6.

7. Onyekaba G, Mauch JT, Patel V, et al. The Abdominal Hernia-Q: a critical analysis of the components that impact quality-of-life. Hernia 2022 Jun;26(3):839–46.

8. Smith OA, Mierzwinski MF, Chitsabesan P, et al. Health-related quality of life in abdominal wall hernia: let's ask patients what matters to them? Hernia 2022 Jun;26(3):795–808.

9. Surek A, Gemici E, Ferahman S, et al. Emergency surgery of the abdominal wall hernias: risk factors that increase morbidity and mortality-a single-center experience. Hernia 2021 Jun;25(3):679–88.

10. Hoffman RD, Danos DM, Lau FH. National health disparities in incisional hernia repair outcomes: An analysis of the Healthcare Cost and Utilization Project National Inpatient Sample (HCUP-NIS) 2012-2014. Surgery 2021 Jun;169(6):1393–9.

11. Liang MK, Holihan JL, Itani K, et al. Ventral Hernia Management: Expert Consensus Guided by Systematic Review. Ann Surg 2017 Jan;265(1):80–9.

12. Hope WW, Tuma F. Incisional Hernia. (Updated 2023 Jan 2). In: StatPearls (Internet). Treasure Island (FL): StatPearls Publishing; 2023 Jan-. Available at: https://www.ncbi.nlm.nih.gov/books/NBK435995/.

13. Tubre DJ, Schroeder AD, Estes J, et al. Surgical site infection: the "Achilles Heel" of all types of abdominal wall hernia reconstruction. Hernia 2018 Dec;22(6):1003–13.

14. Dai W, Chen Z, Zuo J, et al. Risk factors of postoperative complications after emergency repair of incarcerated groin hernia for adult patients: a retrospective cohort study. Hernia 2019 Apr;23(2):267–76.

15. Muysoms FE, Antoniou SA, Bury K, et al, European Hernia Society. European Hernia Society guidelines on the closure of abdominal wall incisions. Hernia 2015 Feb;19(1):1–24.

16. Deerenberg EB, Henriksen NA, Antoniou GA, et al. Updated guideline for closure of abdominal wall incisions from the European and American Hernia Societies. Br J Surg 2022 Nov 22;109(12):1239–50. Erratum in: Br J Surg. 2022 Nov 10;: PMID: 36026550.

17. Burger JW, van't Riet M, Jeekel J. Abdominal incisions: techniques and postoperative complications. Scand J Surg 2002;91(4):315–21.

18. Bickenbach KA, Karanicolas PJ, Ammori JB, et al. Up and down or side to side? A systematic review and meta-analysis examining the impact of incision on outcomes after abdominal surgery. Am J Surg 2013;206:400–9.

19. Brown SR, Goodfellow PB. Transverse verses midline incisions for abdominal surgery. Cochrane Database Syst Rev 2005;4:CD005199.

20. Lee L, Mata J, Droeser RA, et al. Incisional hernia after midline versus transverse specimen extraction incision: a randomized trial in patients undergoing laparoscopic colectomy. Ann Surg 2018;268:41–7.

21. Diener MK, Voss S, Jensen K, et al. Elective midline laparotomy closure: the INLINE systematic review and meta-analysis. Ann Surg 2010 May;251(5):843–56.

22. Patel SV, Paskar DD, Nelson RL, et al. Closure methods for laparotomy incisions for preventing incisional hernias and other wound complications. Cochrane Database Syst Rev 2017 Nov 3;11(11):CD005661.

23. Jenkins TP. The burst abdominal wound: a mechanical approach. Br J Surg 1976 Nov;63(11):873–6.

24. Israelsson LA, Jonsson T, Knutsson A. Suture technique and wound healing in midline laparotomy incisions. Eur J Surg 1996 Aug;162(8):605–9.
25. Deerenberg EB, Harlaar JJ, Steyerberg EW, et al. Small bites versus large bites for closure of abdominal midline incisions (STITCH): a double-blind, multicentre, randomised controlled trial. Lancet 2015;386:1254–60.
26. Millbourn D, Cengiz Y, Israelsson LA. Effect of stitch length on wound complications after closure of midline incisions: a randomized controlled trial. Arch Surg 2009;144:1056–9.
27. Luijendijk RW, Hop WC, van den Tol MP, et al. A comparison of suture repair with mesh repair for incisional hernia. N Engl J Med 2000;343(6):392–8.
28. Burger JW, Luijendijk RW, Hop WC, et al. Long-term follow-up of a randomized controlled trial of suture versus mesh repair of incisional hernia. Ann Surg 2004;240(4):578–85. https://doi.org/10.1097/01.sla.0000141193.08524.e7.
29. Chevrel JP. Traitement des grande éventrations médianes par plastie en paletot et prothèse. Nouv Presse Med 1979;24:695–6.
30. Stoppa RE. Wrapping the visceral sac into a bilateral mesh prosthesis in groin hernia repair. Hernia 2003 Mar;7(1):2–12.
31. Pans A, Elen P, Dewé W, et al. Long-term results of polyglactin mesh for the prevention of incisional hernias in obese patients. World J Surg 1998;22:479–82.
32. Strzelczyk JM, Szymański D, Nowicki ME, et al. Randomized clinical trial of postoperative hernia prophylaxis in open bariatric surgery. Br J Surg 2006;93:1347–50.
33. Abo-Ryia MH, El-Khadrawy OH, Abd-Allah HS. Prophylactic preperitoneal mesh placement in open bariatric surgery: a guard against incisional hernia development. Obes Surg 2013;23:1571–4.
34. Sarr MG, Hutcher NE, Snyder S, et al. A prospective, randomized, multicenter trial of Surgisis Gold, a biologic prosthetic, as a sublay reinforcement of the fascial closure after open bariatric surgery. Surgery 2014;156:902–8.
35. García-Ureña MÁ, López-Monclús J, Hernando LA, et al. Randomized controlled trial of the use of a large-pore polypropylene mesh to prevent incisional hernia in colorectal surgery. Ann Surg 2015;261:876–81.
36. Jairam AP, López-Cano M, Garcia-Alamino JM, et al. Prevention of incisional hernia after midline laparotomy with prophylactic mesh reinforcement: a meta-analysis and trial sequential analysis. BJS Open 2020 Jun;4(3):357–68.
37. Tansawet A, Numthavaj P, Techapongsatorn S, et al. Mesh position for hernia prophylaxis after midline laparotomy: A systematic review and network meta-analysis of randomized clinical trials. Int J Surg 2020 Nov;83:144–51.
38. Hassan MA, Yunus RM, Khan S, et al. Prophylactic Onlay Mesh Repair (POMR) Versus Primary Suture Repair (PSR) for Prevention of Incisional Hernia (IH) After Abdominal Wall Surgery: A Systematic Review and Meta-analysis. World J Surg 2021 Oct;45(10):3080–91.
39. Ahmed J, Hasnain N, Fatima I, et al. Prophylactic Mesh Placement for the Prevention of Incisional Hernia in High-Risk Patients After Abdominal Surgery: A Systematic Review and Meta-Analysis. Cureus 2020 Sep 16;12(9):e10491.
40. Lima HVG, Rasslan R, Novo FCF, et al. Prevention of fascial dehiscence with onlay prophylactic mesh in emergency laparotomy: a randomized clinical trial. J Am Coll Surg 2020;230:76–87.
41. Glauser PM, Brosi P, Speich B, et al. Prophylactic Intraperitoneal Onlay Mesh Following Midline Laparotomy-Long-Term Results of a Randomized Controlled Trial. World J Surg 2019 Jul;43(7):1669–75 [Erratum in: World J Surg. 2019 Mar 29;: PMID: 30824961].

42. Jakob MO, Haltmeier T, Candinas D, et al. Biologic mesh implantation is associated with serious abdominal wall complications in patients undergoing emergency abdominal surgery: A randomized-controlled clinical trial. J Trauma Acute Care Surg 2020 Dec;89(6):1149–55.

43. Kokotovic D, Bisgaard T, Helgstrand F. Long-term Recurrence and Complications Associated With Elective Incisional Hernia Repair. JAMA 2016 Oct 18;316(15): 1575–82.

44. Timmermans L, Eker HH, Steyerberg EW, et al. Short-term results of a randomized controlled trial comparing primary suture with primary glued mesh augmentation to prevent incisional hernia. Ann Surg 2015;261:276–81.

45. Jairam AP, Timmermans L, Eker HH, et al. Prevention of incisional hernia with prophylactic onlay and sublay mesh reinforcement *versus* primary suture only in midline laparotomies (PRIMA): 2-year follow-up of a multicentre, double-blind, randomised controlled trial. Lancet 2017;390:567–76.

46. Bali C, Papakostas J, Georgiou G, et al. A comparative study of sutured versus bovine pericardium mesh abdominal closure after open abdominal aortic aneurysm repair. Hernia 2015;19:267–71.

47. Pizza F, D'Antonio D, Arcopinto M, et al. Safety and efficacy of prophylactic resorbable biosynthetic mesh following midline laparotomy in clean/contemned field: preliminary results of a randomized double blind prospective trial. Hernia 2020;24:85–92.

48. Fischer JP, Basta MN, Wink JD, et al. Cost-utility analysis of the use of prophylactic mesh augmentation compared with primary fascial suture repair in patients at high risk for incisional hernia. Surgery 2015 Sep;158(3):700–11.

Primary Tissue Repair for Inguinal Hernias

The Shouldice Repair Technique and Patient Selection

Divyansh Agarwal, MD, PhD[a,1], Robert D. Sinyard III, MD, MBA[a,2], Lauren Ott, PA-C[b,3], Michael Reinhorn, MD[b,*]

KEYWORDS

- Inguinal hernia • Shouldice • Ilioinguinal • Iliohypogastric • External oblique
- Cremaster • Transversalis fascia

KEY POINTS

- All Shouldice repairs should encounter three critical nerves: the iliohypogastric, the ilioinguinal, and the genital branch of the genitofemoral nerve. Although either of the nerves may warrant preservation or ligation depending on their location, care must be taken to prevent their entrapment during the repair.
- In most settings, but especially the emergency setting, it is important to cut the external oblique all the way through the external ring, as this is the point of incarceration for inguinal hernia. By opening up the ring, an incarcerated hernia is more easily reduced, facilitating exposure of the normal anatomy.
- Overtightening the internal ring is a technical complication of a suture only repair, results in cord ischemia, and can be avoided by checking that a surgical instrument can easily slide along the new internal ring and into the preperitoneal space.
- Division of the lateral cremaster fibers, along with the genital branch of the genitofemoral nerve, is critical in providing excellent exposure in the dissection and for repair. In addition, it reduces recurrence and risk of chronic pain.
- Prescription opioids can be avoided in the vast majority of patients through a combination of administration of local anesthetic at the time of surgery and patient education about multimodal pain management strategies.

---

[a] Department of Surgery, Massachusetts General Hospital, Harvard Medical School, Boston, MA, USA; [b] Mass General Brigham, Newton-Wellesley Hospital, Boston Hernia, Tufts University School of Medicine, Boston, MA, USA
[1] Present address: 21 Beacon Street, Apartment 11-L, Boston, MA 02108.
[2] Present address: 44 Martin Street, Apartment 2, Cambridge, MA 02138.
[3] Present address: 20 Walnut Street, Suite 100, Wellesley, MA 02481.
* Corresponding author. 20 Walnut Street, Suite 100, Wellesley, MA 02481.
E-mail address: mreinhorn@gmail.com
Twitter: @divyansh_aga (D.A.)

Surg Clin N Am 103 (2023) 859–873
https://doi.org/10.1016/j.suc.2023.04.001
0039-6109/23/© 2023 Elsevier Inc. All rights reserved.
surgical.theclinics.com

BACKGROUND

Inguinal hernia, by definition, pertains to a protrusion in the groin ("inguen" in Latin means groin, whereas "hernios" is Greek for an offshoot/bud). Reports describe inguinal hernias dating back to the ancient Egyptians and Greeks. For instance, the mummified remains of the pharaoh Merneptah (1215 BC) has been noted to have a groin wound with scrotal separation, suggestive of an attempt at hernia surgery.[1] Roman physician Celsus also has accounts of hernia repairs, dating back to the first century AD. The French surgeon Guy de Chauliac (1298–1368) wrote extensively about various techniques for inguinal hernia repair. However, it was not until the 1880s that the first modern approach to inguinal hernia repair was developed by Edoardo Bassini. He devised a surgical approach dissecting the layers of the inguinal canal and then reconstructing its posterior wall with interrupted sutures.[1] In 1945, the Canadian surgeon Earle Shouldice further built on the principles of the Bassini repair by adding more suture lines to the reconstruction of the posterior wall.[2] This Shouldice technique of hernia repair is the focus of this article.

RELEVANT ANATOMY

To understand the important aspects of a Shouldice repair, the authors begin with a brief overview of the anatomy necessary to appreciate for a successful inguinal hernia repair.

Aponeurosis of the external oblique comprises the majority of the inguinal canal, including its most superficial portion, the lateral and part of the inferior canal. As the external oblique curls around caudally, it creates half of a cylinder, terminating in an edge that extends from the pubic tubercle to the anterior superior iliac spine (ASIS). This "shelving edge," reflection of the external oblique aponeurosis, is interchangeably known as the inguinal ligament or Poupart's ligament. The external oblique aponeurosis inserts into the anterior rectus sheath medially, curls above the public tubercle, often splitting into lateral and medial crus and forms the external inguinal ring.

The upper portion of the inguinal canal cephalad is made of the internal oblique and the rectus sheath. The internal oblique transitions to the cremaster muscle at the point where the deep or internal inguinal ring occurs. The cremaster muscle wraps the spermatic cord circumferentially. The transversalis fascia makes up the deepest part of the inguinal canal with the aponeurosis of the transversus abdominis muscle more superficially. These two layers may be distinct, but often are fused into one thin layer. Posterior or deep to these two fascial layers in the retroperitoneum, the surgeon can find the inferior epigastric vessels, Cooper's ligament, the lacunar ligament, and the femoral canal, which may contain a femoral hernia. Care must be taken to minimize the risk of injury to the epigastric vessels when entering the retroperitoneum.

It is also important to recognize the course of three important nerve structures. In the anterior groin, the genital branch of the genitofemoral nerve has a reliable course, perforating the floor of the inguinal canal at or near where the Cremaster vessels perforate the floor, which lends itself to easy identification. This nerve may also enter the inguinal canal through the internal ring, deep to the cord structures, and often courses together with the posterior Cremaster fibers. The ilioinguinal nerve almost always courses along the cord as it emerges from the internal obliques usually at or near the internal ring. Last, the iliohypogastric nerve is found medial to the ilioinguinal nerve, emerging between the fibers of the internal obliques, lateral and superior to the internal ring. The iliohypogastric nerve courses along the internal oblique musculature, traveling medially along the rectus sheath before perforating the external oblique aponeurosis. Although the aforementioned description of the typical course of the three nerves occurs in a large percentage of patients, surgeons must take care to look for branches of these nerves or alternative paths to minimize injury.

Several other anatomical terms are routinely used in various textbooks on inguinal hernias. For instance, Hesselbach's triangle is often described as an important structure, whose borders describe the site where direct hernias occur. Hasselbach's triangle is made from the aponeurosis of the transversus abdominis and transversalis fascia; however, its borders have little impact on the surgical repair of a direct hernia. Certain texts also describe the "conjoint tendon," as either the fusion of the internal oblique, transversus abdominis, and transversalis fascia or as the structure made of the internal oblique laterally and the lateral edge of the rectus medially. Importantly, in a proper anatomical dissection, rectus abdominis, external oblique, internal oblique, transversus abdominis, and the corresponding aponeuroses are all separate and distinct layers. It is important for the surgeon to identify these layers as disparate entities during dissection and use them appropriately when performing a pure tissue hernia repair.

ETIOLOGY AND PATHOGENESIS

In the presence of a hernia, the normal anatomy of the inguinal canal is altered by definition. The three common types of groin hernias include direct, femoral, and indirect, each with differing causes. Direct hernias are often the results of stretching forces on or diastasis of the transversalis fascia and aponeurosis of the transversus abdominis fascia. When approached anteriorly, the aponeurosis of the transversus abdominis projects as an outpouching and looks like a hernia sac. During a posterior dissection, the transversalis fascia is stretched out and often called a "pseudosac." In contrast, femoral hernias are the result of femoral canal widening, which results in protrusion of tissue medially to the femoral vessels and above Cooper's ligament. This is commonly seen after pregnancy, which causes laxity in the pelvic ligaments.[3]

Indirect hernias account for the majority of hernias in adults and virtually all inguinal hernias in the pediatric population. Their pathogenesis is explained by a patent processus vaginalis during embryological development. In adults, stretching and weakness of the internal inguinal ring morphs the inguinal canal architecture from cylindrical to conal, terminating in the external inguinal ring. Indirect hernias can present at any age, mediated by the underlying changes in abdominal wall architecture. During early years of life, the inguinal canal is akin to a wide-angle cylinder, preventing peritoneal contents from reaching the scrotum. With age comes loss of elastin and collagen fibers, resulting in laxity in the inguinal canal and substantial dilation of the internal ring. As the proximal canal widens compared with the narrower distal canal, the geometry changes to a narrow angle cone, propelling the contents of the abdominal cavity through the canal. Patients often report symptoms from an indirect hernia when the abdominal contents reach the external ring, made of the fibrous and rigid external oblique. The internal ring, which is made of flexible muscular tissue, is therefore also almost never the site of incarcerations.

NATURE OF THE PROBLEM

Inguinal hernias can be symptomatic, causing pain either at rest or with activity. They can also be asymptomatic, only noticeable in specific postures or during a careful physical examination. Patients who tend to be symptomatic often report an uncomfortable bulge in their groin region, most evident after prolonged sitting or standing. In some scenarios, gastrointestinal or genitourinary symptoms may accompany the discomfort or may be the only symptoms. Nausea or emesis with significant lower abdominal or pelvic discomfort may be a sign of acute incarceration or strangulation.

A careful history and physical examination are critical to diagnosing an inguinal hernia. A common history of presenting illness involves the patient describing a palpable mass or bulge with coughing or Valsalva. Except in unusual cases, this history is virtually diagnostic of a hernia and does not require any confirmatory testing. If, however, the history and physician examination are not conclusive, a computed tomography scan (CT) or MRI scan can be used to better elucidate the underlying defect. Distinguishing direct from indirect hernias is usually not feasible on a physical examination. On the other hand, femoral hernias tend to present as a protrusion below the inguinal ligament and medial to the femoral vessels, lending themselves to an easier diagnosis on physical examination. Examination for an inguinal hernia can be performed with a single finger through the scrotum or alternatively using the entire hand to cover the inguinal canal and feeling for a sliding of hernia contents through the external ring. Although the latter is minimally less sensitive at finding small hernias, it is significantly more comfortable for patients.

A core muscle injury is another common cause of groin pain, and it is imperative that the surgeon differentiate between core muscle injury and inguinal hernia before recommending surgery. Patients with a core muscle injury tend to have discomfort at the site of the insertion of the rectus to the pubis or along the adductor muscles. This disease has had many historical names, including sports hernia, athletic pubalgia, or osteitis pubis. One can clinically assess for a core muscle injury by palpating the relaxed and activated hip flexor, adductor, oblique, and rectus muscles. Abdominal flexion or adduction often exacerbates this tenderness. Patients should be examined supine first then with knees bent. A posterior hip tilt may also help alleviate the symptoms. If a core muscle injury is suspected, patients warrant physical therapy for abdominal core strength and conditioning; surgery is rarely needed.

PREPROCEDURE PLANNING

A sizable proportion of patients report minimal to no symptoms from their hernia. These individuals should be offered the choice of surgical intervention versus watchful waiting, the latter of which has been described as a success in greater than 50% of asymptomatic patients 10 years after the diagnosis of small inguinal hernia. However, a symptomatic hernia should be surgically repaired, especially if it has been determined that the hernia substantially affects the patient's quality of life. Considerations that can serve as relative contraindications for an elective Shouldice repair include class II or higher obesity, history of anterior mesh repairs, or patients with femoral hernias. On the other hand, patients who are thin, young, and otherwise healthy are excellent candidates for a pure tissue repair such as the Shouldice. Individuals with a prior posterior mesh hernia surgery or significant retroperitoneal surgery may also benefit from an anterior repair with or without mesh.

As is requisite, informed consent should include the pros and cons of a non-mesh repair. As part of this discussion, the onus falls on the surgeon to educate the patient and set intraoperative and postoperative expectations. Beyond the standard risks of infection, blood loss, or injury to nearby structures, patients should be made to understand that historically, anterior inguinal hernia repairs carry approximately a 5% to 15% risk of chronic pain. With care to identify all three nerves—ilioinguinal, iliohypogastric, and genital branch of the genitofemoral—the Shouldice repair has a track record of significantly lower rates of chronic pain, potentially due to the high volume of surgery performed at Shouldice hospital and the avoidance of anterior mesh placement. A neurectomy of one or more of the three nerves may be required to complete a safe repair and decrease the risks of chronic pain or disability.[4-6] Rarely, patients express concern about the transient numbness around the surgical site in their inguinal region postoperatively due to neurectomy; however, most understand that the alternative of leaving the nerves in situ involves a high risk of chronic pain and thus choose to proceed with surgical intervention.

PROCEDURAL APPROACH

The patient is positioned supine on the operating table. After induction of anesthesia and administration of preoperative antibiosis, the abdomen is prepped and draped in a usual fashion with chlorhexidine solution and towels. The exact axis of the inguinal ligament is identified using the ASIS and pubic tubercle as landmarks. We routinely perform a regional ilioinguinal nerve block with 10cc of 1% lidocaine with epinephrine.

After anesthetizing the skin and subcutaneous tissues, a 5 to 7 cm incision is then made near the pubic tubercle, typically extending half to two-thirds of the way toward the ASIS. For a more cosmetic result, Langer lines of skin tension are followed. After the skin incision, dissection is carried down through Scarpa's fascia. The superficial epigastric vessels encountered during this may be tied or coagulated with electrocautery. Subsequently, blunt finger dissection can be used to clear the external oblique. We recommend injecting ~10cc of local anesthetic mixture under the external oblique aponeurosis and subsequently clearing it for approximately 5 to 6 cm above its reflection and for additional 2 to 3 cm below its reflection in the upper thigh while taking care to avoid the femoral vessels. Mobilization of the external oblique aponeurosis is a critical step imperative for a successful repair. It is also a maneuver unique to the Shouldice operation; it results in sufficient external oblique aponeurosis required for the repair while minimizing tension. A femoral hernia can often be identified during this mobilization.

Next, the external oblique is cut sharply along its fibers, approximately 5 cm from its reflection or the inguinal ligament. Medially, this is extended to the external inguinal ring and laterally several centimeters lateral to the internal ring. Between the internal oblique fibers, the surgeon should now see two important nerves emerging—the ilioinguinal and the iliohypogastric—whose identification is critical to preventing inadvertent injury and decreasing the risk of chronic pain postoperatively. Depending on the location of the nerves, their fate could be one of three—transected if they are at obvious risk of entrapment while closing the defect, mobilization if necessary, or left in situ if far enough from the anticipated repair.

Once the ilioinguinal and iliohypogastric nerves have been identified and addressed, the Cremaster muscles are separated along their fibers. The fibers are left intact both medially and laterally to create a new internal ring during a later step of the surgery. Separation of cremasteric fibers will reveal a patent processus vaginalis, corresponding to the hernia sac in an indirect hernia (**Fig. 1**).[7]

In men, we then proceed with dissecting the peritoneal sac off of the cord structures for several centimeters into the retroperitoneal space through the dilated internal inguinal ring. For a long indirect hernia sac, the extra-peritoneum can be ligated. In a smaller hernia sac, it should be dissected back and returned to the retroperitoneal space. Even in a direct inguinal hernia, the peritoneum should always be visualized anterior to the cord and dissected back to the retroperitoneum. Care should also be taken to look for preperitoneal fat that may have herniated through the internal ring. If preperitoneal fat herniation is found, the fat may be excised or simply reduced back into the preperitoneal space.

After completing the dissection of any indirect component of the hernia, we proceed with retracting the spermatic cord structures using a Penrose drain. Superior-medial retraction of the cord helps expose the lateral cremasteric muscles and vessels that

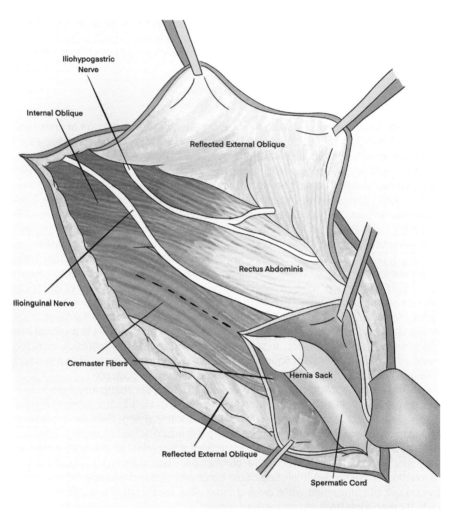

Fig. 1. Anterior view of the inguinal canal after the external oblique aponeurosis is retracted, anterior nerves identified, and cremaster muscles separated to identify an indirect hernia sac. (*Courtesy of* Michael Reinhorn, MD, FACS, Boston, MA.)

penetrate the transversalis fascia in the floor of the inguinal canal. Usually, the genital branch of the genitofemoral nerve is found coursing with the posterolateral cremaster muscles (**Fig. 2**). These muscles, together with the neurovascular bundle, are divided and doubly ligated with the proximal bundle marked with a long suture (**Fig. 3**). This unique maneuver intentionally divides the nerve, thus eliminating all loose tissues superficial to the transversus abdominis aponeurosis. This creates a clear view of the inguinal canal floor. Diligent cleaning of the inguinal canal floor allows the surgeon to easily inspect for a direct or a femoral hernia and improves the precision of the Shouldice repair. Studies from the Shouldice Hospital have observed that the hernia recurrence rate is reduced in half if the cremaster bundle was divided and used to reconstruct the internal ring.

Having divided the cremasters, the spermatic cord is retracted inferolaterally until the repair is complete. We then divide the transversus abdominis and transversalis

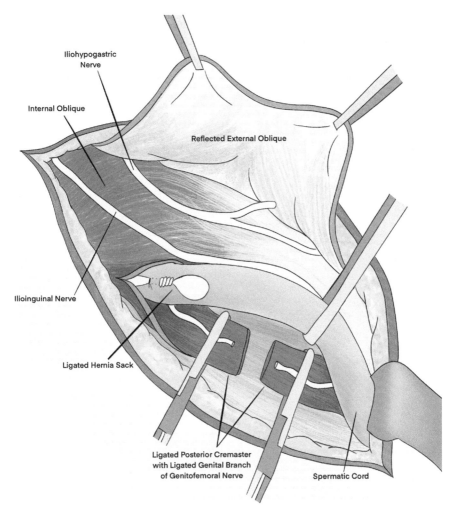

Iliohypogastric
Nerve

Internal Oblique

Reflected External Oblique

Ilioinguinal Nerve

Ligated Hernia Sack

Ligated Posterior Cremaster
with Ligated Genital Branch
of Genitofemoral Nerve

Spermatic Cord

Fig. 2. Dissection demonstrating division of the posterior cremaster muscle with genital branch of the genitofemoral nerve. (*Courtesy of* Michael Reinhorn, MD, FACS, Boston, MA.)

fascia parallel to the reflection of the external oblique aponeurosis (**Fig. 4**); "shelving edge" or "Poupart's ligament" are alternate terms for the latter. This creates an inferior leaflet for the first layer of the Shouldice repair. The medial leaflet is lifted, any retroperitoneal fat or hernia contents are reduced to the preperitoneal space, and the underside of the medial edge of the rectus abdominis muscle is exposed to be used in the repair. Attention is then turned to the femoral canal and if a small femoral hernia is encountered, that defect can be closed using a few interrupted permanent sutures between the inguinal ligament and Cooper's ligament under tension to tighten the femoral canal. Concurrent femoral hernias are found in 2% to 3% of all patients undergoing an inguinal hernia repair.[8,9] In a subset of these individuals, the femoral hernia might be large enough that the tension on the tissue would preclude a Shouldice repair, requiring conversion to a mesh-based repair. For this reason, we always consent patients for a possible conversion to a transrectus preperitoneal/open preperitoneal. We choose this repair as the mesh will cover the entire myopectineal orifice of

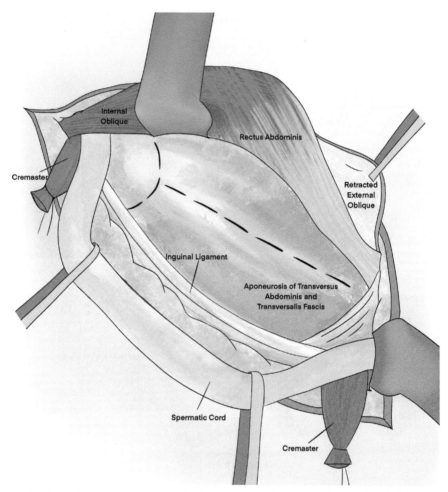

Fig. 3. View of the floor of the inguinal canal after retraction of the cord and division of cremasters. (*Courtesy of* Michael Reinhorn, MD, FACS, Boston, MA.)

Frouchaud, and it can be performed under sedation anesthesia through the same incision.

In women, after the identification of the ilioinguinal and iliohypogastric nerves, longitudinal division of the cremasteric fibers allows the hernia sac to be discernible. As the peritoneal sac in females also contains the round ligament, the ligament should be divided and double-ligated after administration of local anesthesia to minimize the risk of hernia recurrence. We favor ligation of the indirect hernia sac if it is long, and tend to return it to the preperitoneal space if it is small. The posterior cremaster fibers should be divided and can be used to completely close off the internal ring. The genital branch of the genitofemoral nerve is often divided either with the cremaster muscle bundle or the round ligament. Direct and femoral hernias are addressed identically in men and women.

After a thorough assessment of all three potential defects—direct, indirect, and femoral—and the three key aforementioned nerves, a four-layer Shouldice repair can begin. The repair is performed with two long sutures, either 0-0 polypropylene or 32/34

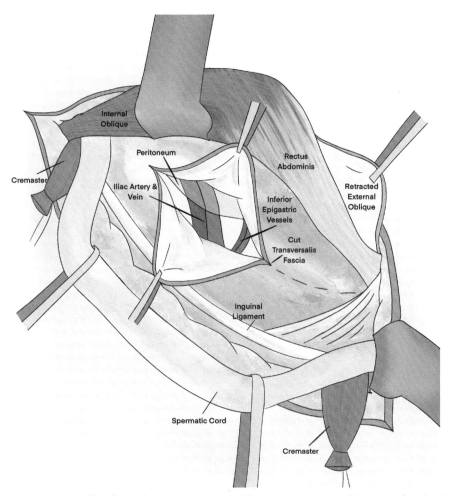

Fig. 4. Incision of the floor of the canal to expose the retroperitoneum. (*Courtesy of* Michael Reinhorn, MD, FACS, Boston, MA.)

gauge stainless steel suture, and each suture is used for two layers of the repair. After obtaining adequate exposure, the first suture is placed in the most inferolateral edge of the rectus, the cut edge of transversalis fascia, and the external oblique aponeurosis reflection at the pubic tubercle. A secure knot is tied, leaving a long tail which will be used again to tie once the second layer of the repair is complete. The goal of the first layer is to recreate a new inguinal canal floor, bringing the underside of the rectus to the transversalis fascia. This is done by running 5 to 10 mm bites of the underside of the rectus to the transversalis fascia that are approximately 5 mm apart (**Fig. 5**). Next, the internal inguinal ring is recreated such that only a Debakey forceps can enter the retroperitoneum along the cord, and a finger can no longer slide into the defect. To achieve this, "a scarf" is created around the cord, using the cremaster stump that was created during the dissection. The cremaster stump is sutured to the underside of the internal oblique muscle, just medial to the spermatic cord, creating a tight internal ring.

At this stage, it is important to verify that forceps can still easily slide into the retroperitoneum; overtightening the new internal ring can result in ischemia to the testicle. It

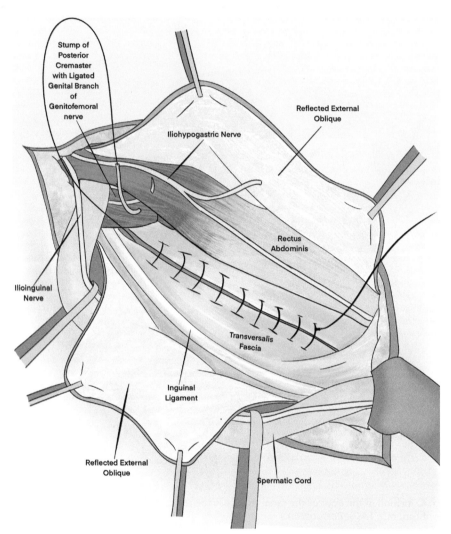

Fig. 5. First layer of Shouldice repair, demonstrating how the underside of the rectus is sutured to the cut edge of transversalis fascia. Laterally, the cremaster stump is sutured to the underside of the internal oblique to recreate the internal ring. (*Courtesy of* Michael Reinhorn, MD, FACS, Boston, MA.)

is possible that the forceps might not slide all the way into the retroperitoneum if the patient had a recurrence after previous posterior mesh hernia repair, as the space gets obscured by the old mesh. The second layer of suturing involves approximately 0.5 to 1 cm bites of the internal oblique laterally and rectus abdominis medially to the external oblique inferiorly (**Fig. 6**). The second layer is performed with the same suture as the first layer and gets tied to the tail of the suture from the first layer. The second layer of the repair is continued until 1 to 2 cm past the pubic tubercle to minimize a medical recurrence. One must also be cautious to expose the inguinal ligament instead of a false fold in the external oblique. If the latter is sutured to, there will not be enough external oblique aponeurosis to complete all four suture layers. In addition,

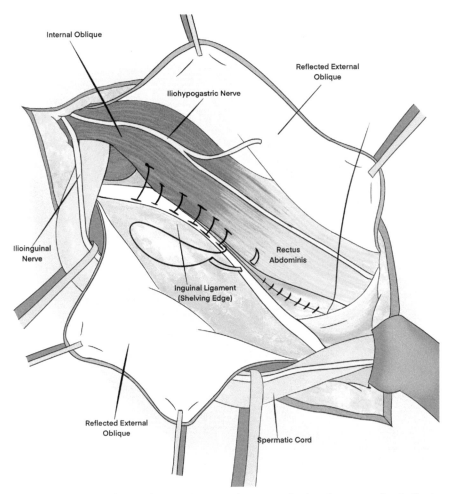

Fig. 6. Second layer of Shouldice repair. A running suture is placed to approximate the internal oblique and rectus with the inguinal ligament. (*Courtesy of* Michael Reinhorn, MD, FACS, Boston, MA.)

the surgeon can consider performing a relaxing incision along the rectus sheath and parallel to the repair if tension is encountered.

The third layer of repair is started just medial to the internal ring and is identical to the second layer. Full-thickness bites of the internal oblique and medially the rectus are sutured to the external oblique (**Fig. 7**) with the tail end of the suture kept long to tie to the fourth layer. Again, 1 cm bites are taken past the pubic tubercle, and the fourth layer is run back. Each bite of the fourth layer strives to juxtapose the rectus and internal oblique to the previously mobilized external oblique. Of note, the second and third layers are the predominant strength layers of the Shouldice repair. Although the fourth and last layer of the repair is underway, there is often minimal amount of external oblique left, thus the sutures from the fourth layer can be visualized on top of the external oblique.[10]

Once all the layers are closed, the surgeon should again verify that DeBakey forceps can still easily fit into the internal ring. Finally, we recreate the roof of the inguinal canal.

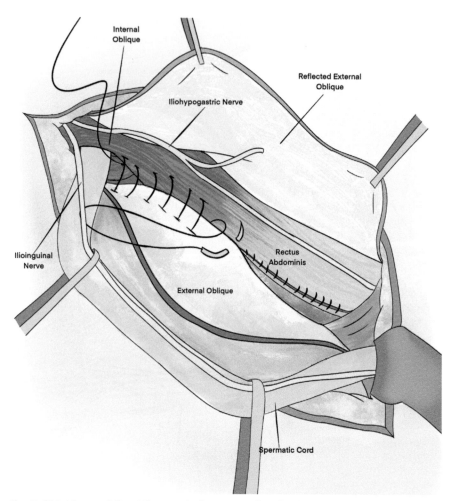

Fig. 7. Third layer of Shouldice repair. (*Courtesy of* Michael Reinhorn, MD, FACS, Boston, MA.)

This is done by suturing the superior leaflet of the external oblique to the inferolateral external oblique with a running absorbable suture while protecting the ilioinguinal and iliohypogastric nerves. Some male patients report a high riding ipsilateral testicle; to circumvent this complaint, the distal end of the cremasteric stump can be left alone, or if some cremaster reflex is desired, sutured to the external oblique.

Finally, simple interrupted sutures can be used to close the Scarpa's fascia, followed by a running vicryl or monocryl intradermal suture for skin closure.

RECOVERY AND REHABILITATION (INCLUDING POSTPROCEDURE CARE)

Patients who have undergone a Shouldice repair are discharged home the same day, often within 1 to 2 hours. Because most only require local anesthesia with intravenous sedation intraoperatively, the use of local pain control together with patient education can help successfully avoid postoperative need for opioids. Postprocedure care for patients typically includes a multimodal pain regimen, including acetaminophen and non steroidal anti inflamatorys (NSAIDs) as well as ice packs for the first few days. Patients are advised to avoid lifting objects heavier than 25lbs for the first 4 weeks to allow for appropriate healing. At that time, they can resume all activities without restriction and are seen in the clinic for routine follow-up.

PATIENT MONITORING AND CHALLENGES

Next, we will briefly summarize some of the most common complications that might be observed during or shortly after a Shouldice repair. As we alluded to in the procedure's description, excessive tightening of the internal ring can result in cord ischemia, which can present with pain in the testicle, possibly accompanied by swelling. In most cases, the testicle atrophies and patients experience resolution of the symptoms, without needing any surgical intervention.

Any dissection plane during a Shouldice can also be a hematoma site. Those that occur superficial to the external oblique are usually because of delayed venous bleeding; they present as areas of induration, tenderness, or pain under the skin incision and are often self-limited, rarely requiring surgical decompression. Scrotal and retroperitoneal hematomas can also present a few hours to days after surgery, and their severity, location, and symptomatic nature often guides the next step in management. Although seromas can occur, they are rare after anterior repairs with suture closure as the potential empty space that serves as the nidus for seroma formation is obliterated.

Importantly, nerve entrapment secondary to a technical error during dissection or while suturing the repair can also occur. The three important nerves mentioned above can all be addressed during the hernia repair by either mobilization, leaving the nerve in situ if the anatomy is favorable, or through a neurectomy. Entrapment of the genital branch of the genitofemoral nerve might occur inadvertently while suturing the posterior layers of the inguinal canal if the posterior cremasteric fibers and vessels are not retracted completely with the cord or not divided. In this complication, patients typically complain of burning pain in their ipsilateral medial thigh and lateral scrotum. To avoid this nerve entrapment, a good strategy is to perform en bloc division and ligation of this posterior cremaster bundle with reimplantation into the internal oblique. If nerve entrapment is recognized in the immediate postoperative period, immediate groin exploration under local anesthesia may allow for identification of and treatment of the problem, avoiding long-term chronic pain for the patient.

Although injury to the ilioinguinal nerve is easily avoided by retraction with the cord or lateral mobilization, it is the iliohypogastric nerve that accounts for a sizable proportion of postoperative chronic pain after anterior inguinal hernia surgery. Beyond recognizing the typical course of this nerve, it is important to appreciate that the iliohypogastric may bifurcate as it travels along the internal oblique. Early identification of this nerve and its branches when performing a suture repair is important to minimizing the risk of its entrapment. Last, when closing the aponeurosis of the external oblique, care must be taken to avoid suturing a branch or the major trunk of the iliohypogastric nerve as it perforates through the external oblique aponeurosis to innervate the skin.

Rarely, a patient may report a burning sensation associated with ejaculation after a Shouldice repair. This dysejaculation is self-limited, and it is important to reassure patients and set expectations that it may take months to years to fully resolve.

OUTCOMES

Several factors including patient selection, surgeon volume, and staff training all play an important role in influencing the outcomes after a hernia repair. The Shouldice

Hospital has maintained the highest level of quality control over the last several decades and has reported a recurrence rate of 1.15% based on their 30-year data.[2] Other centers have reported higher recurrence rates up to ~10%.[11–14]

Beyond recurrence, other clinical and patient-reported outcomes are also important to consider. Chronic pain, urinary retention, and wound complications such as formation of a seroma or hematoma are relatively common after all inguinal hernia repairs and can significantly affect a patient's quality of life. A pure tissue repair such as the Shouldice requires precise anatomical dissection and reapproximation, which helps reduce wound complications, recurrence rates, and the prevalence of chronic pain.

Numerous studies have demonstrated that no one method of hernia repair is best for every patient, and surgeons should be able to offer their patients various approaches to fit each patient's needs. Therefore, before recommending a Shouldice repair, it is important for the surgeon to take into consideration all of the patients' risk factors and motivations for wanting a non-mesh repair. In addition, discussion around the type of hernia repair offered should include consideration of cost and resources used. This becomes particularly important in low-resource settings, where cost of laparoscopic instruments or mesh can be prohibitive for many hospital systems and/or patients. Consequently, tissue-only repairs, which involve little technology, tend to offer high quality at the lowest cost for the appropriately selected patients.[11,15,16]

DISCLOSURE

The authors have nothing to disclose.

REFERENCES

1. Komorowski AL. History of the inguinal hernia repair. Inguinal hernia. Intech; 2014. https://doi.org/10.5772/58533.
2. Shouldice EB. The Shouldice repair for groin hernias. Surg Clin North Am 2003; 83(5):1163–87, vii.
3. Öberg S, Andresen K, Rosenberg J. Etiology of inguinal hernias: a comprehensive review. Frontiers in Surgery 2017;4:52.
4. Bande D, Moltó L, Pereira JA, et al. Chronic pain after groin hernia repair: pain characteristics and impact on quality of life. BMC Surg 2020;20(1):147.
5. Bansal VK, Misra MC, Babu D, et al. A prospective, randomized comparison of long-term outcomes: chronic groin pain and quality of life following totally extraperitoneal (TEP) and transabdominal preperitoneal (TAPP) laparoscopic inguinal hernia repair. Surg Endosc 2013;27(7):2373–82.
6. Melkemichel M, Bringman S, Nilsson H, et al. Patient-reported chronic pain after open inguinal hernia repair with lightweight or heavyweight mesh: a prospective, patient-reported outcomes study. Br J Surg 2020;107(12):1659–66.
7. Agarwal D, Ott L, Reinhorn M. Shouldice Repair for Left Direct Inguinal Hernia. JOMI 2022;(5):2022. https://doi.org/10.24296/jomi/340.
8. Henriksen NA, Thorup J, Jorgensen LN. Unsuspected femoral hernia in patients with a preoperative diagnosis of recurrent inguinal hernia. Hernia 2012;16(4): 381–5.
9. Białecki J, Pyda P, Antkowiak R, et al. Unsuspected femoral hernias diagnosed during endoscopic inguinal hernia repair. Adv Clin Exp Med 2021;30(2):135–8.
10. Chan CK, Chan G. The Shouldice technique for the treatment of inguinal hernia. J Minim Access Surg 2006;2(3):124–8.

11. Amato B, Moja L, Panico S, et al. Shouldice technique versus other open techniques for inguinal hernia repair. Cochrane Database Syst Rev 2012;2012(4): CD001543.
12. Simons MP, Smietanski M, Bonjer HJ, et al. International guidelines for groin hernia management. Hernia 2018;22(1):1–165.
13. Malik A, Bell CM, Stukel TA, et al. Recurrence of inguinal hernias repaired in a large hernia surgical specialty hospital and general hospitals in Ontario, Canada. Can J Surg 2016;59(1):19–25.
14. Martín Duce A, Lozano O, Galván M, et al. Results of Shouldice hernia repair after 18 years of follow-up in all the patients. Hernia 2021;25(5):1215–22.
15. Lorenz R, Arlt G, Conze J, et al. Shouldice standard 2020: review of the current literature and results of an international consensus meeting. Hernia 2021;25(5): 1199–207.
16. Lundström K-J, Holmberg H, Montgomery A, et al. Patient-reported rates of chronic pain and recurrence after groin hernia repair. Br J Surg 2017;105(1): 106–12.

The Minimally Invasive Inguinal Hernia: Current Trends and Considerations

Thomas Q. Xu, MD, Rana M. Higgins, MD*

KEYWORDS

- Inguinal hernia • Laparoscopic • Robotic • Transabdominal preperitoneal
- Totally extraperitoneal

KEY POINTS

- The diagnosis of an inguinal hernia can be made by physical exam alone or in conjunction with imaging.
- A critical area for inguinal hernia repair that requires complete visualization is the myopectineal orifice.
- The majority of patients are candidates for minimally invasive inguinal hernia repair.

INTRODUCTION/HISTORY/DEFINITIONS/BACKGROUND

Inguinal hernias are one of the most common surgical pathologies faced by the general surgeon in modern medicine.[1] One in four adult American men is at risk of developing an inguinal hernia in their lifetime, and the cumulative incidence of an inguinal hernia is around 25% in men and 3% in women.[2] This risk increases as people get older, and with the aging population of the United States, the incidence of inguinal hernias is becoming progressively higher. Inguinal herniorrhaphy is one of the most common operations performed by general surgeons in the United States with roughly 800,000 of these procedures performed each year.[3]

Initially, inguinal herniorrhaphy was described with only tissue repairs, initially by Bassini in 1871 and Shouldice in the 1950s.[4] This was the standard of care until tension-free repairs using mesh were first described by Stock and Usher and then popularized by Lichtenstein in the 1970s.[5] The low rates of recurrence with these tension-free repairs, as well as the easy reproducibility, have seen these described techniques dominate the approach for open repairs since the 1970s.[1]

Minimally invasive techniques for inguinal herniorrhaphy have become more popular and widespread in the past decade.[6] The first approach to repair inguinal hernias

Division of Minimally Invasive and Gastrointestinal Surgery, Medical College of Wisconsin, 8701 Watertown Plank Road, Milwaukee, WI 53226, USA
* Corresponding author.
E-mail address: rhiggins@mcw.edu

Surg Clin N Am 103 (2023) 875–887
https://doi.org/10.1016/j.suc.2023.04.002
0039-6109/23/© 2023 Elsevier Inc. All rights reserved.

laparoscopically was described by Ger in the 1990s.[7] Soon afterward, two major approaches became the most common to fix inguinal hernias laparoscopically: the transabdominal preperitoneal (TAPP) approach and the total extraperitoneal (TEP) approach. These approaches dominated the field of minimally invasive inguinal herniorrhaphy until the rise of the robotic approach, which is performed as a TAPP approach.

Nature of the Problem/Diagnosis

Inguinal hernias are one of the most common hernias seen by general surgeons. They can be categorized as either congenital or acquired hernias. Congenital hernias are typically due to a patent processus vaginalis and are traditionally described as indirect inguinal hernias because they form and protrude through the inguinal canal. As they are congenital, these hernias develop at an early age and are seen in children as well as adults. Acquired inguinal hernias are a result of trauma or disease processes that increase intra-abdominal pressure, such as obesity, chronic coughing, pregnancy, heavy lifting, and chronic constipation.

Inguinal hernias are much more common in men with a 25% lifetime incidence than in women 3%. This is primarily due to anatomic differences, given the spermatic vessels travel through the inguinal canal in men, thus creating a natural opening for part of the peritoneum to herniate through. In women, this space is obliterated and occupied by the round ligament, and thus, there is no true opening past the external ring.

The diagnosis of an inguinal hernia can be made with physical examination alone or in conjunction with imaging findings. Most patients will complain of a bulge in their inguinal region that can be palpated on physical examination. To properly diagnose an inguinal hernia, one should examine the patient standing up as well as lying down. In addition, reducibility of an inguinal hernia should be assessed with every physical examination. Inguinal hernias tend to be easier to reduce sitting down, but easier to identify while the patient is standing up. If palpation of an inguinal hernia is difficult, one can use provocative measures such as asking the patient to perform a Valsava maneuver to elucidate an inguinal hernia. The physical examination for an inguinal hernia is not complete until one documents the presence or absence of testicles in the scrotum and the number of testicles palpable in the scrotum.

If an inguinal hernia is not palpable on examination, but clinical history makes it highly probable, then one can perform adjunct imaging to identify an inguinal hernia. Dynamic testing includes inguinal ultrasound with and without provocative measures to identify an inguinal hernia. Sensitivity for diagnosing inguinal hernias range from 56% to 100% for this image modality.[8] Static imaging options includes CT pelvis as well as MRI pelvis; however, the sensitivity of these imaging studies is lower given their adynamic nature. Studies have demonstrated sensitivities between 48% and 98% in diagnosing inguinal hernias for CT pelvis and 87% to 95% from MRI pelvis.[8] MRI pelvis can also be helpful for the diagnosis of a "sports" hernia or athletic pubalgia and to differentiate that from a true inguinal hernia.

ANATOMY
Layers of the Abdominal Wall

From superficial to deep, the layers of the abdominal wall in the inguinal region include: skin, subcutaneous tissue, Scarpa's and Camper's fascia, external oblique fascia and muscle, internal oblique fascia and muscle, transversus abdominis muscle, transversalis fascia, preperitoneal fat, and peritoneum (**Fig. 1**). The transversalis fascia is the innermost fascial layer of the abdominal wall and it has two distinct layers, the more

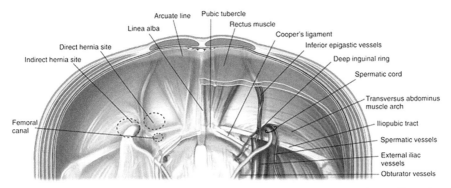

Fig. 1. Layers of the abdominal wall in the inguinal region. (With permission from Tiffany Slaybaugh DaVanzo.)

superficial of which is vascular and the deeper layer is avascular, which makes a beneficial dissection plane into the preperitoneal space.

Myopectineal Orifice

The myopectineal orifice (MPO) was first described by Dr Fruchaud in 1956 as a distinct area of weakness in the pelvic region (**Fig. 2**). It is bordered by the conjoint tendon superiorly, Cooper's ligament inferior, rectus abdominis muscle medially, and iliopsoas muscle laterally. It is divided by the inguinal ligament, which runs diagonally from the pubic tubercle to the anterior superior iliac spine (ASIS). The internal inguinal ring is superior to the inguinal ligament in the MPO, through which the spermatic cord runs in men to penetrate the abdominal wall and into the scrotum. This is the site of an indirect inguinal hernia, which is a pathological weakness in the transversalis fascia allowing the peritoneum to bulge through the internal ring alongside the spermatic cord. The inferior epigastric vessels run medially to the spermatic vessels and create one leg of Hesselbach's triangle. Hesselbach's triangle is defined by the inferior epigastric vessels laterally, the rectus abdominis muscle medially and the inguinal ligament inferiorly. Direct inguinal hernias are defined by hernias through Hesselbach's triangle. Below the inguinal ligament exists the femoral space, medial to the femoral vein, where a femoral hernias develops.

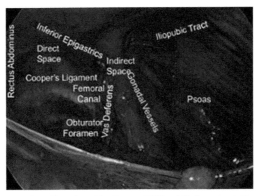

Fig. 2. The myopectineal orifice (MPO). (*From* Miller HJ. Inguinal Hernia: Mastering the Anatomy. Surg Clin North Am. 2018;98(3):607-621; with permission.)

Iliopubic Tract

The iliopubic tract is a thickening of the transversalis fascia that attaches to Cooper's ligament medially and runs parallel and deep to the inguinal ligament. It is an important landmark for the preperitoneal approach to inguinal herniorrhaphy because it is the posterior border of the MPO and marks the superior border of the triangle of pain.

Nerves in the Inguinal Region

Nerves in the inguinal region arise from the lumbar plexus, innervate abdominal musculature, and supply sensation to the skin and peritoneum (**Fig. 3**). The lateral femoral cutaneous nerve enters the abdomen medial and caudal to the ASIS and runs in the lateral aspect of the psoas muscle. It supplies sensation to the upper lateral thigh. The genitofemoral nerve perforates the abdominal wall at the iliopubic tract near and lateral to the internal inguinal ring and runs within the cremasteric fascia with the external genital vessels. The iliohypogastric nerve runs deep to the external oblique just above the inguinal canal and penetrates the external oblique muscle just cranial to the external ring. It provides sensation to the suprapubic region. The ilioinguinal nerve travels within the inguinal canal anterior to the spermatic cord and leaves the canal through the external ring. It provides sensation to the skin at the root of the penis, anterior third of the scrotum, anterior medial thigh and labia majora.

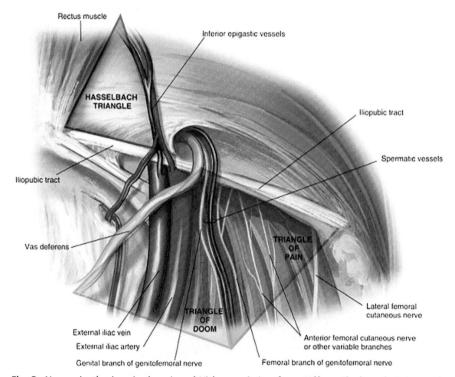

Fig. 3. Nerves in the inguinal region. (With permission from Tiffany Slaybaugh DaVanzo.)

Vasculature in the Inguinal Region

The external iliac artery is the arterial supply to the groin. The deep circumflex iliac and inferior epigastric arteries branch off before becoming the common femoral artery. The obturator artery branches from the internal iliac artery and passes anteroinferiorly on the lateral wall of the pelvis. In up to 80% of pubic rami, there is an aberrant obturator artery, commonly referred to as the *corona mortis* that has an anastomosis with branches of the iliac or epigastric arteries forming a ring that runs directly on Cooper's ligament. There are multiple venous plexi for drainage of the groin, including the pampiniform plexus. Injury to the pampiniform plexus leads to testicular atrophy after herniorrhaphy.

PREOPERATIVE/PREPROCEDURE PLANNING

At the initial consultation, standard history questions should be asked to the patient about their inguinal hernia. Usually, pain or discomfort is the presenting symptom for a clinic visit, whereas an obstructive symptom is usually the presenting symptom for an inpatient consultation. Sometimes, patients notice an inguinal bulge. Questions should be asked about duration of symptoms and whether these symptoms are worsening. In addition, one should try to elicit if there was an inciting event, such as lifting a heavy object or sudden movement. Documentation of reducibility should be included in the initial consultation note as well as the presence or absence of obstructing symptoms including bowel or urinary changes. In addition, physical examination should include the presence or absence of testicles in the scrotum. If the consultation is for a unilateral inguinal hernia, one should always check for and document the presence or absence of a contralateral hernia.

Indications

For primary, unilateral inguinal hernias, the preference of an open approach versus a minimally invasive approach is usually at the discretion of the surgeon. As the population of the United States becomes more obese, this increases the amount of subcutaneous adiposity in patients and thus would favor a minimally invasive approach versus an open approach. However, ultimately this is at the discretion of the surgeon. For primary, bilateral inguinal hernias or primary unilateral inguinal hernias where there is some suspicion of an occult contralateral inguinal hernia, a minimally invasive approach is recommended so that the contralateral side can be evaluated at the same time and repaired if needed. For recurrent inguinal hernias, the approach should be the opposite of what was performed during the last operation. For instance, if an open approach was done for the previous operation, then a minimally invasive approach should be performed for the operation and vice versa.

Contraindications

There are few contraindications for a minimally invasive inguinal herniorrhaphy. Absolute contraindications include an inability to tolerate general anesthesia and an inability to correct an underlying bleeding disorder. Relative contraindications include numerous prior intra-abdominal operations for a TAPP or prior operations in the preperitoneal space, such as a prostatectomy, for a TEP in addition to large, incarcerated scrotal-inguinal hernias.

Preoperative Laboratory Tests and Imaging

Typically, extensive preoperative laboratory tests and imaging is not required. Routine preoperative laboratories include a complete blood count and comprehensive metabolic panel for most patients. If imaging is needed, a dynamic inguinal ultrasound can be performed to help detect hernias that are unable to be palpated on examination or for recurrences. In addition, depending on the patient's functional status, an electrocardiogram (EKG) and a preoperative chest x-ray might be needed. A preoperative anticoagulation plan should be formulated for patients on chronic anticoagulation. Patients should be evaluated in a preoperative medical or anesthesia clinic to medically optimize them for inguinal herniorrhaphy.

OPERATIVE PREPARATION AND PATIENT POSITIONING

Preoperatively, during the day of the operation, the side of the inguinal hernia should be verified. Nothing by mouth (NPO) status should be confirmed. Patients are placed in the supine position, and general anesthesia is then induced. Either a Foley catheter is then placed or patients are required to void immediately preoperatively, within one hour, to ensure the bladder is decompressed. Both arms are then tucked to the sides. The abdomen is prepped with either an alcohol or iodine-based cleaning solution. Preoperative antibiotics are initiated before incision; usually, a first-generation cephalosporin is adequate. The patient is placed in Trendelenburg positioning to allow for the bowel to drop away from the pelvic region (**Fig. 4**).

Procedural Approach

1. Laparoscopic TAPP
   a. Skin incision for first trocar (10–12 mm) periumbilically
   b. Insert 10 mm trocar periumbilically
   c. Insert two more trocars (5 mm) just lateral to rectus sheath on either side just below umbilicus
   d. Create peritoneal flap
      i. Start flap at ASIS and carry to median umbilical ligament
   e. Identify epigastric vessels and keep vessels up
   f. Start medially at pubis and dissect Cooper's ligament to its junction with the iliac vein
   g. Inspect direct hernia space and reduce contents if direct hernia present

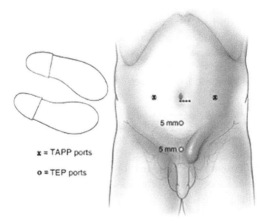

5 mmO

5 mm O

x = TAPP ports

o = TEP ports

Fig. 4. Patient positioning. (*From* Adrales GL, Sacks BC. Management of Inguinal Hernia. In: Cameron JL, Cameron AM. Current Surgical Therapy, Thirteenth ed. Elsevier. 2020; pp. 623-627; with permission.)

h. Skeletonize spermatic cord laterally to inferior epigastric vessels to expose ilio-pubic tract
i. Inspect indirect hernia space and reduce indirect hernia
j. Dissection of preperitoneal space carried out laterally to ASIS
k. Insert mesh through 10 mm port
   l. Open mesh and cover MPO
m. Secure mesh with tacks or sutures if not using a self-adhesive mesh
   i. Ensure one area of fixation is medially to Cooper's ligament
n. Ensure hemostasis
o. Close peritoneal flap, typically using a tacker as more ergonomic than suturing
p. Desufflated abdomen and remove trocars
q. Close 10 mm trocar site fascia
r. Close skin incisions
s. Pull testicle back into scrotum
t. Remove Foley (if placed at the start of the case)

2. Robotic TAPP
   a. Steps similar to laparoscopic TAPP with the following differences
      i. Trocars should be placed 2 to 3 cm above the umbilicus
      ii. Can offset middle trocar to right or left depending on which side inguinal her-nia is located
      iii. Trocars should be placed 8 to 10 cm apart
      iv. Should use all 8 mm trocars
      v. Can use either robotic 0° or 30° scope
      vi. Will always suture close the peritoneal flap instead of tacking

3. Laparoscopic TEP
   a. Skin incision for first trocar (10–12 mm) periumbilically
   b. Open anterior rectus on ipsilateral side and retract muscle laterally to expose posterior sheath
   c. Insert finger over posterior sheath and develop space
   d. Insert balloon trocar and direct trocar toward pubic symphysis
   e. Insert 10 mm 30° and visualize space being created as balloon is inflated
   f. Deflate balloon and insufflate preperitoneal space
   g. Insert two more trocars
      i. First 5 mm trocar just distal to camera port
      ii. Second 5 mm trocar two fingerbreadths away from first 5 mm trocar
   h. Identify epigastric vessels and keep vessels up
   i. Start medially at pubis and dissect Cooper's ligament to its junction with the iliac vein
   j. Inspect direct hernia space and reduce contents if direct hernia present
   k. Skeletonize spermatic cord laterally to inferior epigastric vessels to expose ilio-pubic tract
   l. Inspect indirect hernia space and reduce indirect hernia
   m. Dissection of preperitoneal space carried out laterally to ASIS
   n. Insert mesh through 10 mm port
   o. Open mesh and cover MPO
   p. Secure mesh with tacks or sutures if not using a self-adhesive mesh
      i. Secure mesh medially to Cooper's ligament
   q. Ensure hemostasis
   r. Deflate preperitoneal space and watch mesh positioning as space deflated
   s. Remove trocars
   t. Close anterior rectus sheath

u. Close skin incisions
v. Pull testicle back into scrotum
w. Remove Foley (if placed at the start of the case)

RECOVERY AND REHABILITATION

Most inguinal hernia repairs are performed as outpatient operations. One of the more common immediate postoperative complications is urinary retention with a roughly 10% incidence.[9] This is more common in men over 60 years old or with underlying benign prostatic hyperplasia. Judicious use of fluids intraoperatively as well as postoperatively in the recovery unit can help to mitigate the risk of postoperative urinary retention. Routine Foley catheter placement for bladder decompression is not necessary if patients void immediately before the operation. Recent literature has not demonstrated a reduction in urinary retention rates with Foley catheter placement.[10] Foley catheter placement can be a risk factor for postoperative urinary retention. If postoperative urinary retention does not resolve, this can lead to an overnight observation stay in the hospital.

Pain after surgery is typically well controlled using a multimodal approach, minimizing the use of opioids. Patients are counseled before surgery as well as postoperatively to use scheduled acetaminophen and ibuprofen as well as use ice packs in the groin for the first 24 to 48 hours. Patients are also prescribed 3 days of a muscle relaxer, methocarbamol, for additional pain control if needed. Patients are discharged on a regular diet. The most important activity restriction is no lifting, pushing or pulling more than 10 to 20 pounds for 6 weeks postoperatively to reduce the risk of recurrence. Port site incisions are closed with subcuticular sutures and thus require minimal wound care is required. Patients can shower the day after surgery. They should not immerse incisions underwater for at least 4 to 6 weeks postoperatively, until the incisions are fully healed.

Clinic follow-up is arranged for the patient, and they are seen at approximately 2 weeks postoperatively. Usually, there is no pathology to review as no specimens are routinely sent. At this clinic visit, diet tolerance, pain control, return of bowel function, groin, and testicle pain are assessed. Patients should no longer be requiring pain medication. If patients complain of thigh or groin pain, this should be monitored closely for any progression, but is usually transient from neuropraxia. Typically, no intervention is performed until at least 2 to 3 months postoperatively, once healing is complete. If persistent, additional testing should be performed to evaluate for nerve injury. Scrotal swelling should be monitored and patients should be counseled that these findings will continue to improve and eventually will resolve. Scrotal elevation and supportive underwear are encouraged. Activity restrictions and duration are emphasized to the patient. If there are no persistent concerns, no additional follow-up appointments are needed.

MANAGEMENT
Nonoperative Versus Operative Management

Choosing the optimal time for an operation is one of the most critical decisions in the preoperative period. Watchful waiting is a reasonable choice to give patients if the hernia is asymptomatic and has no signs of incarceration. The rate of strangulation has been shown to be relatively low in this patient population, roughly between 1% and 2%.[11] One should counsel patients that the natural history of inguinal hernias is to gradually enlarge over time and therefore will most likely need a repair in the future. The crossover rate for needing surgical intervention approaches 75% at 10 years.[11]

However, once the hernia is symptomatic and is compromising a patient's quality of life or becomes intermittently incarcerated, then elective repair is recommended. Last, of note, the literature that supports watchful waiting should only be applied to male patients.[11]

Deciding on Which Approach

Once a patient is deemed a candidate for inguinal hernia repair, the next choice in the decision tree is which approach to use for the repair. Choosing an open versus laparoscopic approach for a primary, unilateral inguinal hernia is usually based on a surgeon's preference. If this is a recurrent inguinal hernia, then the surgeon should choose the opposite approach as was performed for the previous operation to avoid scar tissue. In addition, large inguinal hernias that extend down into the scrotum are a relative contraindication for minimally invasive inguinal hernia repair. However, as surgeons become more adept at minimally invasive repairs, this relative contraindication becomes less of a contraindication, and the approach should be based on surgeon experience. If the patient has a known inguinal hernia and a femoral hernia, a minimally invasive approach is recommended, given the full view and dissection of the MPO. If the patient is a poor candidate for general anesthesia, then an open approach is recommended, due to the ability to perform this operation under monitored anesthesia care along with the use of local anesthetics.

Choosing between a TAPP or TEP is usually based on a surgeon's preference. Differences in training patterns typically decide which approach appeals to the surgeon. If a patient has had multiple prior abdominal operations and the intra-abdominal adhesions would seem to be unfavorable, then a TEP is recommended to avoid extensive adhesiolysis.

Inpatient Postoperative Management

This applies to a minority of patients as most inguinal hernia repairs are performed as outpatient operations. However, if a patient requires inpatient admission, it is typically a result of postoperative urinary retention, pain control, or cardiopulmonary monitoring. A regular diet can be ordered to start immediately postoperatively. Intravenous pain medications can be used to supplement oral pain medications. Early ambulation and aggressive pulmonary hygiene with incentive spirometry are ordered and patients should be encouraged to follow these guidelines. Urinary retention usually resolves within a day postoperatively and it is a small minority of patients that require discharge with a Foley catheter.

OUTCOMES

When comparing laparoscopic to open inguinal hernia repair, studies have found that there is a lower rate of postoperative complications in minimally invasive inguinal hernia repair.[12] In addition, rates of readmission were also noted to be lower in laparoscopic inguinal hernia repair.[13] Furthermore, laparoscopic inguinal hernia repair is associated with a reduced incidence of surgical site infection when compared with an open approach for inguinal hernia repair.[14] Utilization of pain medication is also reduced in laparoscopic inguinal hernia repair as opposed to open inguinal hernia repair. In conjunction with this observation, return to work is also shorter in laparoscopic versus open inguinal hernia repair.[14] However, there is a higher incidence of urinary retention in laparoscopic inguinal hernia repair.[2] When looking at length of stay, laparoscopic and open inguinal hernia repairs have similar hospital length of stay.[15]

When comparing laparoscopic TAPP versus TEP repair, the literature demonstrates that there are minimal differences in standard outcomes measures. Rates of hernia recurrence as well as chronic pain were similar between patients who underwent TAPP versus TEP.[16] In addition, operative duration, early postoperative pain, hospital length of stay, rate of wound infection, and time until return of work were similar between the two groups.[16] This would suggest that the choice between TAPP versus TEP ultimately is based on the surgeon's preference. As robotic TAPP becomes more widespread, in studies comparing robotic TAPP versus laparoscopic TEP, operative duration was longer for robotic TAPP but mean pain scores were lower.[17] No difference in clinical recurrence rates have been shown between the two operative approaches.[18–20]

When evaluating laparoscopic versus robotic inguinal hernia repair, outcomes seem to be similar. Studies have demonstrated that the postoperative complication rate as well as chronic pain rate is similar between laparoscopic and robotic inguinal hernia repair.[21] However, operative times were increased when comparing robotic versus laparoscopic inguinal hernia repair.[22] Newer studies have reported that operative times are becoming similar when comparing robotic versus laparoscopic inguinal hernia repair and that the incidence of chronic pain is lower in patients who undergo robotic versus laparoscopic inguinal hernia repair.[23] One of the major purported benefits of robotic inguinal hernia repair is the improved ergonomics; however, the RIVAL trial demonstrated no major ergonomic benefit to surgeons in robotic inguinal hernia repairs.[24] In addition, the RIVAL trial demonstrated that the robotic approach was associated with longer operative times as well as higher median costs and increased surgeon frustration.[24]

SUMMARY

Minimally invasive inguinal hernia repair is safe and effective. A minimally invasive approach to inguinal hernia repair is the procedure of choice for bilateral inguinal hernias, inguinal hernias with associated femoral hernias, as well as recurrent inguinal hernias that were previously fixed with an open approach. As surgeons become more facile at minimally invasive inguinal hernias, the relative contraindications for this approach decreases. If a patient cannot tolerate general anesthesia, they are not a candidate for a minimally invasive approach. For primary inguinal hernia repair, a TAPP versus a TEP is usually based on a surgeon's preference. It provides many benefits in terms of postoperative outcomes, which include decreased postoperative pain, quicker return to work, and decreased surgical site infection rates. Current research does not support much of an advantage for robotic inguinal hernia repair, as there was little improvement in ergonomics with increased associated operative time and costs, though more research is needed at this time to fully delineate potential advantages.

CLINICS CARE POINTS

- Surgeons should provide an option for both an open approach (Lichtenstein) as well as minimally invasive approach (transabdominal preperitoneal [TAPP] or total extraperitoneal) primary inguinal hernia given that the surgeon has the expertise to perform both operations.
- For recurrent inguinal hernias, a minimally invasive approach should be recommended if the prior repair was performed via an open approach and vice versa.

- For bilateral inguinal hernias, a minimally invasive approach should be recommended over an open approach.
- In TAPP, the peritoneal flap should extend from the anterior superior iliac spine to the medial umbilical ligament.
- When performing the initial dissection, it should follow the peritoneal plane and the fatty tissue should be left in contact with the inguinal floor and not the peritoneum.
- Medial dissection should extend to the pubic symphysis and 2 cm below Cooper's ligament, exposing the entire myopectineal orifice, to reduce the incidence of recurrence.
- Lateral dissection needs to be carried far out enough just so that the mesh can lay flat against the abdominal wall.
- Dissection of the peritoneum inferiorly should continue until visualization of vas deferens crosses the external iliac vein and the iliopsoas muscle can be seen. This helps to reduce the chance that the peritoneum slips underneath the mesh, the most common cause of a recurrence.
- The mesh should reach to the pubic symphysis medially and 2 cm below Cooper's ligament, covering the entire myopectineal orifice, to reduce the chances of a recurrence.
- For direct inguinal hernias, 1 to 2 cm of medial mesh crossover to the other side is desired to reduce the risk of recurrence.
- Mesh fixation is usually not necessary except in the cases of large direct inguinal hernias.
- Deflate under direct visualization to confirm final mesh placement.

DISCLOSURE

Dr T.Q. Xu has no conflicts of interest to disclose. Dr R.M. Higgins is a Speaker/Teacher for WL Gore and Intuitive Surgical.

REFERENCES

1. Horne CM, Prabhu AS. Minimally invasive approaches to inguinal hernias. Surg Clin North Am 2018;98(3):637–49.
2. Huerta S, Timmerman C, Argo M, et al. Open, laparoscopic, and robotic inguinal hernia repair: outcomes and predictors of complications. J Surg Res 2019;241: 119–27.
3. Miller HJ. Inguinal hernia: mastering the anatomy. Surg Clin North Am 2018;98(3): 607–21.
4. Marcy H. A new use of carbolized cat guy ligature. Boston Med Surg J 1871;85: 315–6.
5. Lichtenstein IL, Shulman AG, Amid PK, et al. The tension-free hernioplasty. Am J Surg 1989;157(2):188–93.
6. Madion M, Goldblatt MI, Gould JC, et al. Ten-year trends in minimally invasive hernia repair: a NSQIP database review. Surg Endosc 2021;35(12): 7200–8.
7. Ger R. Laparoskopische Hernienoperation [Laparoscopic hernia operation]. Chirurg 1991;62(4):266–70. German. PMID: 1830542.
8. Piga E, Zetner D, Andresen K, et al. Imaging modalities for inguinal hernia diagnosis: a systematic review. Hernia 2020 Oct;24(5):917–26.
9. Roadman D, Helm M, Goldblatt MI, et al. Postoperative urinary retention after laparoscopic total extraperitoneal inguinal hernia repair. J Surg Res 2018;231: 309–15.

10. Fafaj A, Lo Menzo E, Alaedeen D, et al. Effect of intraoperative urinary catheter use on postoperative urinary retention after laparoscopic inguinal hernia repair: a randomized clinical trial. JAMA Surg 2022;157(8):667–74.

11. Schroeder AD, Tubre DJ, Fitzgibbons RJ Jr. Watchful waiting for inguinal hernia. Adv Surg 2019;53:293–303.

12. Fan CJ, Chien HL, Weiss MJ, et al. Minimally invasive versus open surgery in the medicare population: a comparison of post-operative and economic outcomes. Surg Endosc 2018;32(9):3874–80.

13. Sood A, Meyer CP, Abdollah F, et al. Minimally invasive surgery and its impact on 30-day postoperative complications, unplanned readmissions and mortality. Br J Surg 2017;104(10):1372–81.

14. Rana G, Armijo PR, Khan S, et al. Outcomes and impact of laparoscopic inguinal hernia repair versus open inguinal hernia repair on healthcare spending and employee absenteeism. Surg Endosc 2020;34(2):821–8.

15. Aiolfi A, Cavalli M, Ferraro SD, et al. Treatment of inguinal hernia: systematic review and updated network meta-analysis of randomized controlled trials. Ann Surg 2021;274(6):954–61.

16. Aiolfi A, Cavalli M, Del Ferraro S, et al. Total extraperitoneal (TEP) versus laparoscopic transabdominal preperitoneal (TAPP) hernioplasty: systematic review and trial sequential analysis of randomized controlled trials. Hernia 2021;25(5):1147–57.

17. Gundogdu E, Guldogan CE, Ozmen MM. Bilateral inguinal hernia repair: robotic TAPP versus laparoscopic TEP. Surg Laparosc Endosc Percutaneous Tech 2020;31(4):439–43.

18. Peltrini R, Corcione F, Pacella D, et al. Robotic versus laparoscopic transabdominal preperitoneal (TAPP) approaches to bilateral hernia repair: a multicenter retrospective study using propensity score matching analysis. Surg Endosc 2022. https://doi.org/10.1007/s00464-022-09614-y.

19. Rosen, M. J. (Ed.). (2017). Atlas of abdominal wall reconstruction (Second). Elsevier. Available at: https://mcw.on.worldcat.org/search/detail/956648077?queryString=inguinal%20hernia&clusterResults=true&groupVariantRecords=false&format=Book&format=Video&format=Archv&format=Jrnl&format=Map&format=Vis&format=Compfile&format=Object&format=Intmm&format=Web&format=Image&database=all&author=all&year=all&yearFrom=&yearTo=&language=all&scope=wz%3A1698&changedFacet=scope. Accessed January 12, 2023.

20. Cameron, J. L. & Cameron, A. M. (eds). (2020). Current surgical therapy (13th ed., Ser. Current therapy). Elsevier. Available at: https://mcw.on.worldcat.org/search/detail/1126789380?queryString=minimally%20invasive%20inguinal%20hernia&clusterResults=true&groupVariantRecords=false&format=Book&format=Video&format=Archv&format=Jrnl&format=Map&format=Vis&format=Compfile&format=Object&format=Intmm&format=Web&format=Image&database=all&author=all&year=all&yearFrom=&yearTo=&language=all&scope=wz%3A1698&changedFacet=scope&page=2. Accessed January 12, 2023.

21. Solaini L, Cavaliere D, Avanzolini A, et al. Robotic versus laparoscopic inguinal hernia repair: an updated systematic review and meta-analysis. J Robot Surg 2022;16(4):775–81.

22. Qabbani A, Aboumarzouk OM, ElBakry T, et al. Robotic inguinal hernia repair: systematic review and meta-analysis. ANZ J Surg 2021;91(11):2277–87.

23. Vitiello A, Abu Abeid A, Peltrini R, et al. Minimally invasive repair of recurrent inguinal hernia: Multi-institutional retrospective comparison of robotic versus laparoscopic surgery. J Laparoendosc Adv Surg Tech 2022. https://doi.org/10.1089/lap.2022.0209.
24. Prabhu AS, Carbonell A, Hope W, et al. Robotic inguinal vs transabdominal laparoscopic inguinal hernia repair: the RIVAL randomized clinical trial. JAMA Surg 2020;155(5):380–7.

Management of Chronic Postoperative Inguinal Pain

David M. Krpata, MD

KEYWORDS

- Chronic postoperative inguinal pain • Inguinodynia • Inguinal hernia repair
- Neurectomy • Hernia mesh removal

KEY POINTS

- Chronic postoperative inguinal pain (CPIP) can affect all patients regardless of surgical approach including open surgery, minimally invasive surgery, and the use of mesh or primary tissue repairs.
- Initial evaluation of patients with CPIP requires a thorough investigation by the treating physician.
- Nonsurgical therapies include medications, physical therapy, cognitive therapy, and interventional pain management.
- Surgery for CPIP includes neurectomy and/or hernia mesh removal, which results in 90% of patients having an improvement in their pain.

BACKGROUND

Chronic pain after an inguinal hernia repair is the most common long-term complication and the most challenging to manage. Although there has been a recent focus surrounding acute postoperative pain after inguinal hernia surgery with an emphasis on reducing and even eliminating opioid use, it is chronic postoperative inguinal pain (CPIP) that has an equal or even greater potential impact on a patient's life. Many patients suffering from CPIP have reduced activity, limited work capacity, depression, anxiety, and overall reduction in their quality of life.[1]

CPIP is defined as having persistent pain for a minimum of 3 months, for at least 3 months after surgery. For example, a patient who develops pain immediately after an inguinal hernia repair and the pain never resolves can be defined as having CPIP 3 months after the operation. Alternatively, a patient that develops groin pain 3 months after their operation would not technically have a diagnosis of CPIP until 6 months after their operation. Within this definition of CPIP, the characteristics of the pain are not stipulated. The Inguinal Pain Questionnaire developed and validated by Franneby

Cleveland Clinic Lerner College of Medicine, Cleveland Clinic Foundation, 9500 Euclid Avenue, Cleveland, OH 44195, USA
E-mail address: krpatad@ccf.org

Surg Clin N Am 103 (2023) 889–900
https://doi.org/10.1016/j.suc.2023.04.003
0039-6109/23/© 2023 Elsevier Inc. All rights reserved.

and colleagues[2,3] is the most pertinent tool for postoperative inguinal pain (**Box 1**). In a 2018 study, 22,918 Swedish patients were surveyed 1 year after inguinal hernia repair utilizing the Inguinal Pain Questionnaire. In this study, 15.2% of patients reported persistent pain 1 year after the surgery. This specifically meant that patients rated their pain as "pain present, cannot be ignored, impacts concentration on chores or daily activities" or worse. Ten percent rated the pain a 5 or higher on the Inguinal Pain Questionnaire.

In the United States, there are approximately 700,000 inguinal hernias repaired annually. Considering the rate of CPIP is 10% to 15%, more than 100,000 patients will be influenced negatively by an inguinal hernia repair each year in the United States alone. Fortunately, the overall rate of patients seeking medical attention is less than this at 1% to 3% per year. Nevertheless, more than 20,000 patients will seek medical care for CPIP, which is almost half the number of people who will be diagnosed with pancreatic cancer annually. Centers specializing in pancreatic cancer can be found in all major cities; however, CPIP remains an underappreciated disease with limited resources and understanding. The following article will highlight the prevention, diagnosis, medical treatment, and surgical treatment options for CPIP.

RISK FACTORS, NEUROANATOMY, AND PREVENTION

CPIP has several variables that contribute to its cause, including surgical factors and patient factors. As such, completely eliminating CPIP is an unrealistic goal; however, this should not dissuade surgeons from considering options to prevent it. Risk factors for developing CPIP include age younger than 40 years, preoperative pain, earlier groin surgery within 3 years, severe postoperative pain, female gender, an anterior repair and postoperative complications.[4]

All approaches to inguinal hernia repair have the potential for the development of CPIP. This includes anterior approaches with mesh, primary tissue repairs as well as minimally invasive totally extraperitoneal and transabdominal preperitoneal repairs. An anterior approach, or open, inguinal hernia repair is typically considered a greater risk of developing chronic groin pain because of the potential direct contact to inguinal

---

Box 1
Inguinal pain questionnaire (short form)

1. Estimate the worst pain you felt in the operated groin during this past week.
   a. No pain
   b. Pain present but can easily be ignored
   c. Pain present, cannot be ignored but does not interfere with daily activities
   d. Pain present, cannot be ignored, interferes with concentration on chores and daily activities
   e. Pain present, cannot be ignored, interferes with most activities
   f. Pain present, cannot be ignored, necessitates bed rest
   g. Pain present, cannot be ignored, prompt medical advice sought

2. If you have experience groin pain, to what extent has it limited your ability to perform following activities? More than one option may be selected.
   a. Getting up from a low chair
   b. Sitting down (more than 30 minutes)
   c. Standing up (more than 30 minutes)
   d. Going up or down stairs
   e. Driving a car
   f. Exercising or performing sports

nerves. The 3 most important nerves are the iliohypogastric, ilioinguinal, and genitofemoral nerves. These nerves originate from the lumbar plexus with the iliohypogastric nerve from T12-L1, ilioinguinal nerve from L1, and the genitofemoral nerve from L2. Prevention of CPIP is centered on the concept of nerve awareness, which is a respect and understanding of the course of the inguinal nerves to prevent the incorporation of these nerves in the repair as well as avoiding putting these nerves at risk by removing them from their investing fascia.[4]

Importantly for anterior repairs, the iliohypogastric and ilioinguinal nerves pierce through the transversus abdominis muscle in the lateral abdominal wall and run between the transversus abdominis muscle and internal oblique eventually piercing through the internal oblique muscle. The iliohypogastric can most commonly be found 2 to 3 cm above the level of the internal ring while the ilioinguinal will run more inferiorly and travel along the anterior portion of the spermatic cord in the inguinal canal for men and the round ligament for women. The genital branch of the genitofemoral nerve also has the potential for direct injury or contact during an anterior inguinal hernia repair. The genital branch of the genitofemoral nerves runs along the anterior surface of the psoas muscle and through the internal ring along the he inferior portion of the spermatic cord adjacent to the spermatic vein. When performing any inguinal hernia repair, it is best to avoid manipulation of these nerves. Manipulation can result in direct exposure of the nerves to the hernia prosthetics potentially increasing the risk for CPIP. The current recommendation regarding prophylactic neurectomy is to avoid prophylactic neurectomy but practice pragmatic neurectomy, which is to perform selective neurectomy when a nerve is thought to be at-risk.[4]

Regarding hernia-related devices, the anterior approach and minimally invasive approach do not share similar recommendations. For anterior approaches, the use of medium-weight and lightweight mesh has been shown to reduce CPIP when compared with heavyweight synthetic mesh.[5] Unlike anterior repairs, the use of lightweight mesh increases the risk of hernia recurrence while not affecting the rates of CPIP during a minimally invasive approach.[6]

PATIENT EVALUATION OVERVIEW

Evaluation of patients that present with CPIP requires a thorough review of their history, an examination, and imaging. When taking a history of a patient with CPIP, several characteristics of their pain can guide management and provide insight into the potential for a successful treatment. First, an attempt is made to define a patient's pain as either neuropathic or nociceptive. Neuropathic pain is the result of injury to the somatosensory system. Common symptoms include sharp, burning, electrical, and radiating pain. Other paresthesias that are associated with neuropathic pain include numbness, cold sensation, and "pins and needles" sensation. Neuropathic pain can wax and wane and present randomly including waking a patient from sleep. Nociceptive pain is the result of tissue damage or tissue irritation and presents as a dull, aching pain. It commonly can be referred to as mechanical pain or pain that is associated with activity or specific body positions. For example, patients with CPIP who have nociceptive complaints most commonly refer to worsening pain with bending at the waist or sitting with an upright posture. Second, attempts should be made to understand what led to the initial inguinal hernia repair. An expected response is that the patient had a bulge with or without discomfort. Alternatively, patients can describe chronic groin pain without a bulge, which then led to a hernia repair and the pain either failed to improve or worsened. In these instances, it is more important to explore the wide breadth of the differential diagnosis for groin pain because the initial primary cause of their pain may not have been a hernia (**Box 2**). Third, the timing of the pain in relation to the operation can also give clues as to the cause. Severe neuropathic pain that begins immediately after the hernia repair is an indication that a nerve injury has occurred during the operation. This would most often result from fixation directly through a nerve, either suture or tack. Mechanical or nociceptive pain that begins immediately after surgery is suggestive of mesh malposition or meshoma, including perception of mesh plugs. Pain that develops 2 to 6 months after the operation is secondary to scar formation and can be neuropathic or nociceptive. As the duration from the operation increases, the association with the hernia repair and potential for a successful improvement with surgical intervention decrease.

Examination of patients with CPIP begins by ruling out an inguinal hernia recurrence. In the event of a hernia recurrence, the recurrence should be addressed with an operation and the patient should be reassessed for CPIP following recovery. Once a hernia recurrence is ruled out, examination should focus on determining the presence of neuropathic or nociceptive causes of the pain. With experience, hernia prosthetics can be easily assessed with direct examination of the inguinal canal. For example, if direct palpation of a hernia mesh plug may reproduce the patient's nociceptive pain complaints. These patients are most likely to benefit from mesh removal. Alternatively, neuropathic pain can be assessed with dermatomal mapping. Dermatomal mapping is performed by using a skin marker with a felt tip to examine the lower quadrant of the affected side, as well as the upper half of the lower extremity or thigh. The skin marker is gently pressed against the skin, and the patient is asked to assess whether this causes pain, numbness, or invokes a normal sensation. This action is repeated in a grid-like fashion across the lower abdomen and upper half of the lower extremity (**Fig. 1**). At each site of testing, a dot is left for normal sensation, dash (–) for numbness, and plus (+) presence of pain. At the completion of the mapping, the markings

---

Box 2
Differential diagnosis for groin pain

CPIP
  Primary nerve injury
  Secondary nerve injury from scar formation
  Meshoma

Spinal
  Herniated lumbar disk
  Degenerative joint disease
  Sacroiliac joint dysfunction
  Thoracolumbar syndrome

Orthopedic
  Hip labral tears
  Femoral head avascular necrosis
  Acetabular impingement
  Iliopsoas bursitis
  Pelvic fracture

Urologic
  Epididymitis
  Bladder dysfunction

Athletic pubalgia/core injury

Osteitis pubis

Anterior cutaneous nerve entrapment syndrome

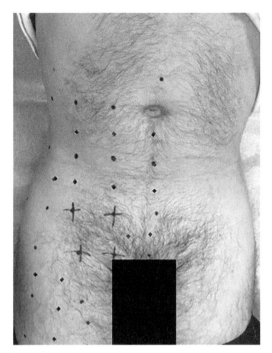

Fig. 1. Dermatomal mapping.

on the skin are assessed for patterns that are consistent with a specific nerve dermatome. Most notable for CPIP are patterns suggestive of iliohypogastric, ilioinguinal, genitofemoral, or lateral femoral cutaneous nerve involvement.

Imaging can be a useful adjunct to evaluation of patients with CPIP. Imaging modality most often depends on the resources available to the surgeon. This author's preference is for dynamic ultrasound evaluation of the groin, which assesses for hernia recurrence, core injuries, neuroanatomy, and any associated neuritis or nerve enlargement, as well as assessment of the any hernia prosthetic and its association with any focal pain. Alternatively, MRI can be used to assess the groin similar to a dynamic ultrasound; however, it comes at a greater cost. Computerized tomography (CT) can be used to rule of mesh related infections and assess the location of a mesh prosthetic during surgical planning for mesh removal. CT scans have limited utility in assessing neuropathic causes of pain.

In patients whom there is a low index of suspicion that the hernia repair has caused the patients complaints, an MRI of the lumbar spine and imaging of the hip should be performed to rule out spinal and orthopedic causes of groin pain. When in doubt, a consultation with an orthopedist and neurosurgeon may be warranted.

MEDICAL TREATMENT OPTIONS

There are several nonsurgical options for the treatment of CPIP including medication, physical therapy, cognitive therapy, and interventional options, such as nerve injections and ablations. Initial postoperative pain should be addressed with acetaminophen, nonsteroidal anti-inflammatory medications, and opioids when appropriate. If pain persists beyond the expected duration of acute postoperative pain or a patient presents months after the initial operation with CPIP, opioids should be avoided and gabapentinoids should be initiated. Gabapentin and pregabalin have multiple functions; however, the treatment of neuropathic pain is the mainstay. Gabapentinoids are gamma-aminobutyric acid (GABA) analogs that function by inhibiting calcium channels. Gabapentin should be initiated at a low dose and titrated to effect, either side effects or the desired effect of pain reduction. The most common side effects associated with gabapentin are somnolence and dizziness. There is a black box warning regarding an increased risk of suicidal thoughts and behaviors, which is the primary reason for initiating this medication at a low dose. The most common starting dosage is 300 mg 3 times daily. Gabapentin can be increased to a total daily dosage of 3600 mg divided over the course of the day (1200 mg, 3 times per day). A more costly alternative to gabapentin is pregabalin. Pregabalin's most common side effects are dizziness and drowsiness. Pregabalin can be started at 50 mg 3 times per day and increased as needed. Studies have demonstrated similar findings to gabapentin, in that, increasing dosage can treat pain in patients who initially have no response to lower dosages of pregabalin.[7] Dosages of up to 600 mg/d divided over 3 daily doses have been used for neuropathic pain. Both gabapentin and pregabalin can exhibit withdrawal symptoms and should be weaned off rather than abruptly stopped.

Other medication adjuncts for the treatment of CPIP include duloxetine hydrochloride, Cymbalta (Eli Lilly & Co, Indianapolis, IN). Duloxetine hydrochloride, a selective serotonin and norepinephrine reuptake inhibitor, received U.S. Food and Drug Administration (FDA) approval for use in treatment of patient with chronic musculoskeletal pain in 2010. Dosing for chronic musculoskeletal pain in CPIP is 60 mg once daily. Duloxetine hydrochloride is most commonly known for its treatment of depression. Patients who are currently being treated for depression at the time of a CPIP diagnosis are encouraged to discuss transitioning their antidepressant medication to duloxetine hydrochloride with the health-care provider who is treating them for depression.

Patients often seek nonmedication therapies to avoid long-term use of prescription medications. Physical therapy may benefit patients with CPIP; however, it should be prescribed with caution because patients with severe mechanical pain from their earlier hernia repair will not tolerate physical therapy well. Physical therapy is reserved for patients with less severe pain that is vague in nature and should be avoided in patients with purely neuropathic pain. Physical therapy should be trialed for a minimum of 3 months and should focus on core strengthening and flexibility. For patients with complaints regarding defecation, urination, and dyspareunia, pelvic floor physical therapy may be more appropriate.

Cognitive behavioral therapy for chronic pain, or chronic pain rehab, has been well studied in pain management. Psychotherapy that relates cognition, emotions, and behaviors to pain likely have a role in treating patients with CPIP. In a study by Miller and colleagues,[1] the authors noted an increased rate of psychological disorders, including anxiety, depression, and pain catastrophizing in patients with CPIP when compared with the general population. Additionally, 18% of patients with CPIP in their cohort reported experiencing emotional or physical abuse. These findings highlight the importance of separating the hernia repair from the patient when treating patients with CPIP. The most important takeaway is that regardless of inguinal hernia repair type, all patients can experience chronic pain, which may be rooted deeper than a prosthetic, fixation or scar formation.

Nonsurgical interventional therapies targeting nerves can be trialed for both therapeutic and diagnostic purposes. Nerve blocks can be performed as field blocks or isolated nerve blocks. A transversus abdominus plane, or TAP, block is an example of a field block. This is a nondirected nerve blockade that can be used for therapeutic purposes to treat or control postoperative pain. Alternatively, isolated nerve blocks targeting specific nerves under image guidance can provide diagnostic information that may guide future surgical interventions. For example, patients with CPIP who are noted to have ilioinguinal nerve changes on ultrasound (US) or have dermatomal mapping suggestive of ilioinguinal nerve distribution will undergo US-guided ilioinguinal nerve block with a local anesthetic. This injection is performed with a low volume (ie, 3 mL) of anesthetic that is injected directly adjacent to the nerve. The intention is to prevent anesthetic from dissipating throughout the groin to other inguinal nerves. If a patient has improvement with this approach, the surgeon can assume the targeted nerve is responsible for the patient's pain. If this injection provides long-term improvement, repeated injections can be performed as needed. If this intervention provides short-term pain relief for less than 48 hours, interventions such as nerve ablation or neurectomy of the targeted nerve should be considered as the next step in management. Other treatment modalities that surgeons should be aware of include dorsal root ganglion blocks or stimulators, transcutaneous electrical nerve stimulations units, and intrathecal pain pumps. These options should be performed by interventional pain management specialist.

SURGICAL TREATMENT OPTIONS

The surgical treatment of CPIP can take many forms including neurectomy and/or mesh removal performed through an open or minimally invasive approach. The decision to perform surgery is equally as challenging as the operations themselves. International organizations have provided treatment algorithms for the management of patients with CPIP.[8] This representation of surgery as another branch point in decision-making is oversimplified. There is no true algorithm for determining if a patient with CPIP should undergo an operation for their pain. It is this author's opinion that the decision to perform surgery is viewed more as a matrix with multiple factors than can influence the decision for or against surgery. This includes quality of life, location of the prosthetic mesh, chronicity of the pain and type of pain, either neuropathic or nociceptive.

Quality of life is paramount when deciding on surgery for CPIP. An in-depth discussion regarding the risk, benefits, and influence on a patient's quality of life centers this decision. Patients with low levels of pain that have minimal impact on their ability to perform daily activities such as self-care, work, and socialization should avoid surgery. Alternatively, patients on the opposite end of the spectrum with limited mobility, loss of work, and loss of relationships have a greater quality of life to regain and are more appropriate candidates for surgery. Mesh and mesh location should also factor into the decision-making. Mesh in the anterior tissue planes have a lower risk of removal compared with mesh placed in the preperitoneal plane; however, with experience performing surgical mesh removal, these risks can be minimized and will have less influence in the decision matrix. The chronicity of a patient's pain is also considered. The longer a patient has experienced pain, the greater the chance their pain has become centralized and peripheral manipulation is less likely to be successful. Equivalent to this concept is the "phantom pain" some patients can experience despite amputation of their limb. Finally, the nature of a patient's pain is used to decide the appropriate operation. For patients with neuropathic pain and abnormalities of the nerves on US, dermatomal mapping suggestive of neuropathic pain or a transient improvement with nerve blocks is considered for neurectomy. Neurectomy is a lower risk operation than mesh removal; however, the changes are permanent and irreversible, which should be considered in the decision-making. Alternatively, patients with nociceptive or mechanical pain are more likely to benefit from mesh removal. Risks associated with mesh removal include, but are not limited to, major vascular injury (iliac vessels), loss of a testicle in men, hernia recurrence, failure to improve pain, and the potential to worsen it. These 4 factors are used to guide shared decision-making between surgeon and patient with CPIP.

Neurectomy

Neurectomy, or transection and segmental resection of a nerve, for CPIP can be performed as a triple neurectomy or selective neurectomy. Triple neurectomy targets the ilioinguinal, iliohypogastric, and genitofemoral nerves as opposed to a selective neurectomy, which targets a specific nerve. Triple neurectomy is performed when patients have neuropathic pain that does not isolate to a single dermatome. Alternatively, when a patient's pain can be isolated to a single nerve, it is this author's preference to perform an isolated neurectomy. Whenever possible, neurectomies are performed through an anterior approach with the nerves transected within the inguinal canal because the nerves traverse through the internal oblique muscle or internal ring. Nerves are transected sharply after suture ligation, and the nerve ending is buried within the muscle bellies of the abdominal wall when possible. Selective genitofemoral neurectomy for patients with preperitoneal mesh after minimally invasive inguinal hernia repair can be addressed laparoscopically. After a diagnostic laparoscopy, isolation and transection of the genitofemoral nerve can be achieved by opening the peritoneum over the psoas muscle with minimal risk. The genital branch can be isolated after bifurcation from femoral branch when appropriate.

Laparoscopic retroperitoneal triple neurectomy provides an alternative approach to triple neurectomy where the surgeon can transect the ilioinguinal, iliohypogastric, and genitofemoral nerves outside of the previous surgical field.[9] This approach is performed with patients in the lateral decubitus position. A balloon dissector is placed into the retroperitoneum and blown up under visualization. The balloon is removed, and the retroperitoneum is insufflated. The ilioinguinal and iliohypogastric nerves are isolated over the quadratus lumborum muscle below the 12th rib after the nerves exit the spine under the psoas muscle (**Fig. 2**). The neurectomy is performed over the quadratus lumborum. Within the retroperitoneum, the genitofemoral nerve is then identified because it pierces through the psoas muscle where a neurectomy can be performed. The laparoscopic retroperitoneal triple neurectomy should only

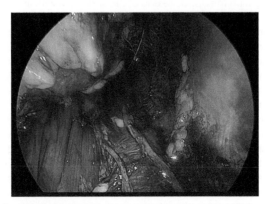

Fig. 2. Laparoscopic retroperitoneal triple neurectomy view of the iliohypogastric and ilioinguinal nerves over the quadratus lumborum muscle.

be performed by surgeons with a thorough understanding of the retroperitoneum and all pertinent anatomy should be delineated before transection of any nerves. Patients should be counseled about the side effects of such a wide neurectomy including possible paresthesia's over the lower quadrant of the abdomen, lateral gluteus, and thigh; potential for lower abdominal wall atrophy and subsequent bulging; and the irreversible nature of a neurectomy. Some have attempted a retroperitoneal triple neurectomy from a supine position; however, the author would caution that proper identification of the appropriate nerves can be more difficult with this approach as the lateral femoral cutaneous nerve can be misinterpreted for the ilioinguinal nerve. Postoperative dermatomal mapping will demonstrate paresthesia along the lateral thigh should this occur.

Mesh Removal

Surgery to remove previously implanted inguinal hernia mesh is an option for patients with CPIP that are refractory to nonsurgical therapy. Performing mesh removal through an open (anterior) approach or a minimally invasive (posterior) approach is determined by the tissue plane of the prosthetic. For mesh placed as a flat sheet within the anterior plane (ie, Lichtenstein repair), removal is approached through an open operation. Alternatively, mesh placed in the preperitoneal plane is addressed from a minimally invasive approach. Biplane meshes, such as hernia plugs and Prolene Hernia Systems (Ethicon; Somerville, NJ), that traverse the inguinal floor and have both anterior and posterior components can be approached either anterior or posterior. It is this author's preference to remove Prolene Hernia Systems through an anterior approach; however, a combined minimally invasive and open approach can be used as well. Hernia mesh plugs are preferentially removed through an anterior approach unless imaging suggests the majority of the mesh plug is within the preperitoneal space. Patients with mesh plugs that have an associated patch (anterior flat sheet) component are carefully assessed to determine if the nociceptive component is thought to be from the plug itself or from the plug and patch. If it is thought that the plug is the cause of the pain and patch is innocent, the plug is removed laparoscopically. For a patient where the plug and the patch are thought to contribute to the CPIP, the plug and patch are removed through an anterior approach.

As with most reoperative surgery, identifying normal anatomy in tissue without scaring is critical. For an anterior approach to mesh removal, the previous incision should be used. The external oblique aponeurosis and the inferior edge of the inguinal ligament is identified and cleared. The external oblique is incised to open the inguinal canal. The mesh prosthetic will most likely be adhered to the external oblique. Careful attention is paid to preserving the external oblique aponeurosis as the shelving edge of the inguinal ligament is identified. The superior flap of the external oblique is then developed by dissecting the mesh off the external oblique aponeurosis, getting beyond the superior portion of the mesh, and exposing the conjoint tendon. After this is complete, the inguinal canal should be completely opened. The spermatic cord is then isolated over the pubis and encircled with a penrose drain. The penrose drain is used to retract the cord because the cord is separated from the mesh until the medial edge of the internal ring is appreciated. The mesh is then dissected off the inguinal floor and underlying muscle beginning at the lateral edge of the mesh working toward the lateral edge of the internal ring. Once the internal ring is identified, a slit is cut in the mesh to create 2 lateral tails. The dissection is continued medially and toward the pubis while unwrapping the mesh from the cord. Finally, the mesh is taken off the final attachments to the shelving edge of the inguinal ligament. During resection of the mesh, the ilioinguinal nerve is commonly encountered and may require neurectomy (**Fig. 3**). Following mesh removal, there may be a recurrent hernia that requires repair. This is typically addressed with the surgeons preferred primary tissue repair of choice. Replacement of prosthetic mesh should be discussed with the patient beforehand to assure they are amenable to additional mesh placement.

Minimally invasive inguinal hernia mesh removal should be addressed as a transabdominal preperitoneal approach. A transverse incision is made along the superior edge of the mesh. The Space of Retzius is entered and the peritoneum is dissected down as the mesh is left on the abdominal wall. The Space of Retzius is opened until the pubic bone and the ipsilateral Coopers ligament are identified. The peritoneum is opened along the inferior edge of the mesh to expose the iliac vessels, gonadal vessels, and vas deferens or round ligament. The lateral edge of the mesh is then dissected off the abdominal wall using cautery. The lateral edge is rolled medially to create tension until the lateral border of the inferior epigastric vessels is encountered. The medial edge of the mesh is then dissected off the overlying muscle working toward the medial edge of the inferior epigastric vessels. Once the medial and lateral edges of the mesh are free, tension is applied to the mesh, and the inferior epigastric vessels are carefully dissected off the mesh. Preservation of these vessels is not critical; however, transecting the vessels can result in these vessels coming down off the abdominal wall with the mesh. Recognizing this is important because the vessels will require ligation again as they come off the iliac vessels. As the dissection progresses toward the iliac vessels, the inferior lateral edge of the mesh is addressed by dissecting the gonadal vessels and the vas deferens from the prosthetic. During this portion of the dissection, the space between the iliac vessels and the mesh is opened obtaining

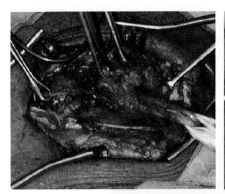
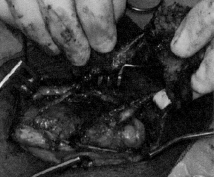
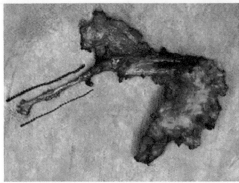

Fig. 3. Open inguinal mesh removal of a previous Lichtenstein inguinal hernia repair.

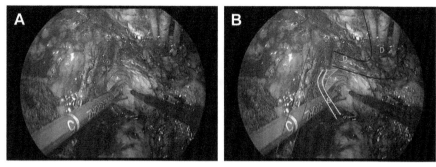

Fig. 4. (*A*) Laparoscopic inguinal mesh removal. (*B*) Laparoscopic inguinal mesh removal with structures (A: gonadal artery and vein, B: vas deferens, C: iliac vein, D: inferior epigastric artery and veins).

a critical view where the inferior epigastric vessels are visualized as they take-off from the iliac vessels (**Fig. 4**). Obtaining this view provides direct access to the proximal epigastric vessels should they require ligation at their take-offs from the iliac vessels during the final dissection of the mesh from the inferior epigastric vessels, which is where the mesh is most adherent. Any final attachments to Coppers ligament and pubis are then addressed, and the mesh is removed from the abdomen once it is fully mobilized. Following mesh removal, if a hernia is identified, it can be addressed with an open primary tissue repair. The most common scenario after mesh removal is that there is no hernia present, which may be the result of scar tissue over the previous defect. If there is no hernia, a prophylactic repair is not performed.

OUTCOMES

When nonoperative therapies fail, surgery can play a significant role in the treatment of CPIP. Fafaj and colleagues[10] reported on the outcomes of surgical intervention for CPIP and found that more than 90% of patients had improvement in their pain and would have mesh removal or neurectomy again. It should be noted that although more than 50% of people will get near resolution of their pain, only 10% achieved complete resolution. It is important to have an informed discussion with patients before surgery to define their expectations regarding their pain. For patients who view complete resolution as the only desired outcome, this author will dissuade these patients from surgery because this is not a realistic expectation.

SUMMARY

CPIP is the most common long-term complication following one of the most common operations performed in the United States every year. Management of any chronic pain can be challenging; however, for surgeons who have no formal training in chronic pain, CPIP, patients can be overwhelming. Referral to hernia centers who specialize in the management of CPIP is equally as important as referral to medical pain management centers. As our understanding of surgical options for CPIP improves, surgery will become a mainstay for refractory pain in CPIP.

CLINICS CARE POINTS

- All inguinal hernia repairs can result in CPIP; however, anterior approaches have shown higher rates compared with laparoscopic approaches.

- Prophylactic neurectomy is not recommended as an attempt to reduce rates of CPIP during inguinal hernia repair.
- Nonoperative options for the treatment of CPIP include medication, physical therapy, cognitive therapy, and interventional pain management.
- Surgical treatment of CPIP with neurectomy and/or mesh removal resulted in pain reduction in 90% of patients.

DISCLOSURE

The author has nothing to disclose.

REFERENCES

1. Miller BT, Scheman J, Petro CC, et al. Psychological disorders in patients with chronic post-operative inguinal pain. Hernia 2023;27(1):35–40.
2. Franneby U, Gunnarsson U, Andersson M, et al. Validation of an inguinal pain questionnaire for assessment of chornic pain after groin hernia repair. Br J Surg 2008;95(4):488–93.
3. Olsson A, Snadblom G, Franneby U, et al. The short-form inguinal pain questionnaire (sf-IPQ): an instrument for rating groin pain after inguinal hernia surgery in daily clinical practice. World J Surg 2019;43(3):806–11.
4. HerniaSurge Group. International guidelines for groin hernia management. Hernia 2018;22(1):1–165.
5. Sajid MS, Leaver C, Baig MK, et al. Systematic review and meta-analysis of the use of lightweight versus heavyweight mesh in open inguinal hernia repair. Br J Surg 2012;99(1):29–37.
6. Bakker WJ, Aufenacker TJ, Boschman JS, et al. Heavyweight mesh is superior to lightweight mesh in laparo-endoscopic inguinal hernia repair: a meta-analysis and trial sequential analysis of randomized controlled trials. Ann Surg 2021; 273(5):890–9.
7. Serpell M, Latymer M, Almas M, et al. Neuropathic pain responds better to increased doses of pregabalin: an in-depth analysis of flexible-dose clinical trials. J Pain Res 2017;10:1769–76.
8. Lange JFM, Kaufmann R, Wijsmuller AR, et al. An international consensus algorithm for management of chronic postoperative inguinal pain. Hernia 2015;19(1): 33–43.
9. Chen DC, Hiatt JR, Amid PK. Operative management of refractory neuropathic inguinodynia by a laparoscopic retroperitoneal approach. JAMA Surg 2013; 148(10):962–7.
10. Fafaj A, Taastaldi L, Alkhatib H, et al. Surgical treatment for chronic postoperative inguinal pain-short term outcomes of a specialized center. Am J Surg 2020; 219(3):425–8.

Primary Uncomplicated Ventral Hernia Repair
Guidelines and Practice Patterns for Routine Hernia Repairs

Matthew Hager, MD[a], Colston Edgerton, MD[b],
William W. Hope, MD[b],*

KEYWORDS

- Umbilical • Epigastric • Hernia • Repair • Mesh • Primary • Laparoscopic • Robotic

KEY POINTS

- Primary ventral hernias usually involve anatomic weaknesses in the midline linea alba at the umbilicus and epigastrium.
- Open, laparoscopic, and robotic repairs each have their own advantages and disadvantages and should be tailored based on clinical characteristics.
- Recent guideline updates characterize hernias as being small (0–1 cm), medium (1–4 cm), and large (over 4 cm) based on diameter of the defect.
- In general, mesh use has been shown to decrease recurrence rates in umbilical hernia repair greater than 1 cm.
- The safest location for mesh is a flat mesh in the preperitoneal or retrorectus space.

INTRODUCTION

Although most surgeons likely understand what defines a primary uncomplicated hernia, it is worthy of discussing as sometimes the definitions can be misunderstood. Primary hernias are defined as hernias that occur where there has not been a previous incision, in contrast to incisional hernias. Primary hernias occur most commonly in the midline at the linea alba due to the abdominal wall anatomy and associated weakness related to a single fascial plane without surrounding muscle. The most common primary hernias are umbilical and epigastric hernias, and of the two, umbilical hernias were found to be present in up to 25% of the population seen on ultrasound (US).[1–5]

No funding was received for this work.
[a] Department of Surgery, Novant/New Hanover Regional Medical Center, 2131 South 17th Street, PO Box 9025, Wilmington, NC 28401, USA; [b] Department of Surgery, Novant/New Hanover Regional Medical Center, University of North Carolina - Chapel Hill, 2131 South 17th Street, PO Box 9025, Wilmington, NC 28401, USA
* Corresponding author.
E-mail address: william.hope@novanthealth.org

https://doi.org/10.1016/j.suc.2023.04.004
0039-6109/23/© 2023 Elsevier Inc. All rights reserved.
surgical.theclinics.com

Although umbilical and epigastric hernias may not be the most technically challenging hernias to repair and often can be referred to as "uncomplicated" these hernias can challenge the surgeon in many ways. Perhaps one of the most challenging parts of treating these hernias is the operating planning. Although most surgeons have a "go to" repair for umbilical and epigastric hernias, the heterogeneity of presentation, patient comorbidities, multiple techniques for repair, decision regarding mesh use, and hopes of avoidance of postoperative complications such as infection, recurrence, and chronic pain often requires careful consideration by the surgeon.

Recently, the European Hernia Society and American Hernia Society (EHS/AHS) published guidelines on the treatment of umbilical and epigastric hernias; although there are certain principles that are supported by evidence for these hernias, there are still many unknowns with debate warranting further research. This article reviews the recent guidelines, controversies, techniques for surgery, and current practice patterns for these common hernias.

Definition, Diagnosis, and Preoperative Considerations

As mentioned earlier, the exact definitions of umbilical and epigastric hernias can be misleading and confusing due to differences in previous classifications. The EHS/AHS guidelines recently suggested a new classification system whereby umbilical hernias are defined as a primary hernia occurring in the midline at the center of the umbilical ring with an epigastric hernia having the center of its defect in the midline above the umbilicus and below the xiphoid process. They further proposed classifying these hernias into small (0–1 cm), medium (1–4 cm), and large (over 4 cm) based on diameter of the defect to better reflect treatment options based on recent research[6] (**Figs. 1–3**)

In general, most cases of umbilical and epigastric hernias can be diagnosed by history and physical alone. There may be some cases where imaging may be useful such as concerns for incarceration/strangulation, patient conditions such as cirrhosis or obesity, or when the hernia defect may be complex, multiple, or large. In these instances, computed tomography (CT) or US may be used based on clinical judgment.

Once an umbilical or epigastric hernia is diagnosed surgeons must discuss treatment options with their patients. The watchful waiting strategy has not been adequately studied for ventral hernias and the studies that do address these hernias usually combine all types of primary and incisional hernias making specific recommendations for umbilical and epigastric hernias difficult. However, due to the high prevalence of umbilical and epigastric hernias, of which many do not seek repair, the strategy of watchful waiting for asymptomatic patients is likely safe, with the recent EHS/AHS recommendations supporting this option.[6]

When surgery is planned, surgeons should evaluate preoptimization strategies that may improve outcomes. Recently, there have been more data focusing on presurgical optimization throughout surgical disciplines. Although they may not be specific to hernia repair, many principles can be extrapolated. As wound complications are some of the most common complications after repair of umbilical and epigastric hernias, it has been suggested to advise smoking cessation for 4 to 6 weeks and weight loss strategies to get the patient to a body mass index (BMI) of 35 kg/m^2 or below before elective surgery.[6]

Prophylactic antibiotic use has also been a topic of research in umbilical and epigastric hernia repair. Although there is insufficient evidence to support routine use, recent guidelines suggest the use of a single perioperative dose when mesh is being used.[6]

Once the patient has been diagnosed, counseled, and optimized for surgery, perhaps the most challenging aspect of planning is consideration of the many technical options for surgical repair.

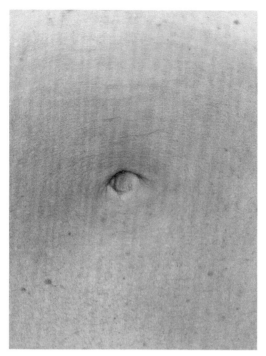

Fig. 1. Small umbilical hernia defined as 0 to 1 cm based on diameter of the defect.

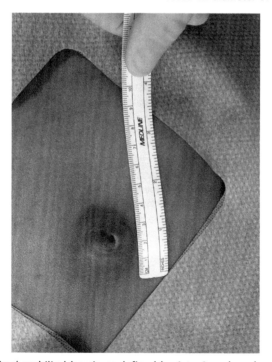

Fig. 2. Medium-sized umbilical hernia as defined by 1 to 4 cm based on diameter of the defect.

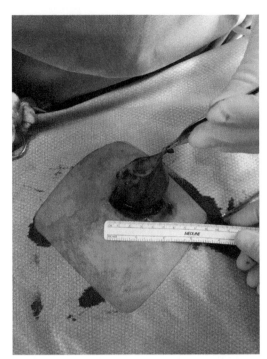

Fig. 3. Large-sized umbilical hernia as defined as great than 4 cm based on diameter of the defect.

SURGICAL CONSIDERATIONS
Primary Suture Repair Versus Mesh Repairs

There continues to be debate about the use of mesh for smaller primary umbilical and epigastric hernias. Although there is substantial evidence that mesh reduces hernia recurrence for larger ventral and incisional hernias,[7] until recently there has not been high-quality evidence for the use of mesh in smaller and primary hernias. Coupled with the concern of the infection and possible chronic pain risk associated with the use of mesh, primary suture repair of umbilical and epigastric hernias remains common.

Recently, there have been five meta-analyses evaluating the use of mesh for umbilical and epigastric hernia with all concluding mesh superior to sutures in reducing recurrence rates.[8–12] The most recent meta-analysis included randomized controlled trial (RCTs), cohort studies, and hernia registries and also concluded decrease in recurrence rate with the use of mesh compared with sutures.[11] Interestingly, it also showed no evidence of higher rates of surgical site infection, hematoma, seroma, or chronic pain with the use of mesh.[11] Secondary to this evidence, the use of mesh was strongly recommended for repair of umbilical and epigastric hernia to reduce recurrence rates in the most recent guidelines.[6] There is, however, continued debate about the use of mesh in hernias less than 1 cm as this group of patients has not been well studied and will likely be difficult to study as these cases can be technically difficult to place mesh in the open fashion without enlarging the defect.

If surgeons do choose to perform suture repair for these hernias, the recent guidelines only have weak evidence to recommend the use of slowly absorbable or nonabsorbable sutures with the exact suture technique being left up to the surgeon[6] (**Fig. 4**).

Open Umbilical/Epigastric Hernia Repairs

There are many different approaches to the open repair of umbilical and epigastric hernias with most relating to plane and technique of mesh placement. There are theoretically five anatomic planes for mesh placement including onlay prefascial plan above the linea able, fascial edges (bridge), retrorectus, preperitoneal, and intraperitoneal onlay mesh (IPOM).[5,13]

Although the evidence is weak relating to which is the ideal plane for mesh placement, the recent EHS/AHS guidelines recommend a flat permanent synthetic mesh in the preperitoneal space[6] (**Figs. 5** and **6**). The guidelines do address specific types of meshes, especially the commonly used preformed meshes specifically designed for intra-abdominal with an anti-adhesive coating (**Fig. 7**). Despite many case series documenting the safety of these meshes, there have been reports of late complications with these meshes including adhesive bowel obstructions or mesh erosions.[14–19] This theoretic advantage of mesh being in the preperitoneal space protected from the viscera as well as the added cost of construction with an anti-adhesive barrier, the guidelines give a weak recommendation for a flat mesh in the preperitoneal position.[6] There has been one RCT comparing flat mesh versus a preformed patch mesh.[15] They reported easier and quicker surgery with the patch mesh with no difference in recurrence rate; however, there was a higher early reoperation rate due to serious complications as well as a higher complication rate at 2 years.[15]

The evidence supporting mesh overlap for epigastric and umbilical hernia repair is also weak, however, suggest that in preperitoneal repair an overlap of 3 cm is needed for hernia defects measuring 1 to 4 cm. Relating to fixation of the mesh and closure of the defect, again there is insufficient evidence to make strong recommendations and

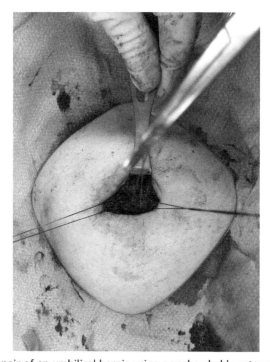

Fig. 4. Primary repair of an umbilical hernia using nonabsorbable sutures.

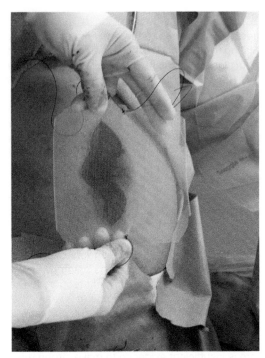

Fig. 5. A flat piece of polypropylene mesh being prepared to be placed in the retromuscular space.

recent guidelines suggest using nonabsorbable suture if fixation is used and closure of the defect in conjunction with mesh placement.[6]

Laparoscopic Umbilical/Epigastric Hernia Repairs

There remains controversy over the benefits of laparoscopy for umbilical hernias. Recent guidelines suggest the use of laparoscopic repair for large (>4 cm) hernias

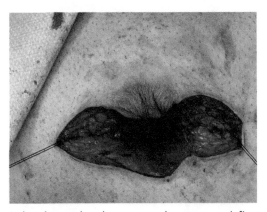

Fig. 6. Mesh after it has been placed retromuscular space and fixated for repair of a medium-sized umbilical hernia.

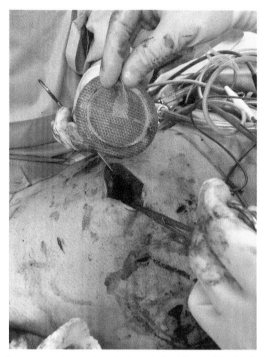

Fig. 7. Placement of a commonly used coated mesh that is specifically designed to be placed for smaller hernias.

or in patients at high risk for wound infection as evidence supports lower infection rates with the use of laparoscopy in these hernias.[6]

There have been six meta-analyses and systemic reviews[20–25] comparing laparoscopic and open repair of ventral hernias but only one[26] specifically related to umbilical hernias. This study evaluated 16,549 patients from three RCTs and seven retrospective reviews and reported increased wound complications, recurrence, and hospital stay but shorter operative time with open repairs.[26] Despite some of the proposed advantages of the laparoscopic repair, it still seems that most umbilical and epigastric hernias are being repaired open with laparoscopy used in about 25% of cases.[27]

The technique for traditional laparoscopic IPOM is well known with gaining of laparoscopic access, lysis of adhesions, reduction of hernia contents with possible sac excision and placement of intra-abdominal mesh[28] (**Fig. 8**). Although there has been recent debate around closure of the defect with laparoscopic IPOM, recent guidelines suggest closing the defect with preperitoneal or retromuscular placement of mesh if possible and at least a 5-cm overlap. If mesh is placed intra-abdominally, guidelines suggest the use of nonabsorbable sutures or tacks.[6]

NEW SURGICAL TECHNIQUES
Robotic Repairs

Robotic platforms have revolutionized surgery and have become very popular in hernia repair. Although there remains debate about where robotic technology is best used in hernia surgery, many surgeons have embraced this technology. Although

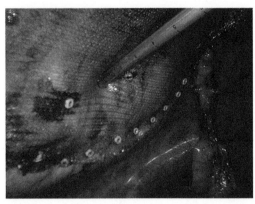

Fig. 8. Traditional laparoscopic IPOM with mesh placement and permanent tack fixation.

there are limited high-quality studies and long-term outcomes associated with robotic hernia repair, many potential advantages are associated with this technology. Specifically related to ventral hernia, there is an improved ability for defect closure and many newer techniques that allow for easier placement of mesh in the preperitoneal or retrorectus space[29] **(Fig. 9)**. Although there is insufficient evidence currently to recommend robotic surgery over any other techniques for repair of umbilical and epigastric hernia, there is no doubt that this technology will find a place in these repairs for certain patients. Critics for the use of robotics in these smaller umbilical and epigastric hernias cite the increased operative time and cost associated with these procedures.[30] Proponents of this technology cite the ability to close defects and place mesh extraperitoneal and often discuss the advantages of gaining expertise with the robotic technology in these smaller and more common hernias[31–33] **(Figs. 10–12)**. Although there likely will be ongoing debate regarding robotic surgery and hernia repair with improved technology, competition in the marketplace, and longer term data regarding outcomes, some answers regarding this technology will be elucidated.

Mini- or Less-Open Sublay and Endoscopic-assisted/Endoscopic Mini- or Less-Open Sublay Repair

One of the potential downsides of open hernia repair relates to the wound complications associated and in some cases the inability to achieve wide overlap of mesh.

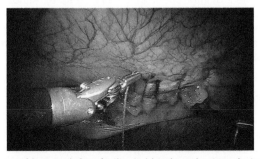

Fig. 9. Suture closure of hernia defect facilitated by the robotic technique.

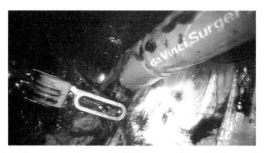

Fig. 10. Expanded totally extraperitoneal (eTEP) access for robotic repair of primary ventral hernia.

Laparoscopic IPOM techniques help solve some of these issues but are hampered by the issue of having mesh placed intra-abdominally with the theoretic disadvantage of adhesions and difficult reoperations even with coated meshes that are made to be placed in this plane.

Recently, a new minimally invasive laparoendoscopic technique has been described with the ability to place a large retromuscular mesh through a small incision using laparoscopic instruments and techniques.[34] This approach has mostly been adopted in Europe but is becoming more popular and can be used for repair of umbilical and epigastric hernias.

Reinpold and colleagues recently reported their experience with mini- or less-open sublay (MILOS) and endoscopic-assisted/endoscopic MILOS (EMILOS) experience in repair of 520 umbilical hernias and 554 epigastric hernias with 1 year follow-up[35] Reported outcomes with this technique showed low recurrence rates of 0% and .5% for umbilical and epigastric hernia, respectively, with low rates or perioperative complications, reoperation, infection, and chronic pain. They concluded that these techniques may be useful for umbilical and epigastric hernias especially in the setting of rectus diastasis.[35]

OUTCOMES

Outcomes associated with umbilical hernia repairs are overall very favorable, however, complications are likely higher than most surgeons appreciate. Recurrence of primary umbilical and epigastric hernias has been cited to be between 1 and 54 depending on the type of repair and follow-up methods.[6,36–39] Aside from recurrences and acute postoperative surgical site occurrences, perhaps the most relevant outcome is patient-reported subjective outcomes. Long-term data addressing chronic

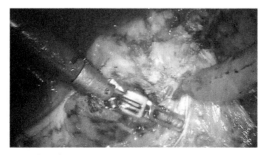

Fig. 11. Robotic eTEP with reducing hernia and dissecting sac.

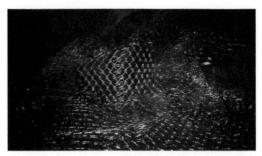

Fig. 12. Robotic eTEP where access was obtained, hernia reduced, and fascial defect closed followed by the placement of mesh.

issues associated with repair come from large national hernia registries. Two good long-term studies come from the Danish hernia registry. One report surveying 295 patients with 5-year follow-up cited chronic complaints in 5.5% of patients that could in part be explained by hernia recurrence.[40] Another study surveyed 132 patients undergoing umbilical hernia repair with a median follow-up of 36 months reporting 12% of patients having moderate/severe pain and a cumulated risk of recurrence of 11.5%.[41] Based on these long-term data, it is important for the surgeon to remember that umbilical and epigastric hernias can cause chronic issues that may be mitigated with appropriate preoperative planning and meticulous surgical technique.

SPECIAL CONSIDERATIONS
Incarcerated/Strangulated

One of the difficulties of making recommendations about treatment for incarcerated or strangulated hernias is the heterogeneity of the patients and cases. Data from the Danish Hernia Database[42] show that emergent hernia surgeries have worse outcomes reporting up to a 15-fold higher readmission, reoperation, and mortality rate compared with elective surgeries. As these studies are not randomized, these results may be confounded by the patient's comorbidities and health status at the time of presentation.[43]

One of the most debated subjects in hernia surgeries relates to the use of mesh in contaminated and clean-contaminated fields and often revolves around whether synthetic mesh, sutures, or biologic/bioabsorbable mesh should be used. Although not definitive, there is evidence to support the use of synthetic mesh in incarcerated umbilical hernias[44,45] with the World Society of Emergency Surgery (WSES) guidelines recommending the use of synthetic mesh for clean and clean-contaminated patients undergoing emergency hernia repair.[46] The most recent EHS/AHS guidelines recommend a tailored approach to incarcerated/strangulated epigastric and umbilical hernias based on patient and hernia characteristics with the consideration of mesh left to surgeon/patient discussion. To date, there is insufficient evidence to support the use of biologic or bioabsorbable mesh in the emergency repair of umbilical or epigastric hernia repair.[6]

Cost

Although cost should not be the first consideration when discussing repair of umbilical and epigastric hernia repair, it requires some attention due to the ubiquitous nature of these procedures. There are limited data about cost specifically related to umbilical and epigastric hernia, but some of the data about hernia in general can be extrapolated. In our current health care system, cost directly attributed to variation in technique and material can be difficult to interpret with many of the contributing factors being out of the control of the surgeon.

Cost of surgical versus nonsurgical treatment options has been compared for umbilical hernia with higher direct financial cost in the first year with surgical treatment; however, with longer term follow-up, cost in the nonsurgical group may surpass those in the surgery group.[47] Relating to surgical care, there are certain areas where cost can be controlled including minimizing wound complications and recurrences, preoperative optimization, utilization of low-cost mesh, and reserving higher cost procedures such as laparoscopic and robotic for those that would see benefit.[6]

Likely cost containment is best served by having the surgeon able to provide good quality care and surgery in an outpatient setting, if appropriate, minimizing complications and recurrence and working in their local environment to achieve cost savings.

Learning Curve and Training

The training and learning curves associated with the repair of umbilical and epigastric hernias are not typically a major focus of the mastery of hernia surgery but deserve attention due to its importance in developing competence for safely performing one of the most common abdominal operations in the world. Furthermore, although these hernias are often thought of as simple, not technically challenging, and often relegated to junior trainees, appropriate training in these hernias is paramount to avoid the viscous cycle of hernia complications that sometimes start with these hernias.[48]

There are minimal data related to the learning curve for open and laparoscopic repair for umbilical and epigastric hernias; however, it is suggested to be around 20 to 30 supervised procedures.[6] Mentorship that stresses to trainees the importance of umbilical and epigastric hernias is that they are not simple/uncomplicated hernias and require meticulous surgical technique and good judgment is an important part of the training process. In addition to this, the use of simulation and structured evidence-based training should allow trainees to successfully perform these repairs.

Practice Patterns

Practice patterns related to umbilical and epigastric hernia vary considerably due to the heterogeneity of patient presentation, comorbidities, and the myriad of techniques available to the surgeon. Older evidence suggests that almost 50% of elective umbilical hernias in the United States are repaired using a primary (suture), even though there has been convincing evidence for the use of mesh.[27]

To help guide surgeons using evidence-based medicine, recent guidelines were published by the EHS/AHS evaluating 18 key questions relating to umbilical and epigastric hernias making recommendations including quality of evidence and strength of recommendation.[6] Two recent studies have help elucidate practice patterns related to umbilical and epigastric hernia in the United States using the Americas Hernia Society/Abdominal Core Health Quality Collaborative (ACHQC). Alkhatib and colleagues evaluated 7030 patients with uncomplicated primary midline ventral hernias reporting overall mesh use of 69% with 98% being synthetic mesh being placed in the intraperitoneal (46%) or preperitoneal (42%) space.[49] They also reported that most of the patients had an open approach (72%) with mesh being used in 58% of these cases and most commonly being patches (70%).[49]

Oyola and colleagues specifically queried the ACHQC to evaluate surgeon's adherence to the recently published guidelines for umbilical and epigastric hernia.[6,50] They reported on 11,088 patients from the ACHQC from 2013 to 2021 and evaluated compliance to selected key questions using a cutoff of 70% for measurement. They concluded that most of the guidelines/recommendations were being followed by surgeons entering data into the ACHQC with noncompliance found for the recommendations of deferring elective surgery for patients with a BMI over 35, preperitoneal placement of mesh, and achieving a 3-cm mesh overlap.[50]

Although these studies shed some light on the current practice patterns, the ACHQC database reports on only a fraction of the total number of umbilical and epigastric hernias performed and therefore firm conclusions cannot be made. As hernia surgery becomes more specialized coupled with the increased knowledge related to these specific hernias, we likely will see improved outcomes and perhaps more adherence to evidence-based guidelines.

SUMMARY

Repair of primary umbilical and epigastric hernias is among the most common abdominal operations performed in the world. Despite being ubiquitous, their management is anything but routine. Recent guidelines can help guide surgeons, whereas evidence for many recommendations remains weak from low-quality data and future well-designed clinical trials addressing key considerations are needed. Nonetheless, there are several guiding principles that surgeons should be familiar with care for these patients most effectively. Ongoing investigation and commitment to understating the role of presurgical optimization and patient selection, meticulous surgical technique, and collecting outcome data will do much to optimize results and minimize morbidity.

CLINICAL CARE POINTS

- Although umbilical hernias are often thought to be uncomplicated, variation in size and patient comorbidiites requires an individualized approach to minimize recurrence and wound morbidity.
- If desired, watchful waiting is generally safe for small uncomplicated fat-containing primary ventral hernias.
- Treatment options, including use of mesh and desired ouctomes should be discussed with patient and shared decision making should be performed for optimal patient outcomes.

DISCLOSURES

Dr W.W. Hope's disclosures (not directly related to the current work): CR Bard: honorarium, speaking, research support; WL Gore: research support, speaking; Lifecell: consulting; Intuitive: speaking, consulting. Medtronic: honorarium consulting/research support.

REFERENCES

1. Bedewi MA, El-Sharkawy MS, Al Boukai AA, et al. Prevalence of adult paraumbilical hernia. assessment by high-resolution sonography: A hospital-based study. Hernia 2011;16:59–62.
2. Nieuwenhuizen J, van Ramshorst GH, ten Brinke JG, et al. The use of mesh in acute hernia: frequency and outcome in 99 cases. Hernia 2011;15:297–300.
3. Christoffersen MW, Rosenberg J, Jorgensen LN, et al. Health-related quality of life scores changes significantly within the first three months after hernia mesh repair. World J Surg 2014;38:1852–9.

4. Bensaadi H, Paolino L, Valenti A, et al. Intraperitoneal tension-free repair of a small midline ventral abdominal wall hernia: randomized study with a mean follow-up of 3 years. Am Surg 2014;80:57–65.
5. Muysoms F, Jacob B. International Hernia Collaboration. consensus on nomenclature of abdominal wall hernia repair. World J Surg 2018;42:302–4.
6. Henriksen NA, Montgomery A, Kaufmann R, et al. Guidelines for treatment of umbilical and epigastric hernias from the European Hernia Society and Americas Hernia Society. Br J Surg 2020;107:171–90.
7. Luijendijk RW, Hop WCJ, van den Tol MP, et al. A comparison of suture repair with mesh repair for incisional hernia. N Engl J Med 2000;343:392–8.
8. Aslani N, Brown CJ. Does mesh offer an advantage over tissue in the open repair of umbilical hernias? A systematic review and meta-analysis. Hernia 2010;14:455–62.
9. Nguyen DH, Nguyen MT, Askenasy EP, et al. Primary fascial closure with laparoscopic ventral hernia repair: systematic review. World J Surg 2014;38:3097–104.
10. Mathes T, Walgenbach M, Siegel R. Suture versus mesh repair in primary and incisional ventral hernias: a systematic review and meta-analysis. World J Surg 2016;40:826–35.
11. Bisgaard T, Kaufmann R, Christoffersen MW, et al. Lower risk of recurrence after mesh repair versus non-mesh sutured repair in open umbilical hernia repair: a systematic review and meta-analysis of randomized controlled trials. Scand J Surg 2018;108:187–93.
12. Shrestha D, Shrestha A, Shrestha B. Open mesh versus suture repair of umbilical hernia: meta-analysis of randomized controlled trials. Int J Surg 2019;62:62–6.
13. Muysoms F. IPOM: history of an acronym. Hernia 2018;22:743–6.
14. Porrero JL, Cano-Valderrama O, Villar S, et al. Umbilical hernia repair with composite prosthesis: a single-centre experience. Hernia 2019;23:143–7.
15. Ponten JEH, Leenders BJM, Leclercq WKG, et al. Mesh versus patch repair for epigastric and umbilical hernia (MORPHEUS Trial); one-year results of a randomized controlled trial. World J Surg 2018;42:1312–20.
16. Berrevoet F, Doerhoff C, Muysoms F, et al. A multicenter prospective study of patients undergoing open ventral hernia repair with intraperitoneal positioning using the monofilament polyester composite ventral patch: interim results of the PANACEA study. Med Devices (Auckl) 2017;10:81–8.
17. Perrakis E, Velimezis G, Vezakis A, et al. A new tension-free technique for the repair of umbilical hernia, using the Prolene Hernia System – early results from 48 cases. Hernia 2003;7:178–80.
18. Vychnevskaia K, Mucci-Hennekinne S, Casa C, et al. Intraperitoneal mesh repair of small ventral abdominal wall hernias with a Ventralex hernia patch. Dig Surg 2010;27:433–5.
19. Tollens T, Den Hondt M, Devroe K, et al. Retrospective analysis of umbilical, epigastric, and small incisional hernia repair using the Ventralex™ hernia patch. Hernia 2011;15:531–40.
20. Castro PM, Rabelato JT, Monteiro GG, al at. Laparoscopy versus laparotomy in the repair of ventral hernias: systematic review and meta-analysis. Arq Gastroenterol 2014;51:205–11.
21. Forbes SS, Eskicioglu C, McLeod RS, et al. Meta-analysis of randomized controlled trials comparing open and laparoscopic ventral and incisional hernia repair with mesh. Br J Surg 2009;96:851–8.
22. Liang MK, Berger RL, Li LT, et al. Outcomes of laparoscopic vs open repair of primary ventral hernias. JAMA Surg 2013;148:1043–8.

23. Sajid MS, Bokhari SA, Mallick AS, et al. Laparoscopic versus open repair of incisional/ventral hernia: a meta-analysis. Am J Surg 2009;197:64–72.

24. Sauerland S, Walgenbach M, Habermalz B, et al. Laparoscopic versus open surgical techniques for ventral or incisional hernia repair. Cochrane Database Syst Rev 2011;3:CD007781.

25. Zhang Y, Zhou H, Chai Y, et al. Laparoscopic versus open incisional and ventral hernia repair: a systematic review and meta-analysis. World J Surg 2014;38: 2233–40.

26. Hajibandeh S, Hajibandeh S, Sreh A, et al. Laparoscopic versus open umbilical or paraumbilical hernia repair: a systematic review and meta-analysis. Hernia 2017;21:905–16.

27. Funk LM, Perry KA, Narula VK, et al. Current national practice patterns for inpatient management of ventral abdominal wall hernia in the United States. Surg Endosc 2013;27:4104–12.

28. Shao JM, Elhage SA, Prasad T, et al. Outcomes of laparoscopic-assisted, open umbilical hernia repair. Am Surg 2020;86:1001–4.

29. Henriksen NA, Jensen KK, Muysoms F. Robot-assisted abdominal wall surgery: a systematic review of the literature and meta-analysis. Hernia 2019;23:17–27.

30. Ye L, Childers CP, de Virgilio M, et al. Clinical outcomes and cost of robotic ventral hernia repair: Systematic review. BJS Open 2021;5.

31. Prabhu AS, Dickens EO, Copper CM, et al. Laparoscopic vs robotic intraperitoneal mesh repair for incisional hernia: An Americas Hernia Society Quality Collaborative Analysis. J Am Coll Surg 2017;225:285–93.

32. Santos DA, Limmer AR, Gibson HM, et al. The current state of robotic retromuscular repairs—a qualitative review of the literature. Surg Endosc 2020;35:456–66.

33. Earle D. Robotic-assisted laparoscopic ventral hernia repair. Surg Clin N Am 2020;100:379–408.

34. Reinpold W, Schröder M, Berger C, et al. Mini- or less-open sublay operation (Milos): A new minimally invasive technique for the extraperitoneal mesh repair of incisional hernias. Ann Surg 2019;269:748–55.

35. Reinpold W, Schröder M, Berger C, et al. Milos and Emilos repair of primary umbilical and epigastric hernias. Hernia 2019;23:935–44.

36. Halm JA, Heisterkamp J, Veen HF, et al. Long-term follow-up after umbilical hernia repair: Are there risk factors for recurrence after simple and mesh repair. Hernia 2005;9:334–7.

37. Arroyo A, García P, Pérez F, et al. Randomized clinical trial comparing suture and mesh repair of umbilical hernia in adults. Br J Surg 2001;88:1321–3.

38. Polat C, Dervisoglu A, Senyurek G, et al. Umbilical hernia repair with the prolene hernia system. Am J Surg 2005;190:61–4.

39. Schumacher OP, Peiper C, Lörken M, et al. Langzeitergebnisse der Nabelhernienreparation nach spitzy. Chirurg 2003;74:50–4.

40. Westen M, Christoffersen MW, Jorgensen LN, et al. Chronic complaints after simple sutured repair for umbilical or epigastric hernias may be related to recurrence. Langenbeck's Arch Surg 2014;399:65–9.

41. Erritzoe-Jervild L, Christoffersen MW, Helgstrand F, et al. Long-term complaints after elective repair for small umbilical or epigastric hernias. Hernia 2013;17: 211–5.

42. Helgstrand F, Jørgensen LN, Rosenberg J, et al. Nationwide prospective study on readmission after umbilical or epigastric hernia repair. Hernia 2013;17:487–92.

43. Li LT, Jafrani RJ, Becker NS, et al. Outcomes of acute versus elective primary ventral hernia repair. J Trauma Acute Care Surg 2014;76:523–8.

44. Abdel-Baki NA, Bessa SS, Abdel-Razek AH. Comparison of prosthetic mesh repair and tissue repair in the emergency management of incarcerated para-umbilical hernia: a prospective randomized study. Hernia 2007;11:163–7.
45. Bessa SS, Abdel-Razek AH. Results of prosthetic mesh repair in the emergency management of the acutely incarcerated and/or strangulated ventral hernias: a seven years study. Hernia 2013;17:59–65.
46. Birindelli A, Sartelli M, Di Saverio S, et al. Update of the WSES guidelines for emergency repair of complicated abdominal wall hernias. World J Emerg Surg 2017;12:37.
47. Strosberg DS, Pittman M, Mikami D. Umbilical hernias: the cost of waiting. Surg Endosc 2017;31:901–6.
48. Liang MK, Berger RL, Li LT, et al. Outcomes of laparoscopic vs open repair of primary ventral hernias. JAMA Surgery 2013;148:1043.
49. Alkhatib H, Fafaj A, Olson M, et al. Primary uncomplicated midline ventral hernias: Factors that influence and guide the surgical approach. Hernia 2019;23: 873–83.
50. Malysz Oyola AM, Faulkner J, Casas B, et al. Are Surgeons of the Abdominal Core Health Quality Collaborative Following Guidelines in Umbilical and Epigastric Hernia Repair? Am Surg 2022;88(9):2163–9.

Preoperative Optimization for Abdominal Wall Reconstruction

Archana Ramaswamy, MD, MBA

KEYWORDS

- Abdominal wall reconstruction • Prehabilitation • Ventral hernia
- Preoperative pneumoperitoneum • Botulinum toxin A

KEY POINTS

- The outcomes of abdominal wall rehabiliation may be improved with prehabiliation of co-morbidities and prehabilitation of the abdominal wall.
- Advanced age, smoking, diabetes, obesity, cirrhosis, and frailty have been identified as risk factors in the population who may benefit from prehabilitation.
- Emerging data from prehabilitaion programs demonstrates mixed outcomes.
- Prehabilitation of the abdominal wall includes mainly usage of botulinum toxin A for chemical component separation, and preoperative progressive pneumoperitoneum, both effective an appropriately selected population.

INTRODUCTION

Despite regional variation, and referral patterns, the prevalence of complex abdominal wall defects and the need for abdominal wall reconstruction continues to increase. The proportion of these patients having serious comorbidities also seems to be increasing. A systematic review and meta-analysis of 22 studies including 5284 patients who underwent open transversus abdominus release (TAR) identified age, gender, body mass index (BMI), comorbidities, and tobacco exposure as being associated with surgical site occurrence (SSO) and with overall complications.[1]

Because of the risk and costs of postoperative complications, especially surgical site infections, some have suggested that preoperative optimization might be more important than operative technique,[2] though in reality it is a combination of the two which likely to provide the best outcomes.

University of Minnesota, Minneapolis VA Medical Center
E-mail address: ramaswam@umn.edu
Twitter: @ArchanaR8 (A.R.)

Surg Clin N Am 103 (2023) 917–933
https://doi.org/10.1016/j.suc.2023.04.022
0039-6109/23/© 2023 Elsevier Inc. All rights reserved.

surgical.theclinics.com

In discussing prehabilitation, we can divide the topic into 2 main sections.

1. Prehabilitation of comorbidities—minimizing preexisting conditions that are associated with increased risks of postoperative complication (both early and late).
2. Prehabilitation of the abdominal wall—preoperative adjuncts that allow restoration of midline and/or allow for the procedure to be completed successfully.

PREHABILITATION OF COMORBIDITIES
Age

With an average life expectancy extending into the mid-80s in many developed nations in the world, patients are being referred for surgical consultation with symptomatic hernias later in life. The perceived risks of surgery stem from both the aging organ systems and from multimorbidity (Charlson Comorbidity Index ≥3, cognitive dysfunction, and frailty). In a pilot study of patients over age 60 years referred for inguinal or ventral hernia to a tertiary care center, high rates of cognitive impairment (29%–47%), frailty (16%) or prefrailty (53%), and multimorbidity (>94%) were present. Surprisingly, there were no significant differences between the age groups of 60 to 64, 65 to 70, or over 70 years. These findings not only suggest that age is just a number, but also that patients not routinely considered elderly may have some significant associated factors that could affect their outcome.[3] Multimorbidity was also seen more commonly in the older population, 55% to 98% of adults over age 65 years, compared with 30% in younger adults. Multimorbidity in ventral hernia patients is associated with increased length of stay, higher mortality, higher rates of emergency surgery, and higher rates of discharge to a care facility. Higher rates of functional dependence can be noted in older patients, and this is also associated with higher rates of complications and mortality. Further data from the pilot study noted that in the 26 patients who did eventually undergo ventral hernia repair, there were similar outcomes when examining readmission, complications, length of stay, and discharge home without any supportive care when stratified into the tertiles of age over 60 years. Of note, the outcomes predicted by age when using risk calculators such as National Surgical Quality Improvement Program (NSQIP) and Charlson Comorbidity Index (CCI) overestimated the expected postoperative complications.[4] It could however be argued that this was a selected population and outcomes in a tertiary care referral center may not be representative of the population undergoing repair elsewhere.

When focusing on the complex abdominal wall population, in a retrospective study examining 300 patients undergoing TAR, no differences were found in readmission at 30 days, in hospital complications, or surgical site infection (SSI) when comparing ages less than 60, 60 to 70, or greater than or equal to 70.[5] These outcomes are also similar to the findings in an NSQIP study including patients from 2005 to 2013 where no differences were found in complications when including patients undergoing both anterior and posterior components separation. Curiously, SSI rate was lower with advancing age.[6] Overall, age could be a proxy for frailty and multimorbidity, but is likely not an independent risk factor for poor outcome. It is most important to note that the above outcomes focus on what is likely a highly selective population who met selection criteria for hernia repair and not the general elderly population with an abdominal wall defect. Prehabilitation for specific associated risk factors can of course be instituted, but these older patients might also benefit from the use of shared decision-making tools. A small randomized study noted improved hernia specific knowledge retention in the experimental arm where the tool was used with high levels of patient satisfaction.[7]

Smoking

Smoking is associated with tissue hypoxia, poor wound healing, and vitamin C deficiency. It is associated with hernia formation and recurrence. Postoperative wound complications are also higher in current smokers[8], and health care costs following inpatient surgical procedures for up to 1 year postoperatively have been shown to be higher in current and former smokers.[9] Current smokers have a higher recurrence rate even with umbilical hernia repair.[10] They have higher rates of respiratory and infectious complications after ventral and incisional hernia repair, and a higher rate of complications, reoperation, readmission, and death.[11]

With higher risk surgical procedures, it is common for requirements to include 4 weeks of preoperative smoking cessation. Randomized evidence notes that smoking cessation 4 weeks preoperatively decreases postoperative complications from 41% to 21%. This group included patients undergoing hernia repair in addition to other procedures, though no subset analysis was performed specifically for hernia patients.[12]

Surgery has been identified as a "teachable moment" to motivate smoking cessation in adults over age 50 years. Even though the highest rates of cessation are associated with those undergoing cardiac or cancer surgery, outpatient procedures are more common and therefore have the largest population impact. Overall, 8% of all "quit events" annually in the United States have been attributed to surgical procedures.[13]

Various methods of smoking cessation have been investigated and almost any type of intervention has been shown to have some efficacy,[14,15] even if started within 2 weeks of surgery. Preoperative advice at the surgical clinic visit to stop smoking prior to hernia surgery has been shown to be effective in almost 20% of individuals, with the rates being improved with a reminder after the clinic visit.[16]

The most effective methods of achieving smoking cessation perioperatively, and maintaining it long term, involve programs that combine pharmacotherapy with counseling sessions.[17] Nicotine replacement is often used, and the possible risks of nicotine replacement therapy are likely outweighed by the benefits,[18] with some evidence that nicotine replacement therapy is not associated with an increased risk of postoperative complications, mortality or readmissions.[19]

Long-term smoking cessation, which may improve long-term hernia recurrence rates, and is a component of whole health, may be associated with timing of preop smoking cessation. In a worldwide cohort of patients undergoing inpatient surgery, almost 40% remained abstinent at 1 year postop. Patients who had quit smoking over 2 weeks before surgery were more likely to be successful long term compared with those who had quit within 2 weeks, or just prior to surgery (day 0 or 1 before surgery).[20]

Diabetes

Perioperative hyperglycemia has been associated with higher rates of postoperative complications and hospital costs in general surgery patients.[21] This has also been noted in patients undergoing complex ventral hernia repair, where perioperative hyperglycemia has been associated with increased length of stay, cost, and higher SSO rates.[22] HbA1C is often used as a marker of assessing hyperglycemia over the 3 months prior and potentially predicting perioperative hyperglycemia. The relationship is complex as perioperative hyperglycemia is associated with a higher rate of readmission following gastrointestinalsurgery, though preop HbA1C does not demonstrate any such correlation. Patients with a higher HbA1c in this study had more frequent postoperative glucose checks and received more frequent insulin doses which may have led to tighter perioperative blood sugar control.[23]

Despite conflicting data on the predictive value of HbA1C, expert consensus in 2017 recommends avoidance of elective ventral hernia repair with HbA1C of greater than 8, with preoperative intervention when greater than 6.5%.[24] Recently, an ACHQC study that looked at outcomes in 2167 patients with diabetes mellitus undergoing ventral hernia repair found no difference in 30-day complication rate, SSI, or composite recurrence at 24 months comparing groups with a HbA1C cutoff of 8%. There was a slightly higher readmission rate (7% vs. 5%) in the group with an HbA1C of greater than or equal to 8%. Since this was a retrospective study, it is impossible to identify whether the group with HbA1C of greater than or equal to 8% had undergone preoperative optimization from an even higher value.[25]

Although it is clear that perioperative glycemic control is of utmost importance, it is difficult to discern whether historical glycemic control via HbA1C affects outcomes. Most recommendations, however, continue to err on the side of caution, and the cutoff of HbA1C of 8 remains.

Obesity

The global obesity epidemic has led to an increased incisional hernia rate, in addition to hernias of increased complexity. BMI is commonly used to estimate body fat content, and cutoffs of 35 or 40 are frequently used. Long-term recurrence rates have also been noted to be increased, even in umbilical hernia repairs, where a BMI increase by 1 point outside of the normal range has been associated with a 9% increased recurrence rate.[10] In more complex hernias, higher rates of wound complications have been noted after parastomal hernia repair,[26] and higher recurrence rates after lateral hernia repairs.[27] In open ventral hernia repairs, an increase in SSI is noted with increasing BMI, as a continuum without a cut point off at a specific BMI.[28] In another study, BMI in the fourth quartile (mean BMI = 43.29) was associated with a higher rate of complications, and was associated with the largest amount of additional spending per complication compared with other factors such as insulin-dependent diabetes, unhealthy alcohol use, and smoking.[29]

BMI, however, may also not be the best measurement of obesity, and some data suggest that visceral fat volume as calculated from preoperative computed tomography (CT) scans may be more informative. In a population undergoing open abdominal wall reconstruction, visceral fat volume above the mean was associated with higher rates of SSO and hernia recurrence, even when BMI did not demonstrate an association.[30]

These associations become less clear when considering minimally invasive abdominal wall reconstruction. In a cohort of 461 patients undergoing laparoscopic or robotic retromuscular abdominal wall reconstruction, there were no differences observed in length of stay, total costs, postoperative complications, or recurrence at 1 year when BMI of greater than 35 was compared with BMI of less than 35. Subgroup analysis with the BMI cutoff being raised to 40 did not alter these findings.[31] These findings have been duplicated by other groups where no differences in short-term complications have been noted between those who underwent minimally invasive retromuscular repair with a BMI cutoff of below or above 35.[32] Even in a heterogenous mix of IPOM (intraperitoneal onlay mesh), TAPP (transabdominal preperitoneal), and retromuscular repairs, no differences in outcomes from the standpoint of complications or recurrence free interval were noted when comparing patients with class II and class III obesity.[33,34]

Achievement of weight loss in patients with complex hernias can be challenging. Less than half of the patients with a BMI of greater than or equal to 35 who were referred to a "weight management navigator" with access to both free and paid programs enrolled in any program. Of those who enrolled, less than half followed up in the hernia clinic at 3 months. Those who participated in the program, however, did lose significantly more weight than those who did not participate (6 kg vs. 1.8 kg).[35]

Given the difficulty of achieving weight loss in some patients, there is a concern about increased hernia complexity developing during this observation period. In a group of patients who underwent open ventral hernia repair, and had 2 preoperative CT scans, several interesting outcomes were noted. Hernia defect size and especially hernia volume increased during the time period of observation regardless of any change in weight. Intra-abdominal volume, subcutaneous volume, and hernia volume were significantly affected by a weight change, both in the 5 kg and the 5 to 10 kg ranges, with less impressive impact over 10 kg. The impact of the weight change was also significantly more in male patients compared with female patients.[36] Similarly, in a group of patients with hernia defects greater than 7 cm horizontally, who underwent observation for various reasons (~50% for operating roomdelays, ~50% for comorbidities, smoking, obesity, lack of symptoms), CT scans over a 6 month time period identified a significant increase in fascial defect area and hernia sac volume. Interestingly, there were no significant changes in hernia-related quality of life scores or physical activity score (The International Physical Activity Questionnaires).[37]

Given the known challenges with achieving weight loss through diet and behavior modification, bariatric surgery is often considered as part of the pathway for the appropriately selected patient. Various studies have demonstrated the safety and benefit of performing a staged bariatric surgery followed by ventral hernia repair to achieve long-term success, even in the complex group of patients with obesity and hernias with loss of domain.[38]

Cirrhosis

Ventral hernias have a high prevalence in individuals with cirrhosis when ascites is present (20%–40%), compared with the noncirrhotic population (2%–3%). This is likely to be multifactorial starting with fascial weakening due to sarcopenia and variceal formation, worsened by increased intra-abdominal pressure from accumulation of ascites. With the risks of skin thinning, breakdown and ascites leak with observation, there are potential benefits to early repair. However, the outcomes from hernia repair can be dismal with recurrence rates as high as 70% to 75% with additional risks of infection and ascites leak when the ascites has not been controlled. Based on the above, watchful waiting has been trialed in patients with cirrhosis. The failure rate of watchful waiting may be 20% to 30%, and the outcomes of urgent repair in this population are worse than in the elective situation, both in prospective and retrospective studies.[39–44]

A VASQIP (The Veterans Affairs Surgical Quality Improvement Program) study has demonstrated a low risk of 30 day and 90 day mortality for umbilical and ventral hernias when performed electively (1%–2%), compared with 13% to 15% when performed on an emergent basis. For all abdominal surgeries, factors associated with poor outcome included MELD (Model For End-Stage Liver Disease) of greater than or equal to 10, low serum albumin, encephalopathy, ascites, and medical comorbidities.[45] Even in umbilical hernias, a systematic analysis of 23 studies with 3229 patients noted that cirrhosis conferred an odd ratio of 8.5 for mortality following repair, with emergency repair being associated with a 2.6 odds ratio compared with elective repair.[46]

With this high rate of failure of observation, and suboptimal outcomes from urgent repair, optimization of the patient with cirrhosis and proceeding with elective repair may be the best pathway to follow. Medical management of ascites should be optimized. In patients where this cannot be achieved, options include paracentesis and Transjugular Intrahepatic Portosystemic Shunt (TIPS). Both have possible associated complications and should be discussed with a multidisciplinary team. If paracentesis is chosen, repeated paracentesis versus placement of a temporary dialysis catheter at the time of surgery can be considered. In a patient with a high MELD (score > 15), thought should be given to whether the patient is a transplant candidate (with hernia repair at time of transplant). If the patient is not a transplant candidate and cannot be optimized via medical management or TIPS, the risk-benefit ratio of high risk surgery versus supportive care should be considered in a patient-centered approach.[39]

Markov modeling suggests that even patients with an MELD-Na score up to 21.3 would benefit from an elective ventral hernia repair.[47] Even in the scenario of refractory ascites, outcomes similar to those in patients without refractory ascites can be achieved.[48]

In our institution, the protocol for these patients includes US-guided paracentesis the day before surgery (with albumin infusion if needed), followed by weekly, or more frequent, outpatient paracentesis based on patient symptomatology. In urgent cases, consideration can be given to leaving a tunneled peritoneal dialysis catheter allowing for continuous drainage and albumin infusion for 7 to 10 days. A trial can then be performed of clamping the catheter to check that the wound is watertight, followed by removal of the catheter. This of course requires an inpatient stay, but is often reasonable as these patients may require a period of inpatient medical management for liver disease stabilization.

Frailty

There is no clearly agreed upon definition, but frailty tends to refer to reduced physiologic function related to age. It renders patients vulnerable to poor outcomes from medical and surgical procedures. Frailty does increase with age, going from 6.5% from age 60 to 69 years up to 65% at age over 90 years.[49] Various tools have been used to identify frailty and vary in complexity. It is interesting to note that "the eyeball test" continues to have a role with initial appearance of frailty being associated with a hazard ratio of 2.14 for mortality in vascular surgery patients.[50]

In a Michigan Surgical Quality Collaborative Hernia Registry Study, using the 5 factor modified frailty index (mF15) scoring system, 4406 patients undergoing ventral hernia repair were studied. Approximately 47% of patients did not have any frailty, with 36% having moderate frailty, and 17% with severe frailty. Those with severe frailty tended to be older, with higher BMI, higher ASA (American Society of Anesthesiology) class, and with larger hernias. When compared with no frailty, severe frailty was associated with higher odds of any complication, serious complication, SSI, and postdischarge adverse events. Any complications and serious complications were also increased in those with severe frailty at smaller (2 cm) and larger (5 cm) hernia sizes. There was also a higher rate of any complication and SSI in the severely frail group when the operation was performed open.[51]

A described method of identifying frailty is by using CT scan identified sarcopenia as a marker. Sarcopenia is a combination of decreased skeletal muscle mass and decreased strength. CT calculations have been described using the area and Housfield units of the psoas muscle. Ventral hernia repair in patients with sarcopenia were noted to have a 5 times higher rate of postoperative complications. Of note, age was not an independent risk factor for postoperative complications.[52] Another study examining sarcopenia and ventral hernia outcomes did not identify any difference in outcome related to sarcopenia. There may be multiple explanations for this, ranging from the methods of calculating sarcopenia to prehabilitation in specialized centers based on other high-risk indicators.[53] As the above studies demonstrate, there is still more research required to identify whether sarcopenia can be consistently used as a proxy for frailty.

As complex as it is to define frailty, identifying which prehabilitation strategies are most effective may be equally challenging. Most studies that have examined prehabilitation focus on patients requiring orthopedics procedures or oncologic resections. Studies that examine a single modality of prehabilitation have focused on nutrition, exercise, or cognitive therapy. Studies that used a multimodality approach often combined some of the above, with some studies also including psychological counseling, and pain management. The outcomes have been heterogeneous with many resulting in no difference between the groups in terms of postoperative outcomes. Some studies have noted lower SSI, decreased overall complication, and decreased length of stay. Many studies seem to lack adequate power.[54] A multicenter RCT is underway to identify whether 3 weeks of a prehabilitation program for individuals over 70 years identified as having frailty or pre-frailty prior to elective general surgery is effective at 1 year follow-up.[55]

Prehabilitation Programs

The individual comorbidities discussed above can be seen in isolation, but are not infrequently seen in combination in an individual patient. An Americas Hernia Society Quality Collaborative (AHSQC) study of open incisional hernia repair using synthetic mesh in a clean field looking at the modifiable comorbidities discussed above (obesity, diabetes, and smoking) demonstrated that patients with any of these were at increased odds of developing a wound complication at 30 days, with the risks increasing with more than 1 comorbidity. More than 1 comorbidity also increased the risks of requiring intervention for a wound complication.[56]

Prehabilitation programs that are not tied to a specific comorbidity have also been described. Though not specifically a prescribed program, increasing levels of preoperative exercise have been associated with a lower postoperative complication rate and lower readmission rate in patients undergoing ventral hernia repair. This finding may be scalable by incorporating increased exercise in preoperative counseling.[57]

Many patients are not referred for preoperative optimization with surgeons identifying barriers including lack of resources, lack of institutional support, and loss of income and referrals.[58] The addition of pay for performance (for prehabilitation referral), surgeon education, and addition of onsite referral facilitators increased the use of prehabilitation prior to hernia repair by 860% in a pilot project.[58]

In patients diverted to the prehabilitation option for smoking, obesity, or frailty screening based on advanced age, a 1 year follow-up was associated with a low rate of emergency surgery (3%), an increase in the number of low-risk patients seen in clinic who went on to hernia surgery, and an increase in RVUs (relative value units) by 58% attributable to hernia operations. In terms of success of prehabilitation, about 9% of patients underwent surgery, and only 1 patient underwent surgery at another facility over the 1 year time period.[59] Another similar study followed patients where the surgeon elected observation based on risk factors—high-risk comorbidities (15.6%), current smoker (18%), HbA1C of greater than 8%, or BMI greater than 33 (68%). Approximately 78% of the patient desired repair, the majority due to pain or functional limitations. At 3 year follow-up, 66% of the patients were reached, with 1/3 of them having visited the emergency department (ED) due to hernia symptoms. Approximately 37% had undergone repair, 75% of which were elective repairs (majority after having reached preoperative requirements such as weight loss). Those who had undergone surgery had a lower median pain score, and improved general satisfaction and cosmesis scores compared with at the start of the study.[60]

Success of prehabilitation in all settings is not that clear. Follow-up of a trial of patients randomized into prehabilitation for obesity with BMI of 30 to 40 noted that 70% assigned to the prehabilitation group completed the program and lost weight with a lower postoperative complication rate. However, at 2 year follow-up there was no difference in percentage of patients who underwent hernia repair, experienced complications, or were hernia-free. There was a high use of minimally invasive surgery (MIS) procedures, and the included patients were in the lower BMI range of obesity, with small to medium sized hernias. Patients in the prehabilitation group did not maintain their weight loss and this may well signal the need to discuss posthabilitation in addition to prehabilitation in this complex group.[61]

Even within a structured program for patients identified as being high risk, 45% did not undergo surgery over a 4 year retrospective study. The causes included inability to meet goals, decrease in symptoms, other medical concerns, and seeking care in a different institution. Of the 65% who did successfully undergo surgery for complex abdominal wall defects, the complications were similar in frequency with the low-risk patients.[62]

While considering the high rate of patients who do not undergo surgery while enrolled in structured or unstructured programs, we should consider the patient-reported outcomes following hernia surgery. In patients with incisional hernias, 63% in one study reported postoperative symptoms of pain, a protrusion, or discomfort, with the same percentage also noting that their abdominal wall seemed better than preoperative.[63] Further data correlating postoperative patient-reported outcomes with preoperative comorbidities and the need for prehabilitation may help us further refine counseling to patients regarding postoperative expectations.

The risks of delay in care during prehabilitation have been noted to be relatively low across several studies with the need for emergency surgery being reported at 3% to 7%. It is important to note that when patients are advised on prehabilitation goals without referral to a structured program, there is a low rate of patient follow-up in the hernia clinic.[59,61,64,65]

Prehabilitation of the Abdominal Wall

Patients with complex abdominal wall defects may benefit from prehabilitation of the abdominal wall prior to undergoing surgical repair. The definition of a complex abdominal wall defect has been varied and has included the width of the defect being greater than 15 cm on CT scan, multiple recurrences, and loss of domain (LOD). Lateral wall retraction in large incisional hernias adds to the disability associated with hernia disease with loss of a functional abdominal wall. Restoration of the abdominal wall with fascial closure during hernia repair reverses these physiologic changes. Adjuncts used preoperatively to help achieve this have been termed "abdominal wall prehabilitation."[66]

Botulinum Toxin

Botulinum toxin A (BTA) is an acetylcholine release inhibitor that has found various uses in medicine, and allows for lateral muscle paralysis in abdominal wall reconstruction. Injection of BTA into external oblique, internal oblique, and transversus abdominus is referred to by some as chemical component separation, and may in some cases allow fascial closure without the need for operative components separation, and in very large hernias, allow for fascial closure in combination with a components separation.[67]

Various injection protocols have been reported, using 100 to 500 units of BTA, diluted with saline, injected with US or CT guidance, with 3 to 5 injections per side using spinal or epidural needles.[68,69] Preoperative timing has also been variable with the majority of studies describing injection at 2 to 4 weeks before surgery.[70,71] Some groups use EMG (electromyelogram) in addition to US during injection to potentially improve the accuracy of the injection sites.[72]

It is unclear whether all 3 layers need to be injected, and there is some suggestion that the outcomes are similar from the standpoint of fascial closure, with the advantage of decreased cost due to a smaller amount of BTA used with 2 layer injection.[73] There is also some thought that if a transversus release is being considered, perhaps preoperative BTA injection to that muscle is unnecessary.

The chemical paralysis leads to elongation of the lateral muscles, with estimates of 3.2 cm per side, 6.3 cm total in a meta-analysis of 4 studies. Conversely, transverse hernia width is decreased by 3.5 cm, in a meta-analysis of 3 studies.[74] A systematic review noted median elongation of 4.0 cm per side, with two-third of patients with large hernias not requiring additional components separation to complete the hernia repair.[66] Another meta-analysis of 14 studies identified at 100% defect closure rate with a median hernia recurrence of 0% (0%–9%) at a median follow-up of 19 months.[74]

As we attempt to identify which patients may benefit from preop BTA, it may be helpful to identify preop those who are likely to require components separation at time of surgery. CT-based measurements of hernia dimensions including volume, area, and ratio of hernia to intra-abdominal volume have been shown to help predict the need for component separation.[75] The next step may be to use image-based deep learning models on preoperative CT image findings. This has demonstrated an accuracy of 81% compared with surgeon prediction of 65% at identifying the need for components separation to achieve fascial closure.[76] A simpler calculation is the rectus width to defect ratio (RDR), calculated by adding the right and left rectus widths and dividing by hernia width. RDR greater than 2 is associated with a fascial closure without the need for myofascial release in 90% of patients.[77] One intriguing idea that will require some study is the idea that BTA should be considered in patients at high risk for recurrence as postoperative laxity may decrease tension on the linea alba.[66]

Preoperative Progressive Pneumoperitoneum

Preoperative progressive pneumoperitoneum (PPP) was first described in the 1940s by Goni Moreno. The original description included repeated access into the peritoneal cavity to instill air with the patient being hospitalized throughout the treatment.[78] It has been initially described for an incarcerated epigastric hernia, but has been adapted over the years to assist in cases of loss of domain to facilitate reduction of contents intraoperatively, achieve fascial closure, and avoid postoperative compartment syndrome.

A generally accepted definition of LOD is when the volume of the hernia sac is greater than 25% of the volume of the abdominal cavity. Two volumetric calculations have been described:the Sabbagh method and the Tanaka method, with the former one being selected as the ideal one in a Delphi consensus in 2020.[79] The Sabbagh method requires volumizing software, whereas the Tanaka method uses the formula for an ellipsoid for calculation.[80]

Techniques for achieving progressive pneumoperitoneum include peritoneal dialysis catheters, central venous catheters, Foley catheters, tunneled venous catheter, or needle access on each occasion. Ambient air and nitrous oxide instillation have been described, with daily injections of 500 to 1000 mL, titrated to symptoms or pressure measurements. Length of time has varied in reports with the majority being in the range of 14 to 30 days. Repeated veress needle access for each session is still used by some groups.[81,82]

Methods of placing temporary catheters to allow for easier access and increased patient tolerance have been described using local anesthesia, or interventional radiology for insertion of the catheter. Using US or CT guidance, a veress or spinal needle is inserted laterally, with creation of pneumoperitoneum, confirmation with radiology, and seldinger technique being used for catheter insertion into a pocket of air.[83]

Various schedules of injections have been described, from as frequently as twice a day to once every 2 to 3 days. The amount insufflated has also varied, from 1 to 2 L to unmeasured quantities based on patient tolerance. Some groups have focused on basing these on the CT measured hernia volume, and instilling the same volume versus up to 3 times the volume, based on patient tolerance.[84,85] When instilling larger quantities, fractionating into 2 equal injections (1 L twice a day) has also been described to allow for improved tolerance while maximizing the effectiveness.[86]

The gas instilled has also varied to include carbon dioxide, oxygen, and ambient air. There are no clear benefits to the use of gases that are more expensive than ambient air, and which are likely also to be more quickly absorbed from the peritoneal cavity. To avoid preferential insufflation of the hernia sac, some recommend the use of an abdominal binder.

The use of PPP is usually in the elective situation, though it has been described in the "semi elective/semi urgent" scenario where a patient presents with an incarcerated hernia, which is urgently reduced, and PPP is undertaken over the following 2 weeks followed by hernia repair.[87]

Postulated benefits of PPP include increasing the abdominal compartment volume, pneumatic adhesiolysis, improving diaphragmatic function, and reducing chronic edema of the mesentery.[88] Venous thromboembolic prophylaxis is almost universally recommended during the PPP administration.[82,83]

Complications related to PPP are common with reported rates of 17% to 60%. Many of these are mild, with nausea, shoulder pain, dyspnea, and pain at the puncture site almost being expected routinely.[86] With the use of imaging, pneumothorax, pneumomediastinum, and subcutaneous emphysema have been noted. Many are reported as incidental findings, which have resolved with deflation of the pneumoperitoneum. Serious complications have also been reported during catheter insertion, including intra-abdominal hematoma and small bowel perforation.[72,82] Rare complications during the administration of PPP following catheter placement include small bowel perforation,[89] and formation of a peritoneocutaneous fistula.[90]

BOTOX AND PREOPERATIVE PROGRESSIVE PNEUMOPERITONEUM

As the benefits of preoperative BTA in complex abdominal wall repair were being realized in achieving fascial closure, the addition of PPP to this technique has been studied more recently. Most of the described techniques involve the administration of BTA 4 to 6 weeks preoperatively, to increase the compliance of the lateral muscles, followed by PPP for a shorter period of time starting at 2 weeks preoperatively. Studies where serial CT scans have been performed demonstrate that there is an additive effect of the 2 modalities. BTA has demonstrated a gain of 3.2 cm per side, with 4.4 cm following PPP.[82] Fascial closure rates of up to 97% have been reported with the combination of PPP and BTA. The benefits of BTA are purported to be with muscular relaxation and PPP with improvement of the hernia to abdominal cavity volume ratio.[72,74,91]

The combination of the 2 techniques has also been shown to have a lower SSO rate in a small study-potentially due to decreased tension on the midline closure with the addition of BTA compared with single modality PPP.[81] The expected lengthening of muscles and decreasing hernia width have however not been consistently noted in the published data,[74] potentially since the increased intra-abdominal pressure from PPP might be counteracting the relaxation from PPP on preoperative imaging. Vigilance should remain high to identify and treat the rare case of postoperative abdominal compartment syndrome.[72]

INDICATIONS FOR BOTULINUM TOXIN A AND/OR PREOPERATIVE PROGRESSIVE PNEUMOPERITONEUM

There are varying recommendations for use of the adjuncts described above. For the use of BTA, some recommendations include scenarios such including a hernia width greater than 10 cm, recurrence after component separation, loss of domain greater than 20%, retracted bulky lateral muscles, and expected difficulty in closing the midline.[67,92] There is some overlap in the indication for PPP with loss of domain over 20% to 25%, hernia width greater than 10 cm, and inability to reduce hernia contents.[92]

The lack of randomized studies and the heterogeneity in the published data make it difficult to make clear recommendations. At a minimum, we can state that BTA seems to be associated with low risk of complications, whereas PPP should only be considered where expertise is available, and appropriate surveillance should be maintained to identify complications early.

SUMMARY

Patients requiring abdominal wall reconstruction often benefit from evaluation of comorbid conditions to attempt preoperative optimization and/or evaluation of the hernia characteristics to consider BTA/PPP. The data regarding prehabilitation for comorbidities are variable, but promising, whereas the data regarding prehabilitation of the abdominal wall are quite consistently supportive of the use of these adjuncts. These complexities are seen in the dichotomy of the systematic analysis of systematic analyses concluding that there is low certainty of possible improvement in outcomes with prehabilitation.[93] However, a Delphi consensus statement identified several statements with over 80% agreement regarding perioperative optimization of the patient with a ventral hernia. These included recommending weight loss via medical management or weight loss surgery when BMI greater than 35, smoking cessation, blood sugar management in diabetics, exercise prehabilitation for those with poor exercise tolerance, treatment of malnutrition, and access to BTA for use when appropriate.[94]

DISCLOSURES

The author does not have any disclosures relevant to the subject matter of this article.

REFERENCES

1. Vasavada BB, Patel H. Outcomes of open transverse abdominis release for ventral hernias: a systematic review, meta-analysis and meta-regression of factors affecting them. Hernia 2022;10 [published online ahead of print, 2022 Aug 3].

2. Joslyn NA, Esmonde NO, Martindale RG, et al. Evidence-Based Strategies for the Prehabilitation of the Abdominal Wall Reconstruction Patient. Plast Reconstr Surg 2018;142(3 Suppl):21S–9S.

3. Kushner BS, Hamilton J, Han BJ, et al. Geriatric assessment and medical preoperative screening (GrAMPS) program for older hernia patients. Hernia : the Journal of Hernias and Abdominal Wall Surgery 2022;26(3):787–94.

4. Kushner BS, Holden T, Han BJ, et al. Perioperative outcomes of the Geriatric Assessment and Medical Preoperative Screening (GrAMPS) program pilot for older hernia patients: does chronological age predict outcomes? Surg Endosc 2022;36(7):5442–50.

5. Kushner BS, Han B, Otegbeye E, et al. Chronological age does not predict postoperative outcomes following transversus abdominis release (TAR). Surg Endosc 2022;36(6):4570–9.

6. Docimo S Jr, Bates A, Alteri M, et al. Evaluation of the use of component separation in elderly patients: results of a large cohort study with 30-day follow-up. Hernia 2020;24(3):503–7.

7. Kushner BS, Holden T, Han B, et al. Randomized control trial evaluating the use of a shared decision-making aid for older ventral hernia patients in the Geriatric Assessment and Medical Preoperative Screening (GrAMPS) Program. Hernia 2022;26(3):901–9.

8. Liu D, Zhu L, Yang C. The effect of preoperative smoking and smoke cessation on wound healing and infection in post-surgery subjects: A meta-analysis. Int Wound J 2022;19(8):2101–6.

9. Warner DO, Borah BJ, Moriarty J, et al. Smoking Status and Health Care Costs in the Perioperative Period: A Population-Based Study. JAMA Surg 2014;149(3):259–66.

10. Donovan K, Denham M, Kuchta K, et al. Predictors for recurrence after open umbilical hernia repair in 979 patients. Surgery 2019;166(4):615–22.

11. DeLancey JO, Blay E Jr, Hewitt DB, et al. The effect of smoking on 30-day outcomes in elective hernia repair. Am J Surg 2018;216(3):471–4.

12. Lindström D, Sadr Azodi O, Wladis A, et al. Effects of a perioperative smoking cessation intervention on postoperative complications: a randomized trial. Ann Surg 2008;248(5):739–45.

13. Shi Y, Warner DO. Surgery as a teachable moment for smoking cessation. Anesthesiology 2010;112(1):102–7.

14. Webb AR, Coward L, Meanger D, et al. Offering mailed nicotine replacement therapy and Quitline support before elective surgery: a randomised controlled trial. Med J Aust 2022;216(7):357–63.

15. Sadek J, Moloo H, Belanger P, et al. Implementation of a systematic tobacco treatment protocol in a surgical outpatient setting: a feasibility study. Can J Surg 2021;64(1):E51–8.

16. Sørensen LT, Hemmingsen U, Jørgensen T. Strategies of smoking cessation intervention before hernia surgery–effect on perioperative smoking behavior. Hernia 2007;11(4):327–33.

17. Iida H, Kai T, Kuri M, et al. A practical guide for perioperative smoking cessation. J Anesth 2022;36(5):583–605.

18. Kim Y, Chen TC. Smoking and Nicotine Effects on Surgery: Is Nicotine Replacement Therapy (NRT) a Safe Option? Ann Surg 2021;273(4):e139–41.

19. Stefan MS, Pack Q, Shieh MS, et al. The Association of Nicotine Replacement Therapy With Outcomes Among Smokers Hospitalized for a Major Surgical Procedure. Chest 2020;157(5):1354–61.

20. Ofori SN, Marcucci M, Mbuagbaw L, et al. Determinants of tobacco smoking abstinence one year after major noncardiac surgery: a secondary analysis of the VISION study. Br J Anaesth 2022;129(4):497–505.
21. Buehler L, Fayfman M, Alexopoulos AS, et al. The impact of hyperglycemia and obesity on hospitalization costs and clinical outcome in general surgery patients. J Diabetes Complications 2015;29(8):1177–82.
22. Won EJ, Lehman EB, Geletzke AK, et al. Association of postoperative hyperglycemia with outcomes among patients with complex ventral hernia repair. JAMA Surg 2015;150(5):433–40.
23. Jones CE, Graham LA, Morris MS, et al. Association Between Preoperative Hemoglobin A1c Levels, Postoperative Hyperglycemia, and Readmissions Following Gastrointestinal Surgery. JAMA Surg 2017;152(11):1031–8 [published correction appears in JAMA Surg. 2018 Aug 1;153(8):782].
24. Liang MK, Holihan JL, Itani K, et al. Ventral Hernia Management: Expert Consensus Guided by Systematic Review. Ann Surg 2017;265(1):80–9.
25. Al-Mansour MR, Vargas M, Olson MA, et al. S-144 lack of association between glycated hemoglobin and adverse outcomes in diabetic patients undergoing ventral hernia repair: an ACHQC study. Surg Endosc, Surg Endosc 2023;37(4): 3180–90.
26. Khan MTA, Patnaik R, Hausman-Cohen L, et al. Obesity Stratification Predicts Short-Term Complications After Parastomal Hernia Repair. J Surg Res 2022; 280:27–34.
27. Köckerling F, Hoffmann H, Adolf D, et al. Potential influencing factors on the outcome in incisional hernia repair: a registry-based multivariable analysis of 22,895 patients. Hernia 2021;25(1):33–49.
28. Tastaldi L, Krpata DM, Prabhu AS, et al. The effect of increasing body mass index on wound complications in open ventral hernia repair with mesh. Am J Surg 2019; 218(3):560–6.
29. Howard R, Thompson M, Fan Z, et al. Costs Associated With Modifiable Risk Factors in Ventral and Incisional Hernia Repair. JAMA Netw Open 2019;2(11): e1916330.
30. Baastrup NN, Jensen KK, Christensen JK, et al. Visceral obesity is a predictor of surgical site occurrence and hernia recurrence after open abdominal wall reconstruction. Hernia 2022;26(1):149–55.
31. Addo A, Lu R, Broda A, et al. Impact of Body Mass Index (BMI) on perioperative outcomes following minimally invasive retromuscular abdominal wall reconstruction: a comparative analysis. Surg Endosc 2021;35(10):5796–802.
32. Ekmann JR, Christoffersen MW, Jensen KK. Short-term complications after minimally invasive retromuscular ventral hernia repair: no need for preoperative weight loss or smoking cessation? Hernia 2022;26(5):1315–23.
33. Kudsi OY, Gokcal F, Chang K. Propensity score matching analysis of short-term outcomes in robotic ventral hernia repair for patients with a body mass index above and below 35 kg/m^2. Hernia 2021;25(1):115–23.
34. Kudsi OY, Gokcal F, Bou-Ayash N, et al. A comparison of outcomes between class-II and class-III obese patients undergoing robotic ventral hernia repair: a multicenter study. Hernia 2022;26(6):1531–9.
35. Maskal SM, Boyd-Tressler AM, Heinberg LJ, et al. Can a free weight management program "move the needle" for obese patients preparing for hernia surgery?: outcomes of a novel pilot program. Hernia 2022;26(5):1259–65.
36. Schlosser KA, Maloney SR, Gbozah K, et al. The impact of weight change on intra-abdominal and hernia volumes. Surgery 2020;167(5):876–82.

37. Jensen KK, Arnesen RB, Christensen JK, et al. Large Incisional Hernias Increase in Size. J Surg Res 2019;244:160–5 [published correction appears in J Surg Res. 2022 Jan;269:142-143].

38. Borbély Y, Zerkowski J, Altmeier J, et al. Complex hernias with loss of domain in morbidly obese patients: role of laparoscopic sleeve gastrectomy in a multi-step approach. Surg Obes Relat Dis 2017;13(5):768–73.

39. Bronswijk M, Jaekers J, Vanella G, et al. Umbilical hernia repair in patients with cirrhosis: who, when and how to treat. Hernia 2022;26(6):1447–57.

40. Licari L, Salamone G, Ciolino G, et al. The abdominal wall incisional hernia repair in cirrhotic patients. G Chir 2018;39(1):20–3.

41. Salamone G, Licari L, Guercio G, et al. The abdominal wall hernia in cirrhotic patients: a historical challenge. World J Emerg Surg 2018;13:35.

42. Latifi Rifat, Samson David JMS, Smiley Abbas, et al. Complex Abdominal Wall Reconstruction with Biologic Mesh for Ventral/Umbilical Hernias in Patients with Cirrhosis. J Am Coll Surg 2022;235(5):S30.

43. Andraus W, Pinheiro RS, Lai Q, et al. Abdominal wall hernia in cirrhotic patients: emergency surgery results in higher morbidity and mortality. BMC Surg 2015; 15:65.

44. Pinheiro RS, Andraus W, Waisberg DR, et al. Abdominal hernias in cirrhotic patients: Surgery or conservative treatment? Results of a prospective cohort study in a high volume center: Cohort study. Ann Med Surg (Lond) 2019;49:9–13.

45. Johnson KM, Newman KL, Green PK, et al. Incidence and risk factors of postoperative mortality and morbidity after elective versus emergent abdominal surgery in a national sample of 8193 patients with cirrhosis. Annals of surgery 2021; 274(4):e345–54.

46. Snitkjær C, Jensen KK, Henriksen NA, et al. Umbilical hernia repair in patients with cirrhosis: systematic review of mortality and complications. Hernia 2022; 26(6):1435–45.

47. Mahmud N, Goldberg DS, Abu-Gazala S, et al. Modeling Optimal Clinical Thresholds for Elective Abdominal Hernia Repair in Patients With Cirrhosis. JAMA Netw Open 2022;5(9):e2231601.

48. Kim SW, Kim MA, Chang Y, et al. Prognosis of surgical hernia repair in cirrhotic patients with refractory ascites. Hernia 2020;24(3):481–8.

49. Gale CR, Cooper C, Sayer AA. Prevalence of frailty and disability: findings from the English Longitudinal Study of Ageing. Age Ageing 2015;44(1):162–5.

50. O'Neill BR, Batterham AM, Hollingsworth AC, et al. Do first impressions count? Frailty judged by initial clinical impression predicts medium-term mortality in vascular surgical patients. Anaesthesia 2016;71(6):684–91.

51. Solano QP, Howard R, Mullens CL, et al. The impact of frailty on ventral hernia repair outcomes in a statewide database. Surg Endosc 2022;1–9 [published online ahead of print, 2022 Nov 7].

52. Barnes LA, Li AY, Wan DC, et al. Determining the impact of sarcopenia on postoperative complications after ventral hernia repair. J Plast Reconstr Aesthet Surg 2018;71(9):1260–8.

53. Schlosser KA, Maloney SR, Thielan ON, et al. Sarcopenia in Patients Undergoing Open Ventral Hernia Repair. Am Surg 2019;85(9):985–91.

54. Sadlonova M, Katz NB, Jurayj JS, et al. Surgical prehabilitation in older and frail individuals: a scoping review. Int Anesthesiol Clin 2023;61(2):34–46.

55. Schaller SJ, Kiselev J, Loidl V, et al. Prehabilitation of elderly frail or pre-frail patients prior to elective surgery (PRAEP-GO): study protocol for a randomized,

controlled, outcome assessor-blinded trial. Trials 2022;23(1):468 [published correction appears in Trials. 2023 Feb 14;24(1):111].

56. Alkhatib H, Tastaldi L, Krpata DM, et al. Impact of modifiable comorbidities on 30-day wound morbidity after open incisional hernia repair. Surgery 2019;166(1): 94–101.

57. Renshaw SM, Poulose BK, Gupta A, et al. Preoperative exercise and outcomes after ventral hernia repair: Making the case for prehabilitation in ventral hernia patients. Surgery 2021;170(2):516–24.

58. Howard R, Delaney L, Kilbourne AM, et al. Development and Implementation of Preoperative Optimization for High-Risk Patients With Abdominal Wall Hernia. JAMA Netw Open 2021;4(5):e216836.

59. Delaney LD, Howard R, Palazzolo K, et al. Outcomes of a Presurgical Optimization Program for Elective Hernia Repairs Among High-risk Patients. JAMA Netw Open 2021;4(11):e2130016.

60. Martin AC, Lyons NB, Bernardi K, et al. Expectant Management of Patients with Ventral Hernias: 3 Years of Follow-up. World J Surg 2020;44(8):2572–9.

61. Bernardi K, Olavarria OA, Dhanani NH, et al. Two-year Outcomes of Prehabilitation Among Obese Patients With Ventral Hernias: A Randomized Controlled Trial (NCT02365194). Ann Surg 2022;275(2):288–94.

62. de Jong DLC, Wegdam JA, Berkvens EBM, et al. The influence of a multidisciplinary team meeting and prehabilitation on complex abdominal wall hernia repair outcomes. Hernia 2023;1–8 [published online ahead of print, 2023 Feb 14].

63. van Veenendaal N, Poelman MM, van den Heuvel B, et al. Patient-reported outcomes after incisional hernia repair. Hernia 2021;25(6):1677–84.

64. Liang MK, Bernardi K, Holihan JL, et al. Modifying Risks in Ventral Hernia Patients With Prehabilitation: A Randomized Controlled Trial. Ann Surg 2018;268(4): 674–80.

65. Casson CA, Clanahan JM, Han BJ, et al. The efficacy of goal-directed recommendations in overcoming barriers to elective ventral hernia repair in older adults. Surgery 2023;173(3):732–8.

66. Wegdam JA, de Vries Reilingh TS, Bouvy ND, et al. Prehabilitation of complex ventral hernia patients with Botulinum: a systematic review of the quantifiable effects of Botulinum. Hernia 2021;25(6):1427–42.

67. Deerenberg EB, Shao JM, Elhage SA, et al. Preoperative botulinum toxin A injection in complex abdominal wall reconstruction- a propensity-scored matched study. Am J Surg 2021;222(3):638–42.

68. Marturano MN, Ayuso SA, Ku D, et al. Preoperative botulinum toxin A (BTA) injection versus component separation techniques (CST) in complex abdominal wall reconstruction (AWR): A propensity-scored matched study. Surgery 2023; 173(3):756–64.

69. Mandujano CC, Lima DL, Alcabes A, et al. Preoperative botulinum A toxin as an adjunct for abdominal wall reconstruction: a single-center early experience at an Academic Center in New York. Rev Col Bras Cir 2022;49:e20213152.

70. Kurumety S, Walker A, Samet J, et al. Ultrasound-Guided Lateral Abdominal Wall Botulinum Toxin Injection Before Ventral Hernia Repair: A Review for Radiologists. J Ultrasound Med 2021;40(10):2019–30.

71. Hipolito Canario DA, Isaacson AJ, Martissa JA, et al. Ultrasound-Guided Chemical Component Separation with Botulinum Toxin A prior to Surgical Hernia Repair. J Vasc Interv Radiol 2021;32(2):256–61.

72. Bueno-Lledó J, Carreño-Saenz O, Torregrosa-Gallud A, et al. Preoperative Botulinum Toxin and Progressive Pneumoperitoneum in Loss of Domain Hernias-Our First 100 Cases. Front Surg 2020;7:3.

73. Deerenberg EB, Elhage SA, Shao JM, et al. The Effects of Preoperative Botulinum Toxin A Injection on Abdominal Wall Reconstruction. J Surg Res 2021;260:251–8.

74. Timmer AS, Claessen JJM, Atema JJ, et al. A systematic review and meta-analysis of technical aspects and clinical outcomes of botulinum toxin prior to abdominal wall reconstruction. Hernia 2021;25(6):1413–25.

75. Schlosser KA, Maloney SR, Prasad T, et al. Three-dimensional hernia analysis: the impact of size on surgical outcomes. Surg Endosc 2020;34(4):1795–801.

76. Elhage SA, Deerenberg EB, Ayuso SA, et al. Development and Validation of Image-Based Deep Learning Models to Predict Surgical Complexity and Complications in Abdominal Wall Reconstruction. JAMA Surg 2021;156(10):933–40.

77. Love MW, Warren JA, Davis S, et al. Computed tomography imaging in ventral hernia repair: can we predict the need for myofascial release? Hernia 2021; 25(2):471–7.

78. Goni Moreno I. Pneumoperitoneum applied to the surgical preparation of large chronic eventrations. Prensa Med Argent 1971;58(21):1037–41 [in Spanish].

79. Parker SG, Halligan S, Liang MK, et al. Definitions for Loss of Domain: An International Delphi Consensus of Expert Surgeons. World J Surg 2020;44(4):1070–8.

80. Adams ST, Slade D, Shuttleworth P, et al. Reading a preoperative CT scan to guide complex abdominal wall reconstructive surgery. Hernia 2022;10 [published online ahead of print, 2022 Jan 5].

81. Tashkandi A, Bueno-Lledó J, Durtette-Guzylack J, et al. Adjunct botox to preoperative progressive pneumoperitoneum for incisional hernia with loss of domain: no additional effect but may improve outcomes. Hernia 2021;25(6):1507–17.

82. Elstner KE, Moollan Y, Chen E, et al. Preoperative Progressive Pneumoperitoneum Revisited. Front Surg 2021;8:754543.

83. Allart K, Sabbagh C, Regimbeau JM. Intraperitoneal catheter introduction for preoperative progressive pneumoperitoneum for abdominal hernia with loss of domain (Goni-Moreno technique). J Visc Surg 2020 Aug;157(4):335–40.

84. Tanaka EY, Yoo JH, Rodrigues AJ, et al. A computerized tomography scan method for calculating the hernia sac and abdominal cavity volume in complex large incisional hernia with loss of domain. Hernia 2010;14:63–9.

85. Bueno-Lledó J, Torregrosa A, Jiménez R, et al. Preoperative combination of progressivepneumoperitoneum and botulinum toxin type A in patients with loss of domain hernia. Surg Endosc 2018;32:3599–608.

86. Cunha LAC, Cançado ARS, Silveira CAB, et al. Management of complex hernias with loss of domain using daily and fractioned preoperative progressive pneumoperitoneum: a retrospective single-center cohort study. Hernia 2021;25(6): 1499–505.

87. Polanía-Sandoval CA, Velandia-Sánchez A, Pérez-Rivera CJ, et al. Early preoperative progressive pneumoperitoneum for a symptomatic giant abdominal incisional hernia. Int J Surg Case Rep 2022;94:107028.

88. Toma M, Oprea V, Grad ON, et al. Incisional hernias with loss of abdominal domain: a new look to an older issue or the elephant in the living room. Literature review. Chirurgia (Bucur) 2022;117(1):5–13.

89. Hajjar R, Badrudin D, Bendavid Y. Spontaneous Small Bowel Perforation during Preoperative Progressive Pneumoperitoneum for Incisional Hernia Repair: Risk Zero Does Not Exist. Am Surg 2019;85(12):599–601.

90. Guerrero-Antolino P, Pous-Serrano S, Bueno-Lledo J, et al. Accidental peritoneum-cutaneous fistula after insufflation of preoperative progressive pneumoperitoneum in a large incisional hernia with loss of domain. BMJ Case Rep 2022;15(5):e248984.

91. Tang FX, Ma N, Huang E, et al. Botulinum Toxin A Facilitated Laparoscopic Repair of Complex Ventral Hernia. Front Surg 2022;8:803023.

92. van Rooijen MMJ, Yurtkap Y, Allaeys M, et al. Fascial closure in giant ventral hernias after preoperative botulinum toxin a and progressive pneumoperitoneum: A systematic review and meta-analysis. Surgery 2021;170(3):769–76.

93. McIsaac DI, Gill M, Boland L, et al. Prehabilitation in adult patients undergoing surgery: an umbrella review of systematic reviews. Br J Anaesth 2022;128(2):244–57.

94. Grove TN, Kontovounisios C, Montgomery A, et al. Perioperative optimization in complex abdominal wall hernias: Delphi consensus statement. BJS Open 2021;5(5):zrab082.

Ventral Hernia Repair
Does Mesh Position Matter?

Nir Messer, MD[a],*, Michael J. Rosen, MD[b]

KEYWORDS

- Plane • Mesh • Onlay • Inlay • Sublay • Underlay

KEY POINTS

- Mesh position has 4 classic planes: onlay, inlay, sublay, and underlay.
- Different types of hernias require different surgical repairs. There is no ideal plane for all types of hernias.
- All mesh planes carry risks and benefits that should be weighed on a case-by-case basis.
- Sublay repair has low surgical site occurrence and recurrence rates but requires high surgical skills and may cause devastating abdominal wall complications. Proper patient selection can minimize the differences in outcomes between onlay, sublay, and underlay.

INTRODUCTION

Similar to most things in hernia surgery, when there are less data, there are significant opinions and anecdotes that drive our practice. Mesh positioning is a commonly discussed detail in ventral hernia repair and is often cited as a major contributor to the outcome of the operation. However, there is a paucity of data that establishes one plane as superior to others.

We are often left to extrapolate from expert centers publishing single-arm studies, reporting their long-term outcomes from retrospective analysis, that rarely have a comparator arm. Moreover, although proponents of each mesh location cite advantages, they often neglect to acknowledge the deleterious effects of accessing that unique plane and the complications that can occur with neurovascular injuries and fascial disruptions. In this article, we will provide an overview of all potential planes to place prosthetic material and review the relevant literature supporting each option as well as the complications associated with accessing each anatomic plane. We will summarize this discussion with our approach to mesh positioning. In our opinion, a true abdominal core health surgeon should master all mesh planes and be able to

[a] Department of Surgery, Cleveland Clinic Foundation, Cleveland, OH, USA; [b] Lerner College of Medicine, Cleveland Clinic Center for Abdominal Core Health, Cleveland Clinic, Cleveland, OH, USA
* Corresponding author.
E-mail address: masrinir@gmail.com

Surg Clin N Am 103 (2023) 935–945
https://doi.org/10.1016/j.suc.2023.04.005

apply the appropriate technique based on hernia and patient characteristics. Mesh position has 4 classic planes: onlay, inlay, sublay, and underlay (**Table 1**).

Onlay repair places the mesh ventral (superficial) to the sutured anterior fascia and deep into the subcutaneous tissue. The main advantage of this technique is its ease of application. The anatomical landmarks are evident and easy to reveal, and the hernia sac may stay intact, avoiding intraperitoneal dissection and adhesiolysis. If the fascia repair stays intact, the mesh is theoretically unexposed to the abdominal viscera, thus thought to prevent mesh erosion, fistulas, and bowel obstruction. Nevertheless, onlay mesh placement may hold some significant disadvantages. This technique can involve extensive subcutaneous dissection and wide skin flaps to develop that plane, particularly for larger, more complex hernias. This may lead to higher rates of skin ischemia, seromas, and increased surgical site infection (SSI) and mesh infection compared with other anatomic planes.

Inlay repair, also called interposition or bridging technique, places the mesh between the medial edges of the hernia defect and secures the mesh to the edges of the anterior fascia without fascial approximation. The main advantage of this technique is its simplicity. This surgery can be done rapidly without needing adhesiolysis or plane development but it is thought to have the highest recurrence rate given the lack of mesh overlap.

This technique is often reserved for "bailout" procedures, in which the hernia is not formally repaired due to intraoperative challenges, and an absorbable mesh can be secured to the fascial edges to prevent evisceration. A subsequent formal staged repair can be accomplished in the future.

Sublay repair places the mesh dorsal (deep) to the sutured anterior fascia, either in the retromuscular or in the preperitoneal space. One of the most popular sublay surgery is the Rives-Stoppa repair. In this technique, the posterior rectus plane and the preperitoneal space below the arcuate line are developed for the placement of the mesh. In cases of substantial defects where a large mesh is needed or when the posterior fascial approximation is impossible, posterior component separation and transversus abdominis release can be performed. In recent years, minimally invasive approaches have been described, and it is becoming increasingly common. This technique holds some significant advantages when performed by experts. It is a reconstructive surgery that restores the abdominal wall components to their natural position. The mesh is placed in a deep plane, which theoretically reduces the recurrence rate but does not expose it to intraperitoneal organs, which are thought to reduce mesh erosion, fistulas, and bowel obstruction. Nevertheless, the sublay mesh placement may also hold some disadvantages. It is a complex procedure that can result in nerve damage, rectus abdominis atrophy, disruption of the linea semilunaris, interstitial hernias, bowel obstructions, and hemorrhage. In a case series describing outcomes after 65 redo-TAR cases, more than a quarter (28%) had linea semilunaris injuries, 15% had posterior sheath breakdown, 9% had mesh displacement, 17% had mesh infection requiring mesh excision, and 12% had bowel obstructions as the precipitating cause of redo-transversus abdominis release (TAR).[1]

Underlay repair places the mesh in the intraperitoneal space and attaches the mesh to the parietal peritoneum and the abdominal wall. It is also called "intraperitoneal onlay mesh—IPOM" repair. The main advantages of this technique are that it does not require myofascial releases and extensive intramuscular dissection and can frequently be conducted in a minimally invasive approach. As with sublay repair, the mesh is placed in a deep plane, which theoretically reduces the recurrence rates and SSI. Another advantage of the minimally invasive approach is the ability to expose a large abdominal wall surface and inspect for other defects. For those reasons, this

Table 1
Common assumptions on mesh plains

	Mesh Plane	Surgical Method	Technical Difficulty	Suitable for	Main Assumption Advantage	Main Assumption Disadvantage
Onlay repair	Mesh is positioned ventral to anterior fascia	Usually, open surgery	Low	Hostile abdomen Low risk of wound morbidity	Technically simple	High SSI and recurrence rate
Inlay repair	Mesh is positioned between the medial edges of the hernia defect	Usually, open surgery	Low	Unapproximated linea alba	Technically simple	High SSI and recurrence rate
Sublay repair	Mesh is positioned dorsal to anterior fascia (retromuscular or preperitoneal space)	Usually, open surgery Can be done laparoscopically or robotic	High	Elective surgeries with a wide defect	Low recurrence rate, lower mesh complications	Technically challenging Associated complications
Underlay repair	Mesh is positioned in the intraperitoneal space	Usually laparoscopically or robotic	Low	Elective surgeries with a small defect	Low recurrence rate	Long-term mesh complications

technique became very popular in the last 2 decades, particularly for minimally invasive approaches. However, this approach places a permanent prosthetic material in the intraperitoneal cavity, which theoretically may cause bowel erosion that may lead to an abdominal abscess, fistula, and bowel obstruction. Another controversy surrounding IPOM repair stems from the concern for high recurrence rates if the fascia has not been reapproximated. However, a study based on data from the prospectively maintained Abdominal Core Health Quality Collaborative (ACHQC) found no association between primary facial closure and SSO.[2] Moreover, in a blinded, multicenter randomized control trial, 129 patients with a ventral hernia (3–10 cm) were randomized to laparoscopic IPOM mesh repair with fascial closure versus laparoscopic IPOM mesh repair without facial closure; in 2 years follow-up, neither differences in SSO nor hernia recurrence was found. However, the fascial closure group demonstrated a statistically significant improvement in quality of life.[3]

LITERATURE REVIEW ON KEY OUTCOMES
Recurrence

Assessing recurrence rates in hernia surgery is notoriously challenging. Given the lack of an agreed-on classification system for hernia complexity, it is difficult to make an apples-to-apples comparison of retrospective data. However, ample literature compares the outcomes of various mesh positions, and we will summarize the results of these limited trials in **Tables 2–5**. Generally, the inlay position carries the highest risk of recurrence and should not be used as a definitive repair.

In an extensive systematic review by Sosin, and colleagues, they demonstrated a significant difference in recurrence rates by mesh location with lower recurrence rates in the sublay (5.8%) and underlay (10.9%) repair than onlay (12.9%) and inlay (21.6%) repair, $(P = .02)$.[4] Another systematic review found that the recurrence rates were 5% in the sublay repair, 7.5% in the underlay repair, and 17% in the onlay repair $(P = .01)$.[5] Although most updated and thoroughly edited, those systematic reviews have several limitations. The vast majority of the studies are retrospective; assumably, 4 out of 51 and 5 out of 62, respectively, are prospective. Reviewed studies have mixed elective, urgent, clean, dirty, primary, and incisional hernia cases. In addition, they incorporate multiple surgical techniques using different synthetic and biological materials. Long-term follow-up rates are often not reported and rarely are patients lost to follow-up accounted for in the analysis, and several publications had a follow-up of only

Table 2
Reviewed outcomes of onlay plane

		Onlay			
	Author, Year	n	Study Type	Rate (%)	P
Recurrence rate	Sosin et al,[4] 2018	6227	Systematic review	9.9	.023
	Albino et al,[5] 2013	5824	Systematic review	17.0	.01
	Chevrel and Rath,[6] 1997	426	Prospective	5.5	NA
SSI	Albino et al,[5] 2013	5824	Systematic review	4	<.001
	Sosin et al,[4] 2018	6227	Systematic review	14	.276
	Haskins et al,[8] 2017	93	Retrospective	5.5	.3
	Bessa et al,[9] 2015	80	Prospective	0	1.0
SSO	Sosin et al,[4] 2018	6227	Systematic review	17.4	.288
	Haskins et al,[8] 2017	93	Retrospective	15.2	.08
Mesh excision	Sosin et al,[4] 2018	6227	Systematic review	0.3	.929
	Albino et al,[5] 2013	5824	Systematic review	5.0	.8

Table 3
Reviewed outcomes of inlay repair

			Inlay		
	Author, Year	n	Study Type	Rate (%)	P
Recurrence rate	Sosin et al,[4] 2018	6227	Systematic review	21.6	.023
	Albino et al,[5] 2013	5824	Systematic review	17.0	<.01
SSI	Albino et al,[5] 2013	5824	Systematic review	25	<.001
	Sosin et al,[4] 2018	6227	Systematic review	12	.276
SSO	Sosin et al,[4] 2018	6227	Systematic review	12.2	.288
Mesh excision	Sosin et al,[4] 2018	6227	Systematic review	0.3	.929
	Albino et al,[5] 2013	5824	Systematic review	1.0	.8

6 months. Finally, a significant amount of the studies is from a single-center or a single surgeon experience.

Despite the limitations mentioned above, many surgeons assume that the retromuscular space is the ideal place in terms of recurrence rate. Nevertheless, this assumption is not supported by other similar data that is often not included in the earlier systematic review. In fact, evaluation of high volume dedicated hernia surgeons collecting prospective data often reports contrasting findings. Looking at Chevrel's series, who developed an onlay mesh repair and followed his 426 patients for up to 20 years, the recurrence rate was 5.5%.[6] Those outcomes were verified by several studies that found similar results.[7,8] A fairly small randomized control study compared onlay and sublay repair enrolled 80 patients with ventral hernia defect sizes ranging from 4 to 10 cm and a 22-month median follow-up. They reported a comparable recurrence rate between the 2 groups.[9] In multiple comparisons between sublay and

Table 4
Reviewed outcomes of sublay plane

			Sublay		
	Author, Year	n	Study Type	Rate (%)	P
Recurrence rate	Sosin et al,[4] 2018	6227	Systematic Review	5.8	.023
	Albino et al,[5] 2013	5824	Systematic review	5.0	<.01
	Bessa et al,[9] 2015	80	Prospective	5.0	1.0
	Fafaj et al,[26] 2020	4211	Retrospective	15.9	.884
SSI	Albino et al,[5] 2013	5824	Systematic review	4	<.001
	Sosin et al,[4] 2018	6227	Systematic review	10.2	.276
	Haskins et al,[8] 2017	93	Retrospective	2.9	.3
	Bessa et al,[9] 2015	80	Prospective	1	1.0
	Petro et al,[28] 2022	100	Randomized clinical trial	0	NA
	Fafaj et al,[26] 2020	4211	Retrospective	3.3	.772
SSO	Sosin et al,[4] 2018	6227	Systematic review	11	.288
	Haskins et al,[8] 2017	93	Retrospective	7.7	.08
	Petro et al,[28] 2022	100	Randomized clinical trial	16	.004
Mesh excision	Sosin et al,[4] 2018	6227	Systematic review	0.5	.929
	Albino et al,[5] 2013	5824	Systematic review	0.5	.8
	Fafaj et al,[26] 2020	4211	Retrospective	0.1	1.0
	Petro et al,[28] 2022	100	Randomized clinical trial	1	.32
Pain and recovery	Petro et al,[28] 2022	100	Randomized clinical trial	5[a]	.66

[a] Numeric rating pain scale.

Table 5
Reviewed outcomes of underlay plane

			Underlay		
	Author, Year	**n**	**Study Type**	**Rate (%)**	**P**
Recurrence rate	Sosin et al,[4] 2018	6227	Systematic review	10.9	.023
	Albino et al,[5] 2013	5824	Systematic review	7.5	.01
	Bessa et al,[9] 2015	80	Prospective	5.0	1.000
	Fafaj et al,[26] 2020	4211	Retrospective	15.0	.884
SSI	Albino et al,[5] 2013	5824	Systematic review	7	<.001
	Sosin et al,[4] 2018	6227	Systematic review	17.7	.276
	Petro et al,[28] 2022	100	Randomized clinical trial	0	NA
	Fafaj et al,[26] 2020	4211	Retrospective	2.7	.772
SSO	Sosin et al,[4] 2018	6227	Systematic review	11.5	.288
	Petro et al,[28] 2022	100	Randomized clinical trial	0	.004
Mesh excision	Sosin et al,[4] 2018	6227	Systematic review	0.5	.929
	Albino et al,[5] 2013	5824	Systematic review	3	.8
	Fafaj et al,[26] 2020	4211	Retrospective	0.5	1
	Petro et al,[28] 2022	100	Randomized clinical trial	0	.32
Pain and recovery	Petro et al,[28] 2022	100	Randomized clinical trial	5[a]	.66

[a] Numeric rating pain scale.

underlay repair for small-size hernia defects, there is no clinical significant difference in the recurrence rates or postoperational complications.[10–12] Even when comparing the new laparoscopic retromuscular repair, also called enhanced totally extraperitoneal approach (eTEP), in a recent systematic review and meta-analysis, there was no significant difference in recurrence rates between eTEP and IPOM in up to 28 months follow-up.[13] That drove SAGES, EAES, and European Hernia Society (EHS) to recommend laparoscopic IPOM to repair incisional hernia defects up to 8 to 10 cm on their guidelines.[14–16] However, for a defect size greater than 8 to 10 cm, the recurrence rate increases sharply following laparoscopic IPOM.[16]

In summary, hernia recurrence rates of each of the mesh locations remains heterogenous and suffers from multiple biases. It is likely that onlay, sublay, and underlay mesh positions are indicated for different types of hernias and thus attempting to compare them head-to-head only leads to further confusion. We think that an abdominal core health surgeon should be facile in each technique and use them based on underlying patient and hernia characteristics, and a perceived superiority in hernia recurrence rates should not drive this decision.

Surgical Site Occurrence

The term surgical site occurrence (SSO) was first introduced by the Ventral Hernia Working Group in 2010.[17] It includes SSI, seroma, wound dehiscence, and enterocutaneous fistulae at the hernia repair site. Correlations between SSO and mesh position have been described vastly. Although most studies report that the inlay position has the highest SSO rate, followed by the onlay position[4,5]; it is thought that the high SSO rates in the onlay position are related to vast subcutaneous dissection and the large skin flaps made during surgery. However, as described above, most knowledge is based on limited studies that enrolled urgent surgeries or contaminated cases with clean wounds undergoing elective surgeries.[18–22] There are strong indications that with the proper patient selection and surgical technique, onlay SSO rates are much lower than reported at large. A recent study compared 93 patients with an average hernia width of 6 cm who underwent onlay repair and matched to patients with sublay repair, found no statistically significant difference concerning 30-day SSI, SSO, or surgical site occurrences requiring procedural intervention (SSOPI).[8] Likely the onlay repair requires careful patient selection. As a large skin flap is required to place the mesh, patients at particularly high risk for wound complications should likely not undergo this approach. This can include obese, smokers, diabetics, and those needing early postoperative anticoagulation.

Several authors taut the advantage of minimally invasive retromuscular repairs versus IPOM mesh. However, a recent metanalysis compared minimally invasive surgery (MIS) IPOM versus MIS retromuscular repair, 11 studies were evaluated in which 2320 patients were enrolled, and it was found that there was no statistically significant difference between patients who received intraperitoneal mesh versus extraperitoneal mesh for SSI, seroma, and hematoma outcome.[13]

As previously mentioned, each anatomic plane for mesh placement carries different SSO rates based largely on the dissection required to access that plane and the resultant wound ischemia and potential space created. However, our summary of the literature suggests that in properly selected patients, similar outcomes can be achieved with each location. As such, it is likely too simplified to conclude that the onlay approach carries a "higher" rate of SSOs as compared with sublay/underlay repairs. In properly selected patients without excessive risk of wound morbidity and relatively small defects, it is a viable option and should always be considered.

Mesh Contamination and Mesh Excision

Although there is often assumed to be a correlation between SSI and mesh contamination, in most cases, SSI does not progress into mesh contamination, and depending on mesh configuration, mesh contamination does not automatically require mesh removal. In addition to surgical wound classification and surgical method (open vs MIS),[23–25] mesh position poses a significant risk factor for mesh contamination and mesh excision. By the nature that mesh is placed superficial to the fascia in an onlay repair, it carries the highest risk of mesh infection and exposure if there is a superficial skin infection. A systematic review of 62 studies with 5824 patients made by Albino and colleagues evaluated the frequency of mesh excision and found statistically significant differences between the onlay mesh position (5%) and the sublay position (0.5%).[5] They attributed this difference to the poorly vascularized fat layer and the large subcutaneous flaps, which constitute a breeding ground for bacterial overgrowth.[4,5] Other data have suggested that most of the mesh in an onlay repair can be salvaged even if exposed. Particularly medium weight uncoated polypropylene meshes have been salvaged even if exposed with proper wound care.[23,24,26] Comparisons of the sublay and underlay positions for mesh infection rates are fairly limited. However, a recent systemic review found no significant difference between the 2 planes, with a mesh removal frequency of 0.5% in the sublay repair and 1.1% in the underlay repair.[5] A study based on the ACHQC database compared 587 cases of open underlay mesh repair with 3624 cases of sublay mesh repair, discovered that mesh position does not affect short-term or long-term outcomes, including SSI, SSOPI quality of life measured by hernia-related quality-of-life survey scores or long-term recurrence rates.[26]

Mesh Erosion

One of the most devastating complications of mesh-based ventral hernia repairs is mesh erosion into the bowel, bladder, or other intra-abdominal viscera. Uncoated intraperitoneal synthetic mesh positioning was attempted at the beginning of the twentieth century, leading to high mesh-erosion rates. That drove hernia surgeons to develop multiple surgeries that positioned the mesh outside the peritoneal cavity to prevent mesh exposure to abdominal viscera. A recent systematic review found that only 89 cases concerning mesh erosion were published between 1996 and 2017; 62.9% were inguinal hernias, 28.1% were incisional/ventral hernias, 6.7% were umbilical, and 2.2% were lumbar or obturator hernia cases. Of all cases described, in 46%, the mesh was initially positioned in extraperitoneal space, 10% were intraperitoneal, and 44% were unknown positions.[27] Although many cases probably have not been published, the low number of published cases compared with the enormous amount of hernia surgeries with mesh indicates that this complication is rare.

Given the recent vigor to utilize advanced surgical techniques to place mesh outside of the abdominal cavity, even for small defects, the absence of high-quality data suggesting that underlay mesh is associated with unacceptably high long-term complication rates should be carefully considered. It is likely that the purported rates of mesh erosion from IPOM mesh are overstated and the suggested benefits of placing mesh outside of the peritoneal cavity are equally overstated.

Pain and Recovery

Although laparoscopic surgeries generally tend to cause less pain than open surgeries, the IPOM procedure is thought to be as painful as an open surgery. That is often another reason that surgeons promote abandoning MIS IPOM for more advanced MIS eTEP type procedures. However, the REVEAL trial is a multicenter clinical trial that randomized 100 patients with midline ventral hernias 7 cm or lesser, 49 to robotic IPOM and 51 to robotic eTEP. The results showed no differences in pain on the day of surgery, 7, and 30 days after surgery. The length of stay, opioid consumption, and 30-day quality of life were also comparable.[28] Conversely, a meta-analysis published in 2022 compared eTEP with MIS IPOM found significantly less pain in the eTEP group.[29] However, this analysis suffers from significant methodologic flaws including that it is based on 5 studies, 4 retrospectives and 1 prospective; of which, postoperative pain was evaluated in 4 of them, 2 studies did not report the SDs, 1 study reported no significant difference in pain severity, and 1 reported a lower acute pain score in the eTEP group.

DISCUSSION

When exploring the ideal plane for all hernia surgeries, we must acknowledge that a hernia is not a single disease. Therefore, different types of hernias require different management. Moreover, even when comparing the same defects in different patients (obese vs thin, young vs old) or a specific defect in different situations (elective vs urgent, only a hernia surgery vs combined surgery), the management will be different. Therefore, we must accept that *there is no holy plane!* Currently, one of the common thoughts is that the retromuscular plain is the ideal plane for most hernias. Between the high SSI and recurrence rates in the onlay repair and the devastating complication of mesh erosion in the underlay repair, the sublay plane logically seems to be the ideal plane. However, this entire line of reasoning neglects the complications associated with accessing this plane. Given the limitations of the literature to truly encompass the heterogenous nature of hernias and hernia surgery, we think it is most beneficial to summarize our approach to mesh positioning considering the unique aspects of the hernia defect and patient characteristics. Inherent to this discussion is a firm understanding of anatomy and surgical dissection of the abdominal wall.

Our approach to heavily contaminated, complex defects, in nonoptimized patients, often undergoing urgent/emergent surgery is to offer a staged approach. In the initial operation, we often will try closure with interrupted figure of 8 slowly absorbable sutures. In cases in which the defect is too large, or excessive tension, we perform an "inlay" repair of a rapidly absorbable synthetic mesh. This serves 2 main purposes, to prevent evisceration, and provide a granulation bed for early skin grafting in the event of superficial skin breakdown. This utilization of the inlay repair is specifically done as a staged approach, accepting a hernia, for subsequent repair in a more elective fashion.

Our approach to definitive repair of the abdominal wall utilizing mesh in various anatomic planes is approached in the following manner. For patients with small defects (<7 cm width), we determine mesh positioning based on patient characteristics and risks for wound morbidity. In obese, diabetic, smokers, we offer a minimally invasive IPOM repair, with or without defect closure. In patients with a hostile abdomen, we will offer an onlay type approach. For these smaller defects, a formal anterior component separation is not necessary, and the size of the skin dissection can be limited to the actual size of the prosthetic required. In our hands, that typically involves 5 cm of coverage. If the surgeon has advanced reconstructive skills, a retromuscular dissection can be performed. If the rectus muscles are wide enough, and the posterior sheath can be closed without tension, that often suffices. However, in certain cases, a formal posterior component separation will need to be performed. We have concerns performing this amount of dissection for relatively small defects, and thus try and avoid sublay type repairs in this type of hernia.

For defects that are 7 to 15 cm, we typically do not perform a minimally invasive approach. Although newer robotic retromuscular repairs are gaining popularity, we believe the data are limited evaluating these repairs, and we have seen a sharp increase in devastating complications associated with these types of repairs in unskilled surgeons' hands. Our approach for these defects is a standard posterior component separation. In these larger defects, the advantage of sublay mesh is likely realized and at least has theoretical advantages. However, as previously mentioned, these approaches should not be performed casually and can result in major postoperative complications and destruction of the abdominal wall neurovascular anatomy.

Finally, defects more than 15 cm should only be approached in expert abdominal core health centers. These defects require significant ancillary support, including intraoperative monitoring, intensive care unit stays, and postoperative support. Often normal anatomic planes are disrupted, and these defects should not be considered by the casual reconstructive surgeon.

In conclusion, the association of mesh plane to surgical outcomes is likely overstated. We believe the abdominal core health surgeon should spend more time mastering all anatomic planes, than worrying about what plane is superior and related to better outcomes. Being proficient at all aspects of mesh deployment will ultimately allow the reconstructive surgeon the ability to customize the operation for the patient, based on what is best for their individual outcome, and not based on the only approach they feel comfortable performing.

CLINICS CARE POINTS

- Each mesh plane possesses advantages and disadvantages, and it is essential to recognize that all mesh planes are legitimate options.
- Proper patient selection is necessary to determine the optimal plane for mesh placement, as using an inappropriate plane can lead to significant complications.

- The sublay repair technique holds significant advantages but is a complex procedure that can result in nerve damage, rectus abdominis atrophy, disruption of the linea semilunaris, interstitial hernias, bowel obstructions, and hemorrhage.

DISCLOSURE

Dr M. Rosen: ACHQC-salary support, Ariste-stock options.

REFERENCES

1. Montelione KC, Zolin SJ, Fafaj A, et al. Outcomes of redo-transversus abdominis release for abdominal wall reconstruction. Hernia J Hernias Abdom Wall Surg 2021;25(6):1581–92.
2. Papageorge CM, Funk LM, Poulose BK, et al. Primary fascial closure during laparoscopic ventral hernia repair does not reduce 30-day wound complications. Surg Endosc 2017;31(11):4551–7.
3. Bernardi K, Olavarria OA, Holihan JL, et al. Primary Fascial Closure During Laparoscopic Ventral Hernia Repair Improves Patient Quality of Life: A Multicenter, Blinded Randomized Controlled Trial. Ann Surg 2020;271(3):434–9.
4. Sosin M, Nahabedian MY, Bhanot P. The Perfect Plane: A Systematic Review of Mesh Location and Outcomes, Update 2018. Plast Reconstr Surg 2018;142(3 Suppl):107S–16S.
5. Albino FP, Patel KM, Nahabedian MY, et al. Does mesh location matter in abdominal wall reconstruction? A systematic review of the literature and a summary of recommendations. Plast Reconstr Surg 2013;132(5):1295–304.
6. Chevrel JP, Rath AM. The use of fibrin glues in the surgical treatment of incisional hernias. Hernia 1997;1(1):9–14.
7. Mommers EHH, Leenders BJM, Leclercq WKG, et al. A modified Chevrel technique for ventral hernia repair: long-term results of a single centre cohort. Hernia J Hernias Abdom Wall Surg 2017;21(4):591–600.
8. Haskins IN, Voeller GR, Stoikes NF, et al. Onlay with Adhesive Use Compared with Sublay Mesh Placement in Ventral Hernia Repair: Was Chevrel Right? An Americas Hernia Society Quality Collaborative Analysis. J Am Coll Surg 2017; 224(5):962–70.
9. Bessa SS, El-Gendi AM, Ghazal AHA, et al. Comparison between the short-term results of onlay and sublay mesh placement in the management of uncomplicated para-umbilical hernia: a prospective randomized study. Hernia J Hernias Abdom Wall Surg 2015;19(1):141–6.
10. Al Chalabi H, Larkin J, Mehigan B, et al. A systematic review of laparoscopic versus open abdominal incisional hernia repair, with meta-analysis of randomized controlled trials. Int J Surg Lond Engl 2015;20:65–74.
11. Awaiz A, Rahman F, Hossain MB, et al. Meta-analysis and systematic review of laparoscopic versus open mesh repair for elective incisional hernia. Hernia J Hernias Abdom Wall Surg 2015;19(3):449–63.
12. Awaiz A, Rahman F, Hossain MB, et al. Reply to comment to Meta-analysis and systematic review of laparoscopic versus open mesh repair for elective incisional hernia. Jensen K, Jorgensen LN. Hernia J Hernias Abdom Wall Surg 2015;19(6): 1027–9.
13. Yeow M, Wijerathne S, Lomanto D. Intraperitoneal versus extraperitoneal mesh in minimally invasive ventral hernia repair: a systematic review and meta-analysis. Hernia J Hernias Abdom Wall Surg 2022;26(2):533–41.

14. Bittner R, Bingener-Casey J, Dietz U, et al. Guidelines for laparoscopic treatment of ventral and incisional abdominal wall hernias (International Endohernia Society (IEHS)-part 1. Surg Endosc 2014;28(1):2–29.
15. Earle D, Roth JS, Saber A, et al. SAGES guidelines for laparoscopic ventral hernia repair. Surg Endosc 2016;30(8):3163–83.
16. Silecchia G, Campanile FC, Sanchez L, et al. Laparoscopic ventral/incisional hernia repair: updated Consensus Development Conference based guidelines [corrected]. Surg Endosc 2015;29(9):2463–84.
17. Ventral Hernia Working Group, Breuing K, Butler CE, Ferzoco S, et al. Incisional ventral hernias: review of the literature and recommendations regarding the grading and technique of repair. Surgery 2010;148(3):544–58.
18. Lamont PM, Ellis H. Incisional hernia in re-opened abdominal incisions: An overlooked risk factor. Br J Surg 2005;75(4):374–6.
19. Santora TA, Roslyn JJ. Incisional Hernia. Surg Clin North Am 1993;73(3):557–70.
20. Shaikh FM, Giri SK, Durrani S, et al. Experience with porcine acellular dermal collagen implant in one-stage tension-free reconstruction of acute and chronic abdominal wall defects. World J Surg 2007;31(10):1966–72 [discussion: 1973-1974, 1975].
21. Bellows CF, Albo D, Berger DH, et al. Abdominal wall repair using human acellular dermis. Am J Surg 2007;194(2):192–8.
22. Luijendijk RW, Lemmen MH, Hop WC, et al. Incisional hernia recurrence following "vest-over-pants" or vertical Mayo repair of primary hernias of the midline. World J Surg 1997;21(1):62–5 [discussion: 66].
23. Li J, Wang Y, Shao X, et al. The salvage of mesh infection after hernia repair with the use of negative pressure wound therapy (NPWT), a systematic review. ANZ J Surg 2022;92(10):2448–56.
24. Warren JA, Love M, Cobb WS, et al. Factors affecting salvage rate of infected prosthetic mesh. Am J Surg 2020;220(3):751–6.
25. Boettge K, Azarhoush S, Fiebelkorn J, et al. The negative pressure wound therapy may salvage the infected mesh following open incisional hernia repair. Ann Med Surg (Lond) 2020;61:64–8.
26. Fafaj A, Petro CC, Tastaldi L, et al. Intraperitoneal versus retromuscular mesh placement for open incisional hernias: an analysis of the Americas Hernia Society Quality Collaborative. Br J Surg 2020;107(9):1123–9.
27. Cunningham HB, Weis JJ, Taveras LR, et al. Mesh migration following abdominal hernia repair: a comprehensive review. Hernia J Hernias Abdom Wall Surg 2019;23(2):235–43.
28. Petro CC, Montelione KC, Zolin SJ, et al. Robotic eTEP versus IPOM evaluation: the REVEAL multicenter randomized clinical trial. Surg Endosc 2023;37(3):2143–53.
29. Li J, Wang Y, Wu L. The Comparison of eTEP and IPOM in Ventral and Incisional Hernia Repair: A Systematic Review and Meta-analysis. Surg Laparosc Endosc Percutan Tech 2022;32(2):252–8.

Laparoscopic Ventral Hernia Repair

Alexandra Hernandez, MD, Rebecca Petersen, MD, MSc*

KEYWORDS

- Incisional hernia • Ventral hernia • Laparoscopy • Laparoscopic ventral hernia repair
- Fascial defect closure

KEY POINTS

- The laparoscopic approach for ventral hernia repair results in decreased wound complications.
- Laparoscopic ventral hernia repair is preferred for patients with morbid obesity, diabetes, and who are immunosuppressed.
- Laparoscopic closure of fascial defects decreases seroma formation and recurrence.

 Video content accompanies this article at http://www.surgical.theclinics.com.

INTRODUCTION AND BACKGROUND

The approach to surgical repair of ventral hernias remains a much debated topic but laparoscopic ventral hernia repair is a well-established technique. Compared with open repair, the main advantage is the reduced rate of wound infection. Although the robotic platform has become more widely used, to date, there are no studies demonstrating the superiority of one approach over another. Ventral hernias remain a common issue, with more than 600,000 repairs annually in the Unites States alone.[1] Incisional hernias occur in up to 30% of patients following open surgery.[2–4] In selecting the best approach for each patient, knowledge of the anatomic features of the hernia, clinical characteristics, surgical techniques and their limitations, and the recovery process is imperative. Herein, we briefly discuss the laparoscopic approach compared with other approaches and outline the key clinical and technical considerations.

PATIENT SELECTION AND PREPROCEDURE PLANNING FOR LAPAROSCOPIC HERNIA REPAIR

In general, most patients should be considered for minimally invasive surgery. The indication for surgical repair of a ventral hernia is relief of symptoms and

---

Department of Surgery, Division of General Surgery, University of Washington, 1959 Northeast Pacific Street, Box 356410, Seattle, WA 98195, USA
* Corresponding author.
E-mail address: rp9@uw.edu

Surg Clin N Am 103 (2023) 947–960
https://doi.org/10.1016/j.suc.2023.05.009
0039-6109/23/© 2023 Elsevier Inc. All rights reserved.
surgical.theclinics.com

prevention of incarceration and strangulation. Additional benefits include the resto-ration of abdominal wall function, respiratory and pelvic floor mechanics, and cosmesis.

Larger size and number of defects is associated with longer duration of surgery and case complexity.[5] Although there are no strict limitations on defect size for laparoscopic hernia repair, consensus statements have suggested avoiding laparoscopic repair in defects greater than 10 cm.[6] Although some have suggested avoiding laparoscopic repair in defects less than 3 cm in size, more recent clinical studies have demonstrated that mesh reduces the risk of recurrence even among patients with defects less than 2 cm. Thus, a minimum size of hernia defect for laparoscopic hernia repair has not been established.[7]

Compared with open repair, specific patient populations should be highly consid-ered for minimally invasive repair. The laparoscopic approach is preferred in patients with higher rates of wound infection. Specifically, this includes patients with morbid obesity, diabetes, and immunosuppression.

Contraindications to laparoscopic ventral hernia repair include prohibitive cardio-pulmonary disease, loss of domain, large abdominal defects, active enterocutaneous fistula, abdominal skin grafts, and removal of a large previously placed prosthetic mesh.[8] Although laparoscopic repair of hernias involving loss of domain has been described in the literature, this is largely limited to case series and results in a higher rate of conversion to an open approach.

Although an open approach to strangulated ventral hernia continues to be the main-stay of emergent surgical treatment, the laparoscopic approach to urgent ventral her-nia repair is feasible. Several studies have demonstrated reduced length of stay, chronic pain, and reduced analgesic use postoperatively when compared with an open approach,[9–11] including a lower risk of mortality in one study.[12] As experience with minimally invasive approaches to hernia repair becomes more widespread, repair of strangulated hernias has also become more common.[13]

PREOPERATIVE OPTIMIZATION

Modifiable risk factors for postoperative complications in elective hernia repair include smoking, obesity, and poor nutrition. Optimization of these factors is associated with reduced risk of surgical site infection and recurrence. At least 4 weeks of smoking cessation is necessary to reduce the negative effects of tobacco on hernia repair.[14] In addition, patients who participate in greater degrees of preoperative exercise have lower rates of postoperative complications, specifically surgical site infection and occurrences after abdominal wall reconstruction.[15] Unfortunately, a significant proportion of patients do not participate in preoperative exercise regimens, which re-mains an area for perioperative programmatic improvement.[15,16]

SURGICAL TECHNIQUE
Preoperative Preparation

Patients should be treated with a multimodal pain regimen (Tylenol, gabapentin, and so forth) before presenting to the operating room. Regional anesthesia is considered in most laparoscopic hernia repairs as postoperative pain can lead to prolonged hospitalization, recovery, and unnecessary increased use of opioids. Several studies have shown benefits to performing a transversus abdominis plane block in patients undergoing laparoscopic ventral hernia repair. This can be per-formed in the perioperative setting with either ultrasound guidance or during sur-gery under direct visualization.[17]

Preoperative antibiotics are administered within 1 hour of the incision. A first-generation cephalosporin is recommended, and if a patient is colonized with Methicillin-resistant Staphylococcus aureus (MRSA), vancomycin is added.[8] We recommend following the American College of Chest physicians comprehensive updated guidelines for venous thromboembolism (VTE) prophylaxis for nonorthopedic surgery patients.[18–20] All patients receive mechanical prophylaxis with intermittent pneumatic compression unless contraindicated. The addition of pharmacologic prophylaxis with either low-molecular weight heparin or unfractionated heparin is given to patients at moderate or higher risk for VTE.

PATIENT POSITIONING AND SURGICAL PREPARATION

The patient is positioned with both arms tucked and well secured to the operating table with appropriate padding of pressure points to allow for steep tilting. Tilting is often necessary because extensive adhesiolysis is required, especially in the setting of recurrent hernias or earlier other abdominal surgeries. For midline hernias, the patient is placed in a supine position, and for lateral hernias (flank, lumbar), the patient is positioned in a lateral or modified lateral decubitus position with bed flexion. A urinary catheter is placed before positioning for cases with an expected operative time of greater than 2 hours. A wide skin prep is necessary for the placement of lateral ports.

ACCESS AND PORT PLACEMENT

The initial location of access to the peritoneal cavity should be away from the hernia defect and any earlier incisions. The ideal location is typically in the left or right upper quadrant and the type of technique (open Hasson technique, Veress needle followed by blind or optical trocar placement, and so forth) should depend primarily on the surgeon's experience.[21] There is no evidence that one technique is better than the other.[22] Additional ports are strategically placed to optimize ergonomics and the ability to perform adhesiolysis as well as fixate the mesh to the abdominal wall. Typically, this requires ports to be placed as laterally as possible, especially for the placement of larger pieces of mesh. We recommend initially placing a 10 to 12 mm trocar to accommodate mesh insertion at Palmer's point (left subcostal region in the midclavicular line) and 2 additional 5-mm ports in the left mid and lower quadrants to achieve triangulation of the target site if no contraindications (Video 1). Placing the 10 to 12-mm port at Palmer's point allows the fascial incision to recede over the costal margin following deflation, decreasing the risk of a port site hernia. Additional 5 mm ports can easily be placed on the contralateral side if needed. A 5-mm 30-degree camera is recommended because it allows for flexibility to switch from port to port to optimize visualization with the crucial goal of avoiding an inadvertent enterotomy.

ADHESIOLYSIS

The majority of cases require some sort of adhesiolysis. All adhesions should be taken down to allow for generous overlap of the mesh, in addition to clearing the abdominal wall along any earlier incisions to assess for occult hernias.[8,21,23] For hernias located in the midline, the falciform and umbilical ligaments should be taken down. If the hernia is more inferiorly located, dissection should be performed to develop the space of Retzius to allow for appropriate mesh overlap inferiorly. Sharp dissection with judicious, limited cautery is strongly recommended during adhesiolysis to avoid an immediate and more importantly a delayed inadvertent enterotomy. Additional port placement and movement of an angled laparoscope from port to port may be required to optimize exposure, countertraction technique, and ergonomics.[8] In addition, the bed should typically be raised and airplaned away from the surgeon to assist with lysis of adhesions. Inadvertent enterotomies increase the risk of mortality, surgical site infection, enterocutaneous fistula, and recurrence.[24,25] The incidence of enterotomy during laparoscopic adhesiolysis has been reported to occur anywhere from 1% to 11% (Bittner 2019, Earle 2016). Close inspection during and after adhesiolysis is paramount because the mortality rate is significantly increased if the enterotomy is not identified and repaired at the initial surgery (0.05% vs 8%).[25]

REDUCTION OF HERNIA CONTENTS AND MEASURING THE DEFECT

The hernia sac and preperitoneal fat need to be completely reduced from the defect before closure. Typically, dissection is started in the preperitoneal plane surrounding the defect and the fat and sac are reduced together. As mentioned above, it is also important to take down the falciform and umbilical ligaments to promote mesh integration and assess for occult hernias. The dissection is usually performed with scissor-electrocautery to ensure adequate hemostasis before mesh placement to avoid the complication of a hematoma (Video 2).

After the abdominal wall is cleared of adhesions, close inspection is again performed to assess for occult hernia defects. It is important to accurately measure the defect and/or area encompassing more than one defect (**Fig. 1**).[26]

Measurements can vary widely if the surgeon is not familiar with the potential errors that can occur, especially in the setting of obesity.[27] Accurate measurement is crucial so that the mesh can be appropriately sized with sufficient overlap to minimize recurrence risk. Both the width (greatest horizontal distance between the lateral margins of the defect(s)) and length (vertical distance between the cranial and caudal margins of the defect(s)) are measured to determine the total defect area either by an external or internal method. The external method is performed with the use of a spinal needle placed through the skin and visualized laparoscopically while the perimeter of the defect is marked on the skin and subsequently measured with a ruler. It is essential that the spinal needle be inserted at a 90° angle to avoid overestimation of the defect (**Fig. 2**). The internal method is typically performed by placing a ruler inside the peritoneal cavity to measure the defect or area of defects. If the defect is small, an instrument tip with a known length can easily be used for measurement. It is important to reduce pneumoperitoneum (8 mm Hg), especially when using the external method to avoid overestimation of the defect. Overestimation or underestimation of the defect may lead to increased difficulty in handling a larger than necessary piece of mesh, excessive laxity, or more significantly an increased risk of recurrence from insufficient overlap.

FASCIAL CLOSURE

If feasible, the fascial defect(s) should be closed to decrease the risk of seroma formation, recurrence rate, and improve abdominal wall function and cosmesis.[8,21,28,29] A randomized study recently showed improved quality of life for patients undergoing primary fascial closure during laparoscopic ventral hernia repair.[30] The most common technique for fascial closure is an extracorporeal percutaneous technique where small (1 mm) stab incisions are made in the skin along the vertical axis of the defect and a suture passer is used to place sutures (0-polydioxanone) every 1 to 2 cm.[30]

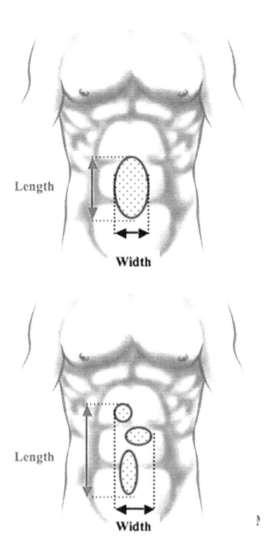

Fig. 1. Measurement of fascial defect(s).

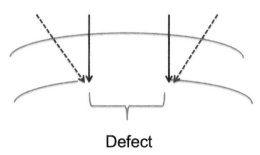

Fig. 2. Errors in defect measurement.

The sutures are then tied down sequentially while holding cross tension on the remaining sutures at reduced pneumoperitoneum (<8 mm Hg) (Video 3). Another percutaneous technique uses a "shoelacing" technique where figure-of-eight sutures are placed every 3 cm.[31] There are a wide array of defect closure techniques that include various suture passers and suture types. Defect sizes that have been closed with the extracorporeal percutaneous technique have ranged from 3 to as large as 12 cm without a concomitant component separation.[29,30] Although laparoscopic intracorporeal closure of the fascial defect with running barbed suture is routinely performed by some surgeons, it is more technically difficult via a laparoscopic approach.[32]

MESH PLACEMENT AND FIXATION

The mesh sizing should focus on mesh area-to-defect area ratio as opposed to the more commonly used single mesh overlap target length of 5 cm. The ratio should be at least 16:1 or more simply stated the radius of the mesh should be 4 times the radius of the defect and more generous overlap should be considered for larger defects.[21,33] In the setting of morbid obesity more studies are needed to truly individualize mesh sizing. When placing the mesh in an intraperitoneal position, a composite synthetic mesh is selected, assuming there are no absolute or relative contraindications such as gross contamination. The mesh is rolled lengthwise and inserted through the 10 to 12 mm trocar and care is taken to ensure the mesh is correctly oriented with the noncomposite side opposing the abdominal wall. The mesh is positioned where it is centered at the midpoint of the closed defect. This step is crucial as malalignment of the mesh will decrease the optimal target mesh area-to-defect area ratio and result in a higher risk of recurrence. The mesh is fixated with transfascial sutures, tacks, or a combination of both. More recent guidelines have recommended all 3 techniques but if tacks are performed alone, a double-crown technique is preferred. There is no strong evidence concerning the use of absorbable versus nonabsorbable tacks but there are studies that have reported a lower cost without increased postoperative pain for nonabsorbable tacks.[21] Intracorporeal fixation with running suture is technically difficult and better accomplished with the robotic platform. Finally, the use of fibrin-based glue or sealant for fixation is currently not recommended due to lack of evidence and concern from limited case series to be associated with a higher risk of recurrence.[8,21] Our preference is to place a combination of transfascial sutures and tacks for fixation. A marker is used to draw an "X" on the mesh to delineate the midpoint and where the 4 equally distanced stay sutures are placed at the perimeter. The stay sutures are then partially tied down, avoiding air-knots with the composite side facing down. If the mesh comes with a paper template, this can be used to draw out the border of the mesh and mark the target suture locations on the skin while deflated. The mesh is then placed in the peritoneal cavity, unrolled verifying the correct orientation after pneumoperitoneum has been reestablished. A 1-mm skin incision is made at the initial marked skin target with an 11 blade. A suture passer is then used to bring the first transfascial suture through. While pulling up on the first suture, the second target site is determined by grasping the suture knot and bringing up the mesh to the estimated target site on the skin at reduced pressure to ensure appropriate tension and alignment of the mesh. This is repeated sequentially for the remaining sutures. The sutures are then tied down with the pressure set at 8 mm Hg. Care is taken to avoid inadvertent injury to the epigastric vessels, which can lead to significant abdominal wall hematoma and increased postoperative pain. Following, a tacking device is used to place tacks every 1 to 2 cm apart at the perimeter of the mesh to decrease the risk of bowel entrapment. Additional tacks are placed in a "quilting pattern" or "double crown" to oppose the mesh to the abdominal wall (Video 4). For larger pieces of mesh, an additional 5-mm port is placed on the contralateral side to assist with placing the tacks under direct visualization.

CLOSURE

Final inspection is performed to assess for inadvertent enterotomies and bleeding. Ports are removed at decreased pressure to ensure that there is no ongoing bleeding to suggest an inadvertent injury to the epigastric vessels. The port-site fascial defects are typically not closed because the larger 10 to 12-mm port is intentionally placed at Palmer's point where the risk of hernia formation is low because it typically recedes over the costal margin on deflation. Skin incisions are closed in the standard fashion and glue is typically applied to the 1-mm skin incisions and port-sites to avoid placement of excessive dressings that are more notable to the patient.

SPECIAL TECHNICAL CONSIDERATIONS
Atypical Hernias

Atypical hernias pose technical challenges when it comes to ensuring appropriate mesh overlap beyond the defect and fixation, which are both crucial to decrease the risk of recurrence.

Suprapubic Hernias

Suprapubic hernias are close to the pubic symphysis and ensuring mesh overlap inferiorly beyond the defect is crucial to avoid recurrence. Dissection should be performed to develop the space of Retzius to allow for appropriate mesh overlap and fixation to the bone and/or Cooper's ligaments should be performed.[21,34]

Subxiphoid Hernias

Subxiphoid hernias are close to the costal margin and optimizing mesh overlap beyond the defect rostrally can be challenging. If the mesh is placed in the intra-abdominal position, the mesh is secured near the costal margin with an intentional overhang to avoid fixation to the diaphragm because this may lead to serious cardiac (tamponade) or pulmonary complications (lung injury, pneumothorax). The option of using nonpenetrating fixation with fibrin-based glues above the costal margin is reasonable but evidence of benefit is lacking.[34] The other option is to develop a pre-peritoneal plane where the mesh can be partially positioned rostrally where the peritoneal flap is then secured to the mesh below the costal margin to avoid an overhang. Preperitoneal dissection and placement of mesh in the preperitoneal position is more easily performed with the robotic platform.[32]

Lateral Hernias

Mobilization of the colon may be required for defects located laterally such as flank or lumbar hernias. Additional caution should be taken to avoid injury to retroperitoneal structures such as nerves, ureters, and vasculature with fixation. In these cases, placement of mesh in the preperitoneal or retromuscular position may be more desirable where fixation is not routinely performed, and greater lateral mesh overlap can be achieved. In these cases, an alternative approach such as an open or robotic approach may be more feasible.

Rectus Diastasis

Rectus diastasis (RD) is an acquired condition characterized by the rectus abdominus muscles being abnormally thinned and separated at the midline often associated laxity of the abdominal muscles. Although RD itself is not a ventral hernia, which is distinguished by a thinned hernia sac, presence of RD is a risk factor for the development of ventral hernias due to the deterioration of connective tissue.[35] Pregnancy is a known risk factor for the development of RD and has a treatment dose effect, with the greater number of pregnancies a woman has had conferring greater risk of the development of RD.[36] Unfortunately, lack of consensus regarding the intrarectus distance (IRD) and measurement method of the IRD required for diagnosis of RD is a barrier to understanding true prevalence and, therefore, risk factors for this pathologic condition beyond pregnancy.[37] The most consistent definition in the literature of RD is an IRD of greater than 2 cm.[38] The presence of RD is a known risk factor of recurrence when present during hernia repair.[39] Mesh reinforcement is currently recommended during hernia repair with a coexisting RD.[21] Several plication techniques exist to address RD at the time of hernia repair but comparison studies are lacking to identify superiority. Potential favorable outcomes when addressing RD at the time of hernia repair include improved cosmesis and abdominal wall function.

Morbid Obesity

A laparoscopic approach is preferred in obese patients because it is associated with decreased risk of wound infection and complication rates.[21] The surgical site infection rate has been reported to be reduced by 70% to 80% in morbidly obese patients with a laparoscopic approach compared with open surgery.[40] Studies have routinely demonstrated a higher risk of recurrence in obese patients; therefore, special consideration should be given in this patient population to performing additional technical steps, including greater mesh overlap, placement of more tacks/sutures for fixation, and closure of defect(s) if feasible.[21] Bariatric-length instruments are also recommended to avoid interference of handles and to optimize maneuverability. Morbidly obese patients without significant symptoms should be strongly advised to lose weight before undergoing definitive repair.

MANAGEMENT OF INADVERTENT ENTEROTOMY

The risk of inadvertent enterotomy during laparoscopic ventral hernia repair ranges between 1% and 11%.[8,21] When an enterotomy is immediately recognized and there is little contamination, it is reasonable to repair the enterotomy and proceed with mesh repair at the time of injury.[41] If there is considerable contamination, the option of repairing the enterotomy laparoscopically, again in experienced hands, and admitting the patient for observation and antibiotic therapy with planned definitive repair with mesh during the same hospitalization is also reasonable.[21,42] The decision for conversion to immediate laparotomy should be based on the extent of contamination, location of injury (small bowel versus colon), and most importantly surgeon's skill and experience. When converting to an open approach to repair a bowel injury, it is also reasonable to proceed with definitive repair of the hernia with mesh. The type of mesh (synthetic, biologic, biosynthetic absorbable) selected should be based on the extent of contamination, mesh position (intra-abdominal, retromuscular, preperitoneal, bridged), and patient characteristics. Several studies have shown reduction in the risk of hernia recurrence with synthetic mesh as compared with biologic mesh in the setting of single-stage repair of clean-contaminated and contaminated settings.[43,44] Synthetic mesh was also associated with lower cost. Ultimately, inadvertent enterotomies are associated with a higher risk of surgical site infection, wound complications, recurrence, and mortality.[21,43,44] These patients should be closely monitored with a low level of suspicion in the postoperative period.

ADVANCED TECHNIQUES

During the past decade, the management of abdominal wall hernias has rapidly evolved. Currently, there is a variety of surgical approach options, which includes an open, laparoscopic, endoscopic, robotic, or hybrid approach combining these modalities. In addition, there are numerous techniques to choose from regarding mesh fixation, mesh placement position, and performance of concomitant component separation. Despite a high volume of studies being published because of a rapidly evolving field, many of these have limited methodology and at times conflicting results. Decision-making regarding the optimal repair strategy continues to rely on societal guidelines, surgeon experience and skillset, and patient characteristics and expectations.

The laparoscopic approach is most commonly associated with an intraperitoneal onlay mesh repair technique as described above and is currently limited in the setting of larger defects, atypical hernias, need for mesh or excessive skin excision, or larger hernia sacs with smaller defects. With the introduction of the robotic platform, extraperitoneal techniques have further been developed and popularized. Although these same techniques have been achieved from a laparoscopic approach, they are often more technically and ergonomically challenging and should only be performed by surgeons with advanced laparoscopic skills and extensive experience. The main advantages of an extraperitoneal technique are a less costly uncoated synthetic mesh is used and the mesh is hidden from intra-abdominal viscera. This potentially decreases the risk of adhesions, trauma from fixation, enterocutaneous fistulae, chronic pain, and mesh infection.

Although there are an increasing number of minimally invasive extraperitoneal techniques, the more commonly performed techniques using laparoscopy include transabdominal preperitoneal and enhanced-view total extraperitoneal techniques. Comprehensive discussion of the majority of novel minimally invasive extraperitoneal techniques is beyond the scope of this article. Laparoscopy has a limited role due to suboptimal ergonomics, instrumentation, and visualization. Moreover, the requirement for a very advanced laparoscopic skillset is necessary, which has become difficult to obtain in the era in which the robotic platform has become popularized with trainees and practicing surgeons.

COMPONENT SEPARATION

Component separation should be considered in the setting of larger defects. Laparoscopic closure of a larger defect may not be possible due to excessive tension. Several minimally invasive component separation techniques have been described, which range from minimally invasive open anterior component separation, endoscopic anterior component separation, and more recently laparoscopic/endoscopic posterior component separation.[45–50] For larger defects, careful preoperative planning of approach and technique should be individualized to patient's clinical characteristics and expectations, in addition to surgeon's experience.

Postoperative Management

Ambulation and increased activity in the perioperative period play a crucial role in rehabilitation of the abdominal wall after hernia repair. The Abdominal Core Surgery

Rehabilitation[SM] Protocol provides guidance for patients and a scaffold for physical therapists working with this patient population to optimize their exercise rehabilitation in the perioperative period. This protocol is available as an application that can be downloaded on a smartphone or on the ACHQC website: https://achqc.org/patients/abdominal-core-surgery-rehabilitation. Historically, weight-bearing precautions have been recommended to reduce intra-abdominal pressure and avoid immediate recurrence. However, there is limited evidence regarding the duration of precautions or restrictions on weightlifting.[51] Further studies in this area are required to more appropriately recommend individualized patient rehabilitation regimens.

Monitoring for complications is critical in the postoperative period. A high index of suspicion is appropriate in cases requiring extensive lysis of adhesions, with prolonged operative times, or in patients with multiple comorbidities and risk factors. Surgical site occurrences are not uncommon, specifically seroma formation, especially if the fascial defect was not closed before mesh reinforcement. Most seromas do not require intervention but should be followed for resolution.[8] Although most iatrogenic enterotomies are identified during the index operation, those that are identified following repair are associated with increased mortality and an increased risk of enterocutaneous fistula, abscess, surgical site infection, mesh infection, and hernia recurrence.[25,41,52,53]

SUMMARY

In recent years, there has been an explosion of information regarding the surgical management of abdominal wall hernias. Advances in minimally invasive techniques have led to improved success and reduced complications. Regardless of the approach or specific techniques, the overall goals of any hernia repair should remain the same, which are to provide relief of symptoms and minimize recurrence. Minimally invasive approaches for ventral hernia repair offer several advantages over an open approach, which include decreased wound complications and faster recovery. Currently, there is no superior minimally invasive procedure for ventral hernia repair. Patient characteristics, type of hernia, defect size, and surgeon experience should play into decision-making regarding optimal approach, along with mesh position, and the various technical aspects for repair.

Beyond the surgical approach, optimization of abdominal wall surgery is contingent on many other factors, including socioeconomics, perioperative nutrition and conditioning, specific anatomic characteristics, closure techniques, and the implications for surrounding organ systems. Alignment of patient and surgeon goals and expectations (elimination of symptoms, bulge, pain, excision of excessive skin, and so forth) before surgery will lead to improved patient satisfaction. Attention to these details will help improve patient outcomes, and further advances and research into these areas will continue to optimize treatment strategies and ultimately outcomes for all.

CLINICS CARE POINTS

- Laparoscopic ventral hernia repair is well established with the main advantage of decreased wound morbidity.
- The laparoscopic approach is preferred in patients at higher risk of infection and should be strongly considered in patients with morbid obesity, diabetes, and immunosuppression.
- Fascial defects should be closed to decrease the risk of seroma formation, reduce recurrence risk, and improve abdominal wall function and cosmesis.

DISCLOSURE

The authors have nothing to disclose.

SUPPLEMENTARY DATA

Supplementary data related to this article can be found online at https://doi.org/10.1016/j.suc.2023.05.009.

REFERENCES

1. Schlosser KA, Renshaw SM, Tamer RM, et al. Ventral hernia repair: an increasing burden affecting abdominal core health. Hernia 2023;27(2):415–21.
2. Bloemen A, Van Dooren P, Huizinga BF, et al. Randomized clinical trial comparing polypropylene or polydioxanone for midline abdominal wall closure. Br J Surg 2011;98(5):633–9.
3. Eker HH, Hansson BME, Buunen M, et al. Laparoscopic vs. open incisional hernia repair: a randomized clinical trial. JAMA Surg 2013;148(3):259–63.
4. van't Riet M, Steyerberg EW, Nellensteyn J, et al. Meta-analysis of techniques for closure of midline abdominal incisions. Br J Surg 2002;89(11):1350–6.
5. Jenkins ED, Yom VH, Melman L, et al. Clinical predictors of operative complexity in laparoscopic ventral hernia repair: a prospective study. Surg Endosc 2010;24(8):1872–7.
6. Cuccurullo D, Piccoli M, Agresta F, et al. Laparoscopic ventral incisional hernia repair: evidence-based guidelines of the first Italian Consensus Conference. Hernia 2013;17(5):557–66.
7. Christoffersen MW, Helgstrand F, Rosenberg J, et al. Lower reoperation rate for recurrence after mesh versus sutured elective repair in small umbilical and epigastric hernias. A nationwide register study. World J Surg 2013;37(11):2548–52.
8. Earle D, Roth JS, Saber A, et al. SAGES guidelines for laparoscopic ventral hernia repair. Surg Endosc 2016;30(8):3163–83.
9. Landau O, Kyzer S. Emergent laparoscopic repair of incarcerated incisional and ventral hernia. Surg Endosc 2004;18(9):1374–6.
10. Olmi S, Cesana G, Erba L, et al. Emergency laparoscopic treatment of acute incarcerated incisional hernia. Hernia 2009;13(6):605–8.
11. Jacob R, Guy SB, Kamila L, et al. Comparison of emergent laparoscopic and open repair of acutely incarcerated and strangulated hernias-short- and long-term results. Surg Endosc 2023;37(3). https://doi.org/10.1007/S00464-022-09743-4.
12. Khorgami Z, Hui BY, Mushtaq N, et al. Predictors of mortality after elective ventral hernia repair: an analysis of national inpatient sample. Hernia 2019;23(5):979–85.
13. Pechman DM, Cao L, Fong C, et al. Laparoscopic versus open emergent ventral hernia repair: utilization and outcomes analysis using the ACSNSQIP database. Surg Endosc 2018;32(12):4999–5005.
14. Petro CC, Prabhu AS. Preoperative Planning and Patient Optimization. Surg Clin North Am 2018;98(3):483–97.
15. Renshaw SM, Poulose BK, Gupta A, et al. Preoperative exercise and outcomes after ventral hernia repair: Making the case for prehabilitation in ventral hernia patients. Surgery 2021;170(2):516–24.

16. Moran J, Guinan E, McCormick P, et al. The ability of prehabilitation to influence postoperative outcome after intra-abdominal operation: a systematic review and meta-analysis. Surgery 2016;160(5):1189–201.

17. Fields AC, Gonzalez DO, Chin EH, et al. Laparoscopic-assisted transversus abdominis plane block for postoperative pain control in laparoscopic ventral hernia repair: a randomized controlled trial. J Am Coll Surg 2015;221(2):462–9.

18. Gould MK, Garcia DA, Wren SM, et al. Prevention of VTE in nonorthopedic surgical patients: antithrombotic therapy and prevention of thrombosis, 9th ed: american college of chest physicians evidence-based clinical practice guidelines. Chest 2012;141(2 Suppl):e227S–77S.

19. Rogers SO, Kilaru RK, Hosokawa P, et al. Multivariable predictors of postoperative venous thromboembolic events after general and vascular surgery: results from the patient safety in surgery study. J Am Coll Surg 2007;204(6):1211–21.

20. Caprini JA. Risk assessment as a guide for the prevention of the many faces of venous thromboembolism. Am J Surg 2010;199(1 Suppl). https://doi.org/10. 1016/J.AMJSURG.2009.10.006.

21. Bittner R, Bain K, Bansal VK, et al. Update of Guidelines for laparoscopic treatment of ventral and incisional abdominal wall hernias (International Endohernia Society (IEHS)): Part B. Surg Endosc 2019;33(11):3511–49.

22. Ahmad G, Gent D, Henderson D, et al. Laparoscopic entry techniques. Cochrane Database Syst Rev 2015;8(8). https://doi.org/10.1002/14651858.CD006583. PUB4.

23. Bittner R, Bingener-Casey J, Dietz U, et al. Guidelines for laparoscopic treatment of ventral and incisional abdominal wall hernias (International Endohernia Society [IEHS])—Part 2. Surg Endosc 2014;28(2):353–79.

24. Krpata DM, Prabhu AS, Tastaldi L, et al. Impact of inadvertent enterotomy on short-term outcomes after ventral hernia repair: An AHSQC analysis. Surgery 2018;164(2):327–32.

25. LeBlanc KA, Elieson MJ, Corder JM. Enterotomy and mortality rates of laparoscopic incisional and ventral hernia repair: a review of the literature. JSLS J Soc Laparoendosc Surg 2007;11(4):408–14. Available at: https://pubmed-ncbi-nlm-nih-gov.offcampus.lib.washington.edu/18237502/. Accessed May 23, 2023.

26. Muysoms FE, Miserez M, Berrevoet F, et al. Classification of primary and incisional abdominal wall hernias. Hernia 2009;13(4):407–14.

27. Cherla DV, Lew DF, Escamilla RJ, et al. Differences of alternative methods of measuring abdominal wall hernia defect size: a prospective observational study. Surg Endosc 2018;32(3):1228–33.

28. Christoffersen MW, Westen M, Rosenberg J, et al. Closure of the fascial defect during laparoscopic umbilical hernia repair: a randomized clinical trial. Br J Surg 2020;107(3):200–8.

29. Bernardi K, Olavarria OA, Liang MK. Primary fascial closure during minimally invasive ventral hernia repair. JAMA Surg 2020;155(3):256–7.

30. Bernardi K, Olavarria OA, Holihan JL, et al. Primary fascial closure during laparoscopic ventral hernia repair improves patient quality of life: a multicenter, blinded randomized controlled trial. Ann Surg 2020;271(3):434–9.

31. Orenstein SB, Dumeer JL, Monteagudo J, et al. Outcomes of laparoscopic ventral hernia repair with routine defect closure using "shoelacing" technique. Surg Endosc 2011;25(5):1452–7.

32. Petro CC, Thomas JD, Tu C, et al. Robotic vs laparoscopic ventral hernia repair with intraperitoneal mesh: 1-year exploratory outcomes of the PROVE-IT randomized clinical trial. J Am Coll Surg 2022;234(6):1160–5.

33. Hauters P, Desmet J, Gherardi D, et al. Assessment of predictive factors for recurrence in laparoscopic ventral hernia repair using a bridging technique. Surg Endosc 2017;31(9):3656–63.

34. Hope WW, Hooks WB. Atypical hernias: suprapubic, subxiphoid, and flank. Surg Clin North Am 2013;93(5):1135–62.

35. Köhler G, Luketina RR, Emmanuel K. Sutured repair of primary small umbilical and epigastric hernias: concomitant rectus diastasis is a significant risk factor for recurrence. World J Surg 2015;39(1):121–6.

36. Werner LA, Dayan M. Diastasis Recti Abdominis-diagnosis, Risk Factors, Effect on Musculoskeletal Function, Framework for Treatment and Implications for the Pelvic Floor. Curr Women s Heal Rev 2018;15(2):86–101.

37. Cavalli M, Aiolfi A, Bruni PG, et al. Prevalence and risk factors for diastasis recti abdominis: a review and proposal of a new anatomical variation. Hernia 2021; 25(4):883–90.

38. Keramidas E, Rodopoulou S, Gavala MI. A proposed classification and treatment algorithm for rectus diastasis: a prospective study. Aesthetic Plast Surg 2022; 46(5):2323–32.

39. ElHawary H, Barone N, Zammit D, et al. Closing the gap: evidence-based surgical treatment of rectus diastasis associated with abdominal wall hernias. Hernia 2021;25(4):827–53.

40. Awaiz A, Rahman F, Hossain MB, et al. Meta-analysis and systematic review of laparoscopic versus open mesh repair for elective incisional hernia. Hernia 2015;19(3):449–63.

41. Sharma A, Khullar R, Soni V, et al. Iatrogenic enterotomy in laparoscopic ventral/ incisional hernia repair: a single center experience of 2,346 patients over 17 years. Hernia 2013;17(5):581–7.

42. Misiakos EP, Patapis P, Zavras N, et al. Current trends in laparoscopic ventral hernia repair. JSLS J Soc Laparoendosc Surg 2015;19(3). https://doi.org/10.4293/ JSLS.2015.00048.

43. Carbonell AM, Criss CN, Cobb WS, et al. Outcomes of synthetic mesh in contaminated ventral hernia repairs. J Am Coll Surg 2013;217(6):991–8.

44. Rosen MJ, Krpata DM, Petro CC, et al. Biologic vs synthetic mesh for single-stage repair of contaminated ventral hernias: a randomized clinical trial. JAMA Surg 2022;157(4):293–301.

45. Harth KC, Rosen MJ. Endoscopic versus open component separation in complex abdominal wall reconstruction. Am J Surg 2010;199(3):342–7.

46. Rosen MJ, Williams C, Jin J, et al. Laparoscopic versus open-component separation: a comparative analysis in a porcine model. Am J Surg 2007;194(3):385–9.

47. Moazzez A, Mason RJ, Katkhouda N. A new technique for minimally invasive abdominal wall reconstruction of complex incisional hernias: totally laparoscopic component separation and incisional hernia repair. Surg Technol Int 2010;20: 185–91. Available at: https://pubmed-ncbi-nlm-nih-gov.offcampus.lib. washington.edu/21082566/. Accessed May 23, 2023.

48. Belyansky I, Zahiri HR, Park A. Laparoscopic transversus abdominis release, a novel minimally invasive approach to complex abdominal wall reconstruction. Surg Innov 2016;23(2):134–41.

49. Tong WMY, Hope W, Overby DW, et al. Comparison of outcome after mesh-only repair, laparoscopic component separation, and open component separation. Ann Plast Surg 2011;66(5):551–6.

50. Dewulf M, Hiekkaranta JM, Mäkäräinen E, et al. Open versus robotic-assisted laparoscopic posterior component separation in complex abdominal wall repair. BJS open 2022;6(3). https://doi.org/10.1093/BJSOPEN/ZRAC057.
51. Loor MM, Shah P, Olavarria OA, et al. Postoperative work and activity restrictions after abdominal surgery: a systematic review. Ann Surg 2021;274(2):290–7.
52. Azin A, Hirpara D, Jackson T, et al. Emergency laparoscopic and open repair of incarcerated ventral hernias: a multi-institutional comparative analysis with coarsened exact matching. Surg Endosc 2019;33(9):2812–20.
53. Thomas JD, Gentle CK, Krpata DM, et al. Comparing rates of bowel injury for laparoscopic and robotic ventral hernia repair: a retrospective analysis of the abdominal core health quality collaborative. Hernia 2022;26(5):1251–8.

Open Complex Abdominal Wall Reconstruction

Clayton C. Petro, MD*, Megan Melland-Smith, MD

KEYWORDS

- Ventral hernia • Component separation • Abdominal wall

KEY POINTS

- Component separation can be performed with either anterior or posterior techniques to alleviate tension on midline fascial closure. Both techniques allow approximately 20 cm of maximum bilateral rectus advancement preoperative cross-sectional imaging can help guide decision making.
- In a posterior component separation, alleviation of midline tension is mostly offered by division of the posterior rectus sheath. The addition of a transversus abdominis release allows for greater than 20 cm of posterior fascial advancement to reduce tension on closure of the posterior fascia while also creating a large retromuscular pocket for wide mesh overlap.
- Preoperative botulinum toxin injection to the abdominal wall can be used to facilitate fascial closure when the hernia volume to peritoneal volume ratio is greater than 20% to 25%. Its benefit in smaller hernias is less well-defined.
- Postoperative respiratory failure requiring reintubation or transfer to a higher level of care can be a manifestation of transient elevations in intra-abdominal pressure that frequently resolve in elective settings within 24 to 48 hours.
- Technical complications of component separation include full thickness injury of the linea semilunaris that can result in iatrogenic hernia defects. Although the incidence is poorly defined, these are likely rare but functionally devastating complications.

INTRODUCTION

Ventral hernia repair remains one of the most common procedures performed by surgeons and more than 600,000 ventral hernias are repaired annually in the United States.[1–3] All repair techniques have limitations to their durability, leading to some inevitable recurrences over time.[4] Repair of recurrent hernias is not only complex but also is associated with progressively higher rates of recurrence after repeated repair. The evolution and refinement of component separation techniques has allowed

Lerner College of Medicine, Cleveland Clinic Center for Abdominal Core Health, 9500 Euclid Avenue A-100, Cleveland, OH 44195, USA
* Corresponding author.
E-mail address: petroc@ccf.org

Surg Clin N Am 103 (2023) 961–976
https://doi.org/10.1016/j.suc.2023.04.006
0039-6109/23/© 2023 Elsevier Inc. All rights reserved.

surgical.theclinics.com

surgeons to address large or complex hernias with the ability to restore abdominal wall contour and function.[5]

For the purposes of this article, complex abdominal wall reconstruction will be defined as the utilization of component separation techniques for ventral hernia repair. Herein, the authors discuss the relevant indications and techniques of component separation, patient selection criteria, preoperative adjuncts that may assist with fascial or soft tissue closure, and complications of component separation.

PURPOSES OF COMPONENT SEPARATION

In contemporary hernia surgery, component separation serves two main purposes.

Relieve Tension on Midline Fascial Closure

The traditional aim of a component separation is to serially and strategically divide myofascial layers of the abdominal wall to alleviate tension on midline fascial approximation.

Historic surgical techniques to relieve tension on midline fascial closure has been pursued as early as 1916 by Dr Charles Gibson,[6] who used relaxing incisions on the medial rectus sheaths parallel to the midline. Chevrel further modified this technique by recreating the linea alba with an overlapping anterior fascia "turnover." These techniques, however, were insufficient for closing larger midline defects.[7,8] In addition, autologous tissue transfers such as the free graft or pedicled tensor fascia lata flaps are also associated with high rates of complications, recurrences, and donor-site morbidities.[9,10]

Oscar Ramirez constructed these historic approaches by adding lateral release. He described a posterior rectus sheath release with the addition of division of the lateral external oblique (EO) that provided additional fascial medialization.[11] Component separation has since evolved to address undue midline tension through strategic and serial division of the rectus and lateral abdominal wall musculofascial layers allowing closure of larger defects.

The benefits of a hernia repair that reestablishes the midline and restores the rectus muscles to a more anatomic midline location allow proper usage of the abdominal wall with improved core muscle function. Little is known about the negative long-term consequences of dividing the lateral abdominal muscles. However, in patients with massive hernia defects, the functional benefits of restoring the midline including strength, stability, respiratory function, and improvements in quality of life outweigh the "sacrifice" of one of these lateral muscles.[5,12,13]

The indications for component separation are not well-defined and variables other than size of the fascial defect must be considered including.

- The compliance of the patient's abdominal wall. A patient with a compliant abdominal wall and a large defect may achieve fascial closure more easily than other patients with smaller defects but more rigid abdominal walls.
- The contents of the hernia sac. The length and width of a fascial defect alone are sometimes not reflective of the contents of the hernia. Small fascial defects can be associated with large, voluminous hernia sacs that contain bowel and other organs leading to the loss of domain.

Retromuscular Mesh Placement

The other purpose of component separation is creation of a large retromuscular pocket for mesh placement. Although the Rives-Stoppa retrorectus dissection facilitates retromuscular mesh, the addition of a transversus abdominis release (TAR) allows wider overlap and alleviation of any tension on the posterior rectus sheath closure for larger hernias. Retromuscular mesh has additional benefits, including.[14]

- A large retromuscular pocket allowing wide overlap and reinforcement of the visceral sac.
- A well-vascularized plane allows for optimal mesh incorporation.
- Mesh placement outside of the peritoneal cavity, away from the viscera and separated from the superficial wound by muscle.
- The ability to use of uncoated monofilament polypropylene mesh which is both inexpensive and resilient to infection.
- Avoidance of excessive subcutaneous flap dissection limiting postoperative wound morbidity.

Because of these benefits offered by retromuscular mesh placement, this technique has become the most versatile approach to complex ventral hernia repair over anterior component separation with onlay mesh.

TECHNIQUES OF COMPONENT SEPARATION

Techniques of component separation can be broadly categorized into anterior and posterior, depending on which of the lateral abdominal wall muscle(s) are divided. For anatomic references, see **Fig. 1**. Both anterior and posterior component separations allow for approximately 20 cm of bilateral rectus and midline fascial advancement. It is important to note that anterior and posterior component separations should not be performed concomitantly during the same operation due to the risk of destabilizing the anterior abdominal wall.

Open Anterior Component Separation

Ramirez originally described his anterior component separation technique with serial division of two myofascial structures on each side of the abdominal wall. His method involved a step-wise approach, whereby after each release, the hernia defect edges

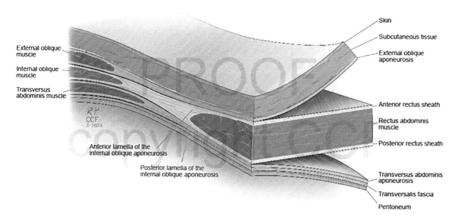

Fig. 1. Anatomy of the abdominal wall. Purple indicates "anterior" abdominal wall components including the external oblique muscle, green indicates internal oblique muscle with anterior and posterior lamella encasing the rectus muscle, and orange indicates the "posterior" components of the transversus abdominis with underlying transversalis fascia and peritoneum. (Reprinted with permission, Cleveland Clinic Foundation ©2023. All Rights Reserved.)

were assessed for tension and further releases only carried out when needed. The operation begins by undermining the subcutaneous tissue and creating large skin flaps to expose the anterior rectus sheath fascia. This subcutaneous dissection is continued lateral, beyond the linea semilunaris to facilitate releases. The first myofascial division is of the medial boarder of the posterior rectus sheath followed by separation from the overlying rectus muscle. This retrorectus dissection allows for medial advancement of 3, 5, and 3 cm in the upper, middle, and lower third of the abdominal wall, respectively, of the bilateral rectus muscles and their associated anterior fascia (6, 10, and 6 cm bilaterally) (**Table 1**).

If medialization of then anterior fascia is still not possible, the external oblique aponeurosis is divided 1 to 2 cm lateral to the linea semilunaris and separated from the underlying internal oblique (IO) muscle. This combined with the posterior rectus sheath division, this allows for 5, 10, and 3 cm of advancement, respectively, in each third of the abdominal wall, totaling 10, 20, and 6 cm of bilateral advancement for an anterior component separation (see **Table 1**).[11] It should be emphasized that mesh can be placed in the retromuscular, intraperitoneal, or onlay positions following an anterior component separation.

Ramirez's operation was initially referred to as a "components separation," however, has since been designated as "anterior component separation" following the initiation of posterior releases. Newer techniques of separating the posterior rectus sheath and transversus abdominis (TA) from the anterior IO, EO, and rectus muscle bodies had been termed a "posterior component separation."

Open Posterior Component Separation

In a posterior component separation, the posterior elements are disconnected from anterior abdominal wall, allowing anterior fascial advancement. The posterior fascial advancement is achieved by dividing the posterior lamella of the IO followed by TAR. The TAR allows for significant posterior fascial advancement greater than 20 cm to create a large visceral sac and retromuscular pocket.

Operative steps include medial division of the posterior rectus sheath and subsequent dissection of the retrorectus space laterally toward the linea semilunaris where the perforating neurovascular bundles are seen; this retrorectus dissection is usually referred to as a "Rives-Stoppa" repair.[15] If further myofascial release is required for posterior rectus sheath closure, the posterior lamella of the IO is divided followed by the TA muscle, which both relieve tension on the posterior fascia. After division of the TA, this dissection is continued laterally into the preperitoneal space and can proceed as far as the medial boarder of the psoas muscle (**Fig. 2**). The posterior rectus sheath is then closed followed by mesh placement in the newly created retromuscular/preperitoneal pocket. The anterior fascia is closed over top of the mesh (**Fig. 3**).

Each of these operative steps offers consistent medial advancement of the anterior and posterior layers. To assess the relative effectiveness of a posterior component separation regarding fascial advancement, quantitative tension changes on the anterior and posterior fascia have been measured in a prospective observational study.[16] This study reported tension in the abdominal wall using a tensiometer after serial release of each component. For the anterior fascia, they found that posterior sheath incision and retrorectus dissection contributed to −82% reduced tension while incision of the posterior lamella of the IO and TAR contributed −18% to tension reduction. For the posterior fascia, the retrorectus dissection contributed only −3%, whereas incision of the posterior lamella of the IO and TAR reduced tension by −53% and −38% from baseline, respectively (see **Table 1**). A posterior rectus sheath closure with minimal tension is important to prevent posterior rectus sheath breakdown, which

Table 1
Component separation advancement and alleviation of tension

	Ramirez Anterior Component Separation		Posterior Component Separation with Transversus Abdominis Release			
	Retrorectus Dissection	External Oblique Division	Retrorectus Dissection	Division of Posterior Lamella of Internal Oblique	Transversus Abdominis Division	Retromuscular Dissection
Maximum unilateral anterior advancement						
Superior 1/3	3 cm	5 cm	4.1 cm	4.2 cm	4.5 cm	5.5 cm
Middle 1/3	5 cm	10 cm	5.9 cm	6.1 cm	6.6 cm	7.9 cm
Inferior 1/3	3 cm	3 cm	7.6 cm	8.0 cm	8.6 cm	9.9 cm
Maximum unilateral posterior advancement						
Superior 1/3	NA	NA	4.4 cm	4.6 cm	5.3 cm	6.9 cm
Middle 1/3			6.2 cm	6.6 cm	7.5 cm	9.6 cm
Inferior 1/3			7.5 cm	7.5 cm	9.5 cm	11.2 cm
Changes in midline tension						
Anterior fascia	NA	NA	−82%	−18%	0%	NA
Posterior fascia			−3%	−53%	−38%	

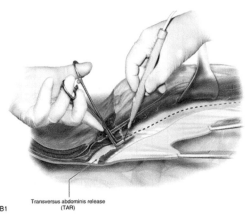

Transversus abdominis release
(TAR)

B1

Fig. 2. Transversus abdominis release. (With permission from Joe Chovan.)

can lead to either intraparietal herniation and associated bowel obstruction, or occult exposure of the retromuscular mesh to the underlying viscera.[17]

Cadaveric studies measuring the amount of fascial advancement after each release further support the tension theory.[18] For the anterior fascia, the retrorectus dissection achieved 7.6 cm of unilateral advancement, 8.0 cm after incision of the posterior lamella of the IO, 8.6 cm after TAR, and 9.9 cm after completion of the entire posterior

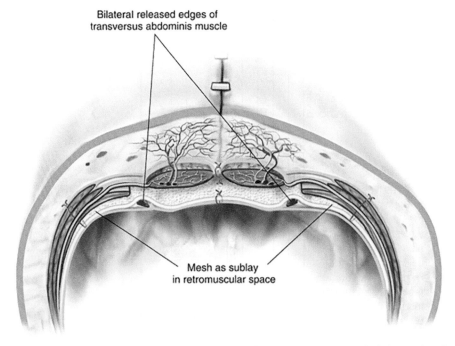

Bilateral released edges of
transversus abdominis muscle

Mesh as sublay
in retromuscular space

Fig. 3. Mesh placement following TAR. (*Reprinted from* Rosen MJ. Atlas of Abdominal Wall Reconstruction. Second ed. Philadelphia PA: Elsevier; 2017; with permission.)

component separation with TAR. Respective posterior sheath advancement was 7.5, 8.3, 9.5, and 11.2 cm after each corresponding step (see **Table 1**). These results are comparable to Ramirez's findings with anterior component separation.

Mesh Reinforcement

Although component separation alleviates tension on midline hernia repair, this alone is associated with early recurrence rates (within 1 year) as high as 53%.[19] Prosthetic reinforcement has become a mainstay and complementary to component separation. In modern abdominal wall reconstruction, mesh is critical for the durability of any hernia repair and contemporary descriptions of any component separation include some prosthetic reinforcement.

Mesh reinforcement in the setting of an anterior component separation has limitations for several reasons. Retrorectus mesh placement is often not possible for large defects because the posterior rectus sheaths are under too much tension for closure. The addition of concomitant posterior component separation to aid posterior sheath closure should not be combined with any anterior component separation at the same time. Wide overlap can be achieved by creating large subcutaneous skin flaps for onlay mesh; however, this comes at the cost of undermining the blood supply of the subcutaneous tissue and predisposing patients to soft tissue necrosis and associated wound morbidity. Minimizing skin flap dissection limits mesh overlap and is impractical. Finally, intraperitoneal mesh is most used during anterior component separation, and these barrier-coated synthetics or bio-prosthetics come at an additional cost.

In comparison to the anterior component separation, the posterior component separation with TAR allows for equivalent myofascial relaxation to approximate the midline. However the latter technique has gained such wide popularity in the field of abdominal wall reconstruction because of the ability to create a reproducible, well-vascularized, retromuscular pocket for mesh placement, all through a midline incision without the need for skin flaps.[20] Creation of this large visceral sac isolated from the peritoneal cavity allows for use of uncoated monofilament polypropylene mesh, which is inexpensive and resilient to infection.

PATIENT SELECTION

When deciding whether a patient requires a component separation, examining the width and length of the fascial defect is a good place to start. This can be measured preoperatively by physical examination or cross-sectional imaging (algorithm 1). In each width category, there are several options for repair and choice is usually based on surgeon experience and preference.

- Hernias less than 7 cm usually do not require a component separation. These can be repaired with either an open, minimally invasive approach with intraperitoneal mesh or a Rives-Stoppa type of with retrorectus mesh. A Rives-Stoppa retrorectus repair can be carried out transabdominally and totally extraperitoneal for hernias less than 7 cm wide.[21] These hernias can also be repaired with onlay mesh using open techniques.
- Hernias 7 to 10 cm may or may not require a component separation for midline fascial approximation. These hernias can be repaired minimally invasively with fascial closure followed by a large piece of intraperitoneal mesh. They can also be repaired with an open retromuscular approach. An open or robotic TAR can be added to achieve posterior rectus sheath closure if necessary. Carbonell proposed that a rectus width to hernia width ratio greater than 2 reliably predicts the ability to reapproximate the fascia with a Rives-Stoppa retromuscular dissection

alone without the need for further myofascial release.[22] Carbonell equation: $2 \times$ RW:DW $\leq$ 2:1 (RW: rectus width, DW: defect width).

- Hernias greater than 10 cm may require either an anterior or posterior component separation for both rectus approximation (midline closure) and posterior fascial approximation depending on abdominal wall compliance. This can be accomplished with either open anterior component separation or open or robotic posterior component separation with TAR.

When dealing with emergency ventral hernias, such as obstruction leading to strangulation and open abdomens, component separation techniques should be avoided. The use of these techniques to achieve fascial closure after an abdominal catastrophe when patients are in a catabolic state is feasible but met with high failure rates. Maintaining native abdominal wall planes leaves reconstruction options for the future when patients have recovered. During emergency operations, our proffered closure techniques include primary closure with interrupted figure-of-eight sutures or bridging the fascial defect with an absorbable prosthetic, such as Vicryl mesh (**Fig. 4**).

PREOPERATIVE ADJUNCTS

In patients with large, loss-of-domain hernias, preoperative adjuncts including botulinum toxin injection or tissue expansion have been used to facilitate fascial and/or abdominal wall closure. Tanaka and colleagues previously published a method using cross-sectional imaging for calculating the hernia sac to abdominal cavity volume ratio (VR). A ratio of less than 25% is thought to be predictive of the loss of abdominal domain. However, there remains of void of evidence supporting the routine use of preoperative adjuncts in abdominal wall reconstruction, especially progressive pneumoperitoneum with its associated severe complications.[23]

Botulinum Toxin

Botulinum neurotoxin type A (BoNT-A) is used in "chemical component separation" or "chemical component paralysis."[24] The BoNT-A is injected preoperatively to

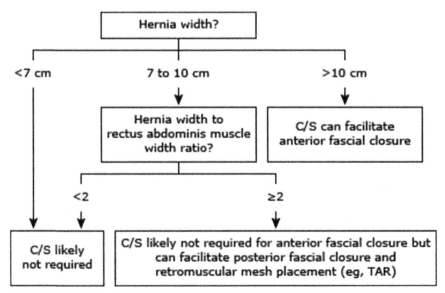

Fig. 4. Determining the need for component separation in ventral hernia repair.

temporarily paralyze the lateral abdominal wall muscles leading to lengthening of these muscles. The ultimate goal is to reduce tension on midline abdominal wall closure and possibly prevent the need of dividing these muscles during repair.

Currently, there is no consensus on which patients would benefit from BoNT-A injections before ventral hernia repair. Many authors have cited Tanaka and colleagues' hernia volume to peritoneal VR greater than 20% to 25%[25] as an indication to consider the use of preoperative BoNT-A [36].

A typical protocol for BoNT-A injection involves three to five injections per side of the abdominal wall, as described below.[26]

- Injections should be given under conscious sedation to minimize patient discomfort.
- Three hundred units of BoNT-A are reconstituted in 150 cc of injectable 0.9% sodium chloride solution (final concentration of 2 units/cc).
- Two syringes are labeled and loaded onto a three-way stopcock: one with the BoNT-A solution and the other with injectable saline. This stopcock is attached to an extension tubing secured to an 18-gauge spinal needle.
- Ultrasound is used to identify the three muscle bellies of the lateral abdominal wall (EO, IO, and TA) at three sites: subcostal, anterior axillary line, and lower quadrant.
- Using ultrasound guidance, the spinal needle is first advanced into the TA muscle belly at each of the three sites. Sterile saline is injected to confirm needle location. Then, 8.3 cc (16.6 units) of BoNT-A is injected into the TA muscle belly.
- The needle is then withdrawn into the IO followed by the EO muscle, injecting a total of 25 cc (50 units) of BoNT-A at each site in each location.
- The same sequence is repeated at each of the six sites.
- Given that it takes 2 weeks for BoNT-A to achieve its maximal effect, injections should be done at least 2 weeks before ventral hernia repair.

There have been systematic reviews and meta-analyses showing BoNT-A pretreatment before ventral hernia repair decreased the width of the abdominal wall defect by approximately 3.5 cm, decreased the thickness of the lateral abdominal wall muscles and increased the length of the abdominal wall by 3.2 cm on either side, for a total of 6.3 cm elongation.[27–29] These studies have also shown an overall increase in peritoneal volume. However, these radiographic changes have not translated into downstaging hernia repair techniques such as reduced need for component separation.[28,30] A propensity score-matched study of 145 patients with an average hernia width of 14.1 cm found that preoperative BoNT-A resulted in a higher percentage of fascial closure (92% vs 81%); however, these patients also received more components separation with preoperative BoNT (61% vs 47%).[31] This would suggest that BoNT-A is an insufficient technique to downstage these large hernias from needing a component separation.

Tissue expanders

When repairing massive ventral hernias, it is important to distinguish whether the defect in the abdominal wall is due to myofascial versus skin/subcutaneous tissue deficiency. Although myofascial defects are typically reconstructed using components separation, skin/subcutaneous defects can be repaired by tissue expansion. Generally, these patients have a concern for loss of domain with soft tissue loss from traumatic injury, soft tissue infection, oncologic resections, or a prior open abdomen. In pediatrics, these scenarios are seen in the setting of gastroschisis and omphalocele.

Tissue expansion is used to expand the local tissue in preparation for a local reconstruction. The process involves placement of a silicone balloon under the subcutaneous tissue or fascia followed by inflation the balloon with serial injections of saline.[32] This ultimately provides well-vascularized skin, subcutaneous tissue, and/or abdominal fascia which can be used to repair large ventral defects.

Tissue expanders are usually placed adjacent to the long axis of the defect and can be inserted in two different planes.

- Expanders can be placed between the subcutaneous tissue and the abdominal wall muscles, and this placement is more common in context of an abdominal wall reconstruction where the component separation is providing sufficient myofascial advancement. The tissue expansion assures that the patient has sufficient soft tissue for wound closure at the end of a case.
- Alternatively, expanders can be placed between the lateral abdominal wall muscles (IO/EO or IO/TA), which is less commonly used as this results in bidirectional expansion and is less effective expansion of the skin and subcutaneous tissue.[33] This placement can also result in unnecessary increased intraperitoneal pressure.

When possible, the balloon implant should match the length of the wound. Incisions are incorporated into one margin of the eventual flap or should be planned perpendicular to the line of expansion to prevent dehiscence. Expansion of the device can begin at the time of implantation or 1 to 3 weeks later, providing sufficient tension for expansion without compromising perfusion or the integrity of the wound through which it was placed. Typically, the devices are injected weekly for 6 to 12 weeks and should be continued until the expanded flap is approximately 20% larger than the size of the defect.

Tissue expansion techniques are not without complications and morbidity. These devices require surgery to place and careful management of expansion while awaiting definitive reconstruction. They should be placed at least 6 to 12 weeks before ventral hernia repair. Complications including device infections, flap ischemia, patient intolerance/pain, and scar widening can occur in 15% of patients.[34]

COMPLICATIONS
Wound Morbidity

Open anterior component separation is associated with wound morbidities in as many as 50% of patients due to the need to create wide subcutaneous skin flaps. These flaps disrupt the perforators from the deep superior and inferior epigastric arteries that supply the central abdominal skin. These patients are at risk of flap necrosis and surgical site infections.[35] Alternatives to traditional open anterior component separation including perforator preservation and endoscopic-assisted techniques have been shown to have a much lower rate of wound complications ranging from 2% to 14%.[36-38]

The overall wound morbidity rates of anterior and posterior component separation techniques are comparable.[35,39] However, posterior component separation eliminates the need for subcutaneous skin flap dissection thus reducing the risk of skin flap necrosis.

Risk factors for wound morbidity and mesh complications include.[40]

- Patient factors such as body mass index, poorly controlled diabetes, and a history of previous surgical site infection.
- Hernia factors including size of the fascial defect and wound class.
- Technical factors related to the surgical approach including open versus minimally invasive as well as mesh type and location.

Pulmonary Complications

Following repair of a massive ventral hernia with the loss of domain, there is the potential for development of postoperative intra-abdominal hypertension/abdominal compartment syndrome. In the setting of elective abdominal wall reconstruction, this commonly manifests as postoperative respiratory complications requiring reintubation and/or transfer to the intensive care unit (ICU). Changes in plateau pressure (PP) after fascial reconstruction during ventral hernia repair have been shown to directly correlate with postoperative respiratory complications (increase in PP $\geq$ 6 mm Hg, odds ratio [OR] 8.67; increase in PP $\geq$ 9 mm Hg, OR 11.5).[41]

For patients who have undergone repair of a massive ventral hernia with a tight abdominal wall closure, the PP should be measured before and after closure of the anterior fascia. This measurement is taken by anesthesia. Recommendations regarding extubation are as follows.

- An increase in PP of less than 6 mm Hg can be safely extubated.
- PP increase of $\geq$6 mm Hg in a young patient but with no pulmonary disease or concern from anesthesia staff is extubated and monitored in the ICU overnight.
- PP increase of $\geq$6 mm Hg with concern for pulmonary compromise (old age, underlying lung disease, or obstructive sleep apnea) will typically remain intubated until they're airway pressures decrease and are deemed ready to extubated by ICU staff.
- PP increase of $\geq$9 mm Hg will remain intubated and paralytics should be considered to help counteract this transient abdominal hypertension, especially if there is difficulty ventilating the patient or decreased urine output that is not due to hypovolemia. Note that bladder pressure measurements are not useful in this setting.

Abdominal compliance improves within 12 to 24 hours, provided myofascial release was performed. Hence, elevations in intra-abdominal pressure after ventral hernia repair are usually transient and can be expected to resolve within 48 hours.[42]

It is important to recognize that patients undergoing elective hernia repair with a myofascial release that results in transient intra-abdominal hypertension/abdominal compartment syndrome are very different from those with traditionally encountered abdominal compartment syndrome following acute abdominal catastrophes. The World Society of the Abdominal Compartment Syndrome has recognized these reconstructions in the elective setting as unique situations that are fundamentally different from critically ill patients.[43]

Linea Semilunaris Injury

Full-thickness transection of the linea semilunaris results in separation of the medial rectus muscle from the lateral oblique muscles.[44] This can occur during the TAR dissection with failure to recognize the linea semilunaris just lateral to the perforating neurovascular bundles. It can also occur from inappropriate posteromedial dissection during an anterior component separation. Following transection, patients usually present with a lateral bulge a few months after their hernia repair. Bilateral linea semilunaris injuries result in a "floating" rectus muscle and are commonly referred to a "Mickey Mouse" hernia defect on cross-sectional imaging (**Fig. 5**).

The incidence of this complications is currently unknown; however, it is typically only encountered by inexperienced surgeons during open or robotic TAR when care is not taken to respect myofascial boundaries.[45] This iatrogenic hernia can be repaired using posterior component separation with TAR.

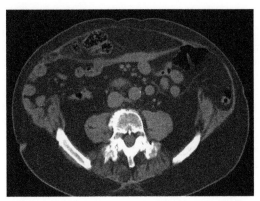

Fig. 5. Axial cross-section demonstrating bilateral linea semilunaris injuries result in a "Mickey Mouse" hernia defect.

SUMMARY AND RECOMMENDATIONS

- In modern abdominal wall reconstruction, component separation serves two purposes: to alleviate tension on midline fascial approximation and to create a large retromuscular pocket to accommodate mesh.
- Component separation can be performed with either anterior or posterior techniques, both of which allow approximately 20 cm of maximum bilateral rectus advancement. In addition, TAR allows for greater than 20 cm of posterior fascial advancement, creating a large retromuscular pocket allowing wide mesh overlap. It should be emphasized that anterior and posterior component separations should not be performed concomitantly due to the risk of destabilizing the anterior abdominal wall.
- Hernia width determined preoperatively by physical examination or cross-sectional imaging typically guides decision-making regarding component separation (algorithm 1):
- Hernias less than 7 cm wide can typically do not require component separation.
- Hernias 7 to 10 cm wide, the decision to use component separation can be predicted when the width of the hernia is greater than twice the width of the rectus muscle. Although such hernias can usually be repaired without component separation, a TAR may be performed to achieve posterior rectus fascia closure following a retromuscular approach.
- Hernias greater than 10 cm wide, usually require repair with component separation. However, component separation may not be necessary for patients with good abdominal wall compliance.
- Preoperative botulinum toxin injection has been used to facilitate fascial closure when the hernia volume to peritoneal VR is greater than 20% to 25%. Tissue expansion can be used to facilitate soft tissue coverage. However, there is a lack of consensus regarding the routine use of preoperative adjuncts in abdominal wall reconstruction.
- Open anterior component separation is associated with high rates of skin flap necrosis and wound infections. However, the wound complication rates of comparable anterior and posterior component separation techniques are similar.
- Postoperative respiratory failure requiring reintubation can be a manifestation of intra-abdominal hypertension/transient abdominal compartment syndrome after

large or complex ventral hernia repair. A change in PP of greater than 6 mm Hg after fascial closure is an indication to leave the patient intubated at the end of surgery. Abdominal wall compliance improves in 12 to 24 hours with resolution of this transient intra-abdominal hypertension in 48 hours.

- Full-thickness injury of the linea semilunaris is a technical complication that causes separation of the medial rectus muscle from the lateral oblique muscles resulting in "Mickey mouse" defects. To avoid this, the surgeon should understand the relevant anatomy and obey myofascial boundaries.

CLINICS CARE POINTS

- When deciding whether a patient requires a component separation, the width and length of the fascial defect should be taken into consideration as well as the abdominal wall compliance.
- Surgeons operating on hernias greater than 10 cm should be prepared to perform a component separation for midline reapproximation.
- The use of preoperative adjuncts, including Botox, should be considered experimental.
- Anterior component separation should be avoided in patients at increased risk of wound morbidity.
- Posterior component separation with TAR should be considered for complex hernias given its ability to provide both facial medialization and wide retromuscular mesh overlap.
- When dealing with emergency ventral hernias, such as obstruction leading to strangulation and open abdomens, component separation techniques should be avoided.

REFERENCES

1. Fischer JP, Basta MN, Mirzabeigi MN, et al. A Risk Model and Cost Analysis of Incisional Hernia After Elective, Abdominal Surgery Based Upon 12,373 Cases: The Case for Targeted Prophylactic Intervention. Ann Surg 2016;263(5):1010-7.
2. Poulose BK, Beck WC, Phillips SE, et al. The chosen few: disproportionate resource use in ventral hernia repair. Am Surg 2013;79(8):815-8.
3. Schlosser KA, Renshaw SM, Tamer RM, et al. Ventral hernia repair: an increasing burden affecting abdominal core health. Hernia 2023;27(2):415-21.
4. Flum DR, Horvath K, Koepsell T. Have outcomes of incisional hernia repair improved with time? A population-based analysis. Ann Surg 2003;237(1):129-35.
5. Criss CN, Petro CC, Krpata DM, et al. Functional abdominal wall reconstruction improves core physiology and quality-of-life. Surgery 2014;156(1):176-82.
6. Gibson CL. OPERATION FOR CURE OF LARGE VENTRAL HERNIA. Ann Surg 1920;72(2):214-7.
7. Köckerling F. What Do We Know About the Chevrel Technique in Ventral Incisional Hernia Repair? Front Surg 2019;6:15.
8. Chevrel JP. [The treatment of large midline incisional hernias by "overcoat" plasty and prothesis (author's transl)]. Nouv Presse Med 1979;8(9):695-6.
9. Williams JK, Carlson GW, deChalain T, et al. Role of tensor fasciae latae in abdominal wall reconstruction. Plast Reconstr Surg 1998;101(3):713-8.
10. Williams JK, Carlson GW, Howell RL, et al. The tensor fascia lata free flap in abdominal-wall reconstruction. J Reconstr Microsurg 1997;13(2):83-90, discussion 90-91.

11. Ramirez OM, Ruas E, Dellon AL. Components separation" method for closure of abdominal-wall defects: an anatomic and clinical study. Plast Reconstr Surg 1990;86(3):519–26.

12. Haskins IN, Prabhu AS, Jensen KK, et al. Effect of transversus abdominis release on core stability: Short-term results from a single institution. Surgery 2019;165(2): 412–6.

13. Licari L, Guercio G, Campanella S, et al. Clinical and Functional Outcome After Abdominal Wall Incisional Hernia Repair: Evaluation of Quality-of-Life Improvement and Comparison of Assessment Scales. World J Surg 2019;43(8):1914–20.

14. Novitsky YW, Elliott HL, Orenstein SB, et al. Transversus abdominis muscle release: a novel approach to posterior component separation during complex abdominal wall reconstruction. Am J Surg 2012;204(5):709–16.

15. den Hartog FPJ, Sneiders D, Darwish EF, et al. Favorable Outcomes After Retro-Rectus (Rives-Stoppa) Mesh Repair as Treatment for Noncomplex Ventral Abdominal Wall Hernia, a Systematic Review and Meta-analysis. Ann Surg 2022;276(1):55–65.

16. Benjamin Miller, Ryan Ellis, Clayton Petro, David Krpata, Ajita Prabhu, Lucas Befffa, et al. Transversus abdominis release does not provide anterior fascial advancement: an observational study of the quantitative tension of the abdominal wall during discrete steps of posterior component separation.

17. Carbonell AM. Interparietal hernias after open retromuscular hernia repair. Hernia J Hernias Abdom Wall Surg 2008;12(6):663–6.

18. Majumder A, Miller HJ, Del Campo LM, et al. Assessment of myofascial medialization following posterior component separation via transversus abdominis muscle release in a cadaveric model. Hernia J Hernias Abdom Wall Surg 2018;22(4): 637–44.

19. de Vries Reilingh TS, van Geldere D, Langenhorst B, et al. Repair of large midline incisional hernias with polypropylene mesh: comparison of three operative techniques. Hernia J Hernias Abdom Wall Surg 2004;8(1):56–9.

20. Zolin SJ, Fafaj A, Krpata DM. Transversus abdominis release (TAR): what are the real indications and where is the limit? Hernia J Hernias Abdom Wall Surg 2020; 24(2):333–40.

21. Santos DA, Limmer AR, Gibson HM, et al. The current state of robotic retromuscular repairs-a qualitative review of the literature. Surg Endosc 2021;35(1): 456–66.

22. Love MW, Warren JA, Davis S, et al. Computed tomography imaging in ventral hernia repair: can we predict the need for myofascial release? Hernia J Hernias Abdom Wall Surg 2021;25(2):471–7.

23. van Rooijen MMJ, Yurtkap Y, Allaeys M, et al. Fascial closure in giant ventral hernias after preoperative botulinum toxin a and progressive pneumoperitoneum: A systematic review and meta-analysis. Surgery 2021;170(3):769–76.

24. Ibarra-Hurtado TR, Nuño-Guzmán CM, Echeagaray-Herrera JE, et al. Use of botulinum toxin type a before abdominal wall hernia reconstruction. World J Surg 2009;33(12):2553–6.

25. Tanaka EY, Yoo JH, Rodrigues AJ, et al. A computerized tomography scan method for calculating the hernia sac and abdominal cavity volume in complex large incisional hernia with loss of domain. Hernia 2010;14(1):63–9.

26. Zendejas B, Khasawneh MA, Srvantstyan B, et al. Outcomes of chemical component paralysis using botulinum toxin for incisional hernia repairs. World J Surg 2013;37(12):2830–7.

27. Timmer AS, Claessen JJM, Atema JJ, et al. A systematic review and meta-analysis of technical aspects and clinical outcomes of botulinum toxin prior to abdominal wall reconstruction. Hernia 2021;25(6):1413–25.

28. Wegdam JA, de Vries Reilingh TS, Bouvy ND, et al. Prehabilitation of complex ventral hernia patients with Botulinum: a systematic review of the quantifiable effects of Botulinum. Hernia J Hernias Abdom Wall Surg 2021;25(6):1427–42.

29. Elstner KE, Read JW, Saunders J, et al. Selective muscle botulinum toxin A component paralysis in complex ventral hernia repair. Hernia J Hernias Abdom Wall Surg 2020;24(2):287–93.

30. Horne CM, Augenstein V, Malcher F, et al. Understanding the benefits of botulinum toxin A: retrospective analysis of the Abdominal Core Health Quality Collaborative. Br J Surg 2021;108(2):112–4.

31. Deerenberg EB, Shao JM, Elhage SA, et al. Preoperative botulinum toxin A injection in complex abdominal wall reconstruction- a propensity-scored matched study. Am J Surg 2021;222(3):638–42.

32. Althubaiti G, Butler CE. Abdominal wall and chest wall reconstruction. Plast Reconstr Surg 2014;133(5):688e–701e.

33. Novitsky YW, Chmielewski L, Lee M, et al. Tissue expansion during abdominal wall reconstruction. In: Novitsky YW, editor. Hernia surgery: current principles. Springer; 2016. p. 307.

34. Paletta CE, Huang DB, Dehghan K, et al. The use of tissue expanders in staged abdominal wall reconstruction. Ann Plast Surg 1999;42(3):259–65.

35. Krpata DM, Blatnik JA, Novitsky YW, et al. Posterior and open anterior components separations: a comparative analysis. Am J Surg 2012;203(3):318–22, discussion 322.

36. Saulis AS, Dumanian GA. Periumbilical rectus abdominis perforator preservation significantly reduces superficial wound complications in "separation of parts" hernia repairs. Plast Reconstr Surg 2002;109(7):2275–80, discussion 2281-2282.

37. Ghali S, Turza KC, Baumann DP, et al. Minimally invasive component separation results in fewer wound-healing complications than open component separation for large ventral hernia repairs. J Am Coll Surg 2012;214(6):981–9.

38. Jensen KK, Henriksen NA, Jorgensen LN. Endoscopic component separation for ventral hernia causes fewer wound complications compared to open components separation: a systematic review and meta-analysis. Surg Endosc 2014;28(11):3046–52.

39. Hodgkinson JD, Leo CA, Maeda Y, et al. A meta-analysis comparing open anterior component separation with posterior component separation and transversus abdominis release in the repair of midline ventral hernias. Hernia J Hernias Abdom Wall Surg 2018;22(4):617–26.

40. Petro CC, O'Rourke CP, Posielski NM, et al. Designing a ventral hernia staging system. Hernia J Hernias Abdom Wall Surg 2016;20(1):111–7.

41. Blatnik JA, Krpata DM, Pesa NL, et al. Predicting severe postoperative respiratory complications following abdominal wall reconstruction. Plast Reconstr Surg 2012;130(4):836–41.

42. Petro CC, Raigani S, Fayezizadeh M, et al. Permissible Intraabdominal Hypertension following Complex Abdominal Wall Reconstruction. Plast Reconstr Surg 2015;136(4):868–81.

43. Kirkpatrick AW, Nickerson D, Roberts DJ, et al. Intra-Abdominal Hypertension and Abdominal Compartment Syndrome after Abdominal Wall Reconstruction: Quaternary Syndromes? Scand J Surg 2017;106(2):97–106.

44. Pauli EM, Wang J, Petro CC, et al. Posterior component separation with transversus abdominis release successfully addresses recurrent ventral hernias following anterior component separation. Hernia J Hernias Abdom Wall Surg 2015;19(2): 285–91.

45. Pauli EM, Juza RM. Managing complications of open hernia repair. In: Novitsky YW, editor. Hernia surgery: current principles. Berlin, Germany: Springer; 2016. p. 207.

The Role of Robotics in Abdominal Wall Reconstruction

Sara Maskal, MD[a], Lucas Beffa, MD[b],*

KEYWORDS

- Robotic • Hernia • TAR • Mesh • Repair

KEY POINTS

- Robotic abdominal wall reconstruction is an exciting and new approach to complex hernia repairs.
- The increased cost and time associated with this new approach needs to be offset with clinical benefit to the patient.
- Current high-quality clinical evidence to support the use of robotic abdominal wall reconstruction is critically lacking; however, several small retrospective series demonstrate favorable outcomes.

INTRODUCTION

Although an open surgical approach to abdominal wall reconstruction (AWR) has traditionally been used for large, complex ventral hernia repair, the robotic platform is increasing in popularity and challenging that paradigm. During the last decade, there has been a rapid uptake of robotic surgical techniques, with particularly high assimilation in the field of hernia repair despite a scarcity of high-level evidence.[1] Here we present a review of the technique of robotic AWR and the current state of evidence.

NATURE OF THE PROBLEM

Techniques in ventral hernia repairs have evolved during the past several decades. For complex ventral hernias requiring AWR, there is substantial evidence for durable repair utilizing placement of mesh in the retromuscular position with transversus abdominis release (TAR).[2,3] As surgical technology advances, general surgeons are increasingly utilizing minimally invasive approaches for many operations.[4,5] Although laparoscopy

[a] Cleveland Clinic Foundation, 9500 Euclid Avenue, Cleveland, OH 44195, USA; [b] Lerner College of Medicine, Cleveland Clinic Foundation, 9500 Euclid Avenue, Cleveland, OH 44195, USA
* Corresponding author.
E-mail address: BeffaL@ccf.org
Twitter: @BeffaLukeMD (L.B.)

Surg Clin N Am 103 (2023) 977–991
https://doi.org/10.1016/j.suc.2023.04.007
0039-6109/23/© 2023 Elsevier Inc. All rights reserved.

is routinely used in ventral hernia repairs, its uptake in more complex AWR has been limited by ergonomic challenges in accessing the retromuscular plane and suturing intracorporeally, leaving open repairs as the only feasible approach for repairing large defects.[6,7] However, the robotic platform has changed the landscape of AWR by offering a new technology that enables AWR to take place via a minimally invasive approach.

Between 2010 and 2017, the estimated annual robotic cases for general surgeons increased from 10,000 to 246,000.[8] For ventral hernia repairs specifically, the use of robotic surgery increased by a 44.8- fold difference between 2012 and 2018.[1,9,10] Although proponents of robotic surgery in general emphasize the benefits of a minimally invasive approach and the perceived ergonomic benefits of the robotic console, critics cite concern for increased costs, operating room time, and lack of clear benefit over existing techniques.[10,11] Despite a lack of high-quality evidence, it is clearly an area of growing interest, yet the question remains as to the clinical benefit.

ANATOMY

The same fundamental anatomy of open surgery applies to robotic AWR. The boundaries of the abdominal wall comprise the costal margin, xyphoid process of the sternum, the pubic symphysis, inguinal ligament, and iliac crest. The paired rectus abdominis muscles are separated by the linea alba in the midline, bounded by the semilunar line laterally and originate from the pubic symphysis and pubic crest and insert on the costal margin. The lateral abdominal wall comprises 3 layered muscles from superficial to deep: the external abdominal oblique, internal abdominal oblique, and the transversus abdominis. Below the arcuate line, the external abdominal oblique, internal abdominal oblique, and the transversus abdominis muscle aponeuroses fuse medially to form the anterior rectus sheath. Above the arcuate line, the aponeurosis of the internal abdominal oblique splits to contribute to both the anterior and posterior rectus sheath (PRS). The posterior lamella of the internal abdominal oblique overlies the transversus abdominis muscle above the arcuate line and deep to that is the transversalis fascia followed by the peritoneum. The pretransversalis or preperitoneal planes can be followed superiorly to the costal margin and inferiorly to the space of Retzius.

The blood supply to the anterior abdominal wall can be divided into 3 zones: (1) zone I in the upper, central abdomen is supplied by the superior and deep inferior epigastric arteries, (2) zone II is the lower abdominal wall and receives blood supply from the epigastric arcade, superficial inferior epigastric, superficial external pudendal, and superficial circumflex iliac arteries as well as perforators from the deep circumflex iliac arteries, and (3) zone III is lateral to the semilunar line and receives blood from the musculophrenic, intercostal, and lumbar arteries.[12]

The sensory and motor innervation of the anterior abdominal wall derives from T7 to L1 spinal levels as well as the ilioinguinal and iliohypogastric nerves. Just medial to the semilunar line, there are perforating neurovascular bundles, which are composed of anterior branches of thoracoabdominal nerves T7 to T12 and associated vessels, which must be preserved during retrorectus dissection to avoid abdominal wall denervation.

Figs. 1–4 represent important anatomical landmarks during robotic TAR.

PREOPERATIVE PLANNING

Preoperative optimization has been a debated in hernia surgery for many years. Too often risk factors and comorbidities are used to deny hernia repairs to patients who fall outside strict and often arbitrary benchmarks. This delays care and places patients

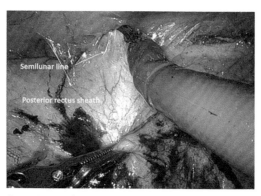

Fig. 1. Retrorectus dissection to the semilunar line.

at risk for incarceration, obstructions, and decrease in quality of life simply for fear of postoperative complications. It is the authors' opinion that the pendulum has swung too far with this preoperative comorbidity optimization and that high-quality data need to be provided before any strong recommendations in this area. This section will focus on 3 preoperative conditions that are modifiable and commonly cited as barrier to hernia repairs: weight, smoking, and diabetes.

Weight

Body mass index (BMI) is cited as one of the most common preoperative relative contraindications for definitive hernia repair. Depending on the study, a "high" BMI can mean anyone more than 30 kg/m^2 or higher than 35 kg/m^2. BMI has been studied extensively as a risk factor for hernia recurrence as well as postoperative wound complications.[13–15] According to a recent analysis of the abdominal core health quality collaborative (ACHQC) evaluating hernia recurrence for those patients less than and those more than BMI 35, they found no difference in hernia recurrence. Additionally, a recent randomized trial where patient were randomized to preoperative weight loss before hernia or standard care, showed no difference in hernia recurrence with preoperative weight loss.[16]

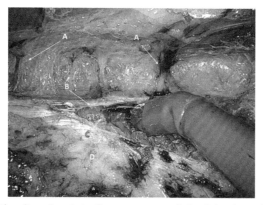

Fig. 2. A view of the dissection into the transversus abdominis plane showing (A) perforating neurovascular bundles, (B) the cut edge of the posterior lamella of the internal oblique, (C) transversus abdominis muscle, and (D) PRS.

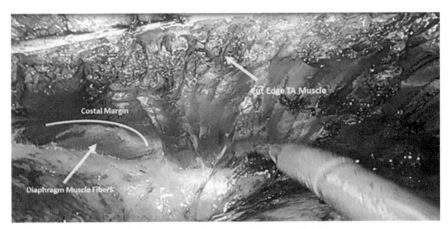

Fig. 3. Superior extent of the dissection in the pretransversalis plane.

Diabetes

Patients with diabetes that is well controlled seem to have similar outcomes to those patients without diabetes. Concerning hernia surgery, it has previously been proposed that patients should delay open complex AWR until a Hgb A1C of less than 8, or even some with less than 6.5, is achieved.[15,17] However, there are several more recent studies that have scrutinized this practice, showing that it may not be as important as previously thought.[18]

Smoking

For patients' overall health, it is always recommended for smoking cessation. Yet, the question remains if active smoking before hernia repair increases postoperative complications. Earlier studies have indicated that active smoking within 12 months of surgery increases postoperative complications after elective hernia repair.[19,20] However, these only show an increase in absolute risk by about 1% to 2% for most complications. There are other large hernia-specific studies that have shown no difference in surgical site occurrences requiring procedural intervention (SSOPI) or surgical site infections (SSI) with active smokers after propensity score matching.[21]

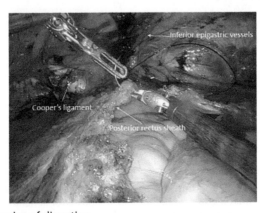

Fig. 4. Inferior margins of dissection.

In summary, the authors advocate for an educated discussion between patient and surgeon surrounding each individual's postoperative risk.

PREOP AND PATIENT POSITIONING

Planning and patient positioning the day of surgery is key to a successful surgery in robotic AWR, including room preparation. Given the relative novelty of robotics in AWR, there is often a knowledge gap, which exists around the procedure and the operating room support staff, thus communicating with those individuals before the case is key. The following are general tips.

- Ensure the proper equipment is available for the case, even if unclear if it will be used
- Positioning of the bed, monitors, and robotic cart within the room
- Robotic instruments available, including specialized instruments (stapler, staple loads, ultrasonic shears, and so forth)
- Drape robotic arms before induction of anesthesia and cover with a sterile gown
- Discuss potential for conversion to laparoscopy or open procedure

Patient Positioning

For midline abdominal wall defects between the semilunar lines.

- Supine with bed flexed at the hips (**Fig. 5**)
- Both arms out on arm boards at 90°. Alternative, arms can be tucked at the patient's side if hernia is located at the subxiphoid or suprapubic location
- Place foley catheter
- Padding over the patients face to protect against robotic arm trauma

For flank and lateral abdominal wall defects.

- Lateral decubitus position with use of axillary roll, arm board, and bean bag, or other appropriate position device
- Bed is flexed at the hips, which opens the angle between the costal margin and the anterior superior iliac spine (**Figs. 6** and **7**)
- Place foley catheter

PROCEDURE APPROACH

These approaches will be broken into 2 main categories. The first being trans-abdominal approaches or those procedure where you intentionally enter in the

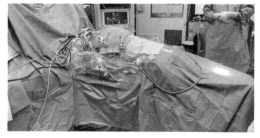

Fig. 5. Patient position with arms out and bed flexed for robotic AWR.

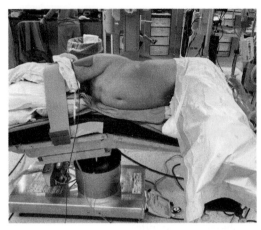

Fig. 6. Patient position for a lateral hernia defect with bed flexed in the lateral decubitus position.

peritoneal cavity. The second being totally extraperitoneal approaches, where the hernia repair is completed without intentionally entering the peritoneal cavity.

I. Transabdominal approaches
  a. Single-dock Rives-Stoppa
    i. Entry is gained in the upper abdomen through a visiport or cut down technique depending on surgeon's preference
    ii. Three robotic ports are placed lateral to the rectus muscle
    iii. Adhesiolysis is completed and hernias reduced. The ipsilateral PRS is incised 5 cm lateral to the ipsilateral edge of the defect
    iv. The PRS is taken off the rectus muscle with cautery and blunt dissection, and this plane is carried to the midline, including at least 8 cm caudad and cephalad to the defect
    v. The PRS is then incised posterior to the linea alba, keeping the linea alba intact anteriorly, and the preperitoneal plane is entered at the midline

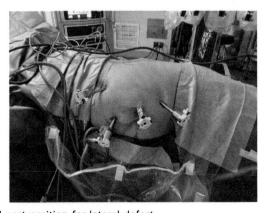

Fig. 7. Patent and port position for lateral defect.

     vi. The peritoneum is swept off the linea alba along the length of the midline dissection, including taking the hernia sac down with the peritoneum if possible

    vii. Preperitoneal dissection is taken to the contralateral PRS

   viii. The contralateral PRS is then incised along the length of entire dissection

    ix. Dissection is taken to the semilunar line on the opposite side of the abdomen as identified by the neurovascular bundles

     x. Anterior fascia is then closed with running barbed #1 slowly absorbable suture

    xi. Any holes in the posterior layer are then closed with a barbed absorbable suture

   xii. The retromuscular pocket is then measured, and an uncoated polypropylene synthetic mesh is selected, cut to the measured dimensions, and placed into the retromuscular pocket centering the mesh on the defect

  xiii. No fixation is necessary and drains are not needed

  xiv. The initial incision on the ipsilateral PRS is then closed with a 2 to 0 or 3 to 0 barbed absorbable suture

b. Double-dock TAR

     i. Entry is again gained in either the right or left upper abdomen through a visiport or cut down technique

    ii. Three robotic ports are placed on the same side of the abdomen as initial entry, exchanging the initial port for a robotic trocar

   iii. One port being adjacent to the costal margin, one being in the midabdomen approximately in line with the umbilicus, and one being lower abdomen lateral to the inferior epigastric vessels

   iv. Robot is docked and complete adhesiolysis is performed

    v. Dissection begins by incising the contralateral PRS along the length of the midline, at least 8 cm caudad and cephalad to the defect

   vi. The PRS is then taken off the rectus muscle with blunt dissection and cautery, carried out to the semilunar line identified by the neurovascular bundles

  vii. The TAR is started in the upper abdomen (can also be started in the lower abdomen) by incising the posterior lamella of the internal oblique approximately 1 cm medial to the perforators

  viii. The transversus abdominis (TA) muscle is then divided by "hooking" the muscle with the monopolar scissor, lifting up, and using cautery

   ix. This will then expose the pretransversalis or preperitoneal plane

    x. Keeping medial traction on the posterior sheath is vital to the development of the lateral plane, which is typically developed by bluntly sweeping the TA muscle anteriorly in a traction-countertraction principle

   xi. The TAR is completed by carrying this dissection under the costal margin cephalad and down to Coopers ligament caudad

   xii. The dissection is carried out lateral as far as possible, which typically goes beyond the midaxillary line

  xiii. Three additional robotic trocars are then placed into the contralateral abdominal wall to mirror the initial ports

  xiv. The defect is then measured intracorporally, and the length and width of the posterior flap is measured as well

   xv. An uncoated polypropylene mesh is then cut to the measured dimensions (doubling the measured width)

      xvi. The mesh is scrolled, leaving a 3-cm "tail" and the scroll is held together with an absorbable suture

      xvii. The mesh is then placed on the opposite side and positioned under the undocked ports

     xviii. The "tail" of the mesh is sutured to the abdominal wall with absorbable suture

      xix. The robot is undocked and the boom is rotated 180° (Xi system), or the patient bed is rotated 180° (Si system) and redocked to the opposite ports

      xx. An equal dissection takes place on the opposite abdominal wall

      xxi. Once the contralateral TAR is completed, the PRS is closed with running 2 to 0 barbed suture, including any holes in the peritoneum

     xxii. Anterior fascia is closed with a running #1 barbed slowly absorbable suture

    xxiii. Mesh is deployed by rolling it out from under the working ports

    xxiv. Drains placed against the mesh are optional

  c. Robotic transabdominal preperitoneal

      i. These work best for flank hernias but can be used in midline as well

      ii. The patient is positioned in lateral decubitus with the defect side up as outlined previously

     iii. Entry is gained through an open cut down or optical entry in the upper abdomen

     iv. Three robotic ports are then placed as close to the midline as possible

      v. A horizontal incision in the peritoneum is made least 5 cm proximal to the defect and 8 cm caudad and cephalad to the defect, entering into the preperitoneal plane and leaving the TA muscle anteriorly

     vi. The peritoneal flap is developed by traction-countertraction principles with blunt and sharp dissection where needed

    vii. This is carried out to the costal margin cephalad, Coopers ligament caudad, and to the medial border of the psoas muscles as evidenced by the iliac artery. This dissection includes reduction of the hernia sac and contents

    viii. The fascial defect is closed with #1 running slowly absorbable barbed suture

     ix. The preperitoneal pocket is measured and an uncoated polypropylene mesh is cut and placed into the pocket filling the dissected space and centered on the closed defect

      x. No fixation is typically performed provided good overlap is achieved posteriorly, if there is concern, then mesh can be sutured to the psoas muscle with interrupted absorbable suture

     xi. The peritoneal flap is then closed over the mesh with running 2 to 0 or 3 to 0 slowly absorbable barbed suture

II. Totally extraperitoneal approaches

  a. Enhanced-view Totally Extraperitoneal

      i. Patient is positioned as previously described

      ii. Initial entry is gained over the rectus muscle in the upper abdomen; we prefer an optical trocar using a 0° laparoscope; however, a cut down is also acceptable

     iii. The retrorectus space is entered, making sure to leave the PRS intact

     iv. The PRS is bluntly mobilized off the rectus muscle using the tip of the trocar or with the end of the laparoscope

      v. Two additional robotic ports are then placed into the retrorectus space

vi. The initial port is exchanged for a robotic port and the robot is docked to the ports

vii. Any remaining retromuscular attachments are divided, and the PRS is incised typically in the upper abdomen posterior to the linea alba entering the preperitoneal plane

viii. The peritoneum is swept off the linea alba, and a "crossover" is performed by reaching the contralateral PRS

ix. The peritoneum is taken down in the midline 8 cm caudad and cephalad to the defect, and the hernia sac is reduced

x. The contralateral PRS is mobilized as previously described

xi. Anterior and PRS are closed as previously described

xii. Mesh is deployed to fill this space

POSTOPERATIVE CARE

Enhanced recovery protocols vary widely from institution to institution; however, we typically apply multimodal oral analgesia postoperative day one while trying to limit systemic IV narcotics. Early enteral feeding is highly recommended. Decreased length of stay is one of the potential benefits of robotic AWR surgery, which is augmented by ERAS pathways. Often these procedures can be performed as an outpatient or be discharged after an overnight stay. If a drain is used, we typically remove it within 1 week with close outpatient follow-up.

We do not limit activity or place weightlifting restrictions after hernia repair given the lack of evidence to suggest activity causes hernia recurrence. We do recommend that we let the patients' pain guide their activity. On average, 2 to 4 weeks of postoperative convalescence is considered plenty of time to recover without significant risk in our experience.

OUTCOMES AND CURRENT EVIDENCE
Intraoperative Complications

With any advances in surgical technology, ensuring safety is paramount. A large case control study found no difference intraoperative complications between robotic and open TAR (8.9% vs 16.5%, $P = .137$) and an 8.9% conversion rate to open.[22] Adhesions were the most common reason cited for conversion. Other studies have reported lower estimated blood loss for robotic AWR compared with open AWR but no difference in transfusion requirements.[23] Although reports of intraoperative complications are low, it is worth noting that robotic AWR can lead to similar complications to open AWR.[23,24]

Operative Time

Operative times are consistently longer in robotic surgery. Despite a higher rate of concomitant procedures in the open TAR group, Bittner and colleagues reported longer average operating times for robotic TAR (rTAR; 365 ± 78 min vs 287 ± 121, $P < .01$), which is similar to other retrospective studies.[22,23,25,26] Additionally, randomized controlled trials have shown increased operative times for robotic ventral hernia repair (VHR) compared with laparoscopic intra-peritonesl onlay mesh (IPOM) VHR.[27,28]

Ergonomics

The robotic platform is generally thought to improve ergonomics compared with traditional laparoscopy due to articulating instruments, three-dimensional stereoscopic displays, motion scaling, and tremor reduction.[29] Multiple studies have demonstrated lower cognitive and physical stress for task-completion using robotic trainers over laparoscopy, especially for complex tasks.[30–32] Laparoscopy can be physically demanding and has been reported to cause physical symptoms in up to 86.9% of surgeons.[33] Although robotic surgery is often cited to improve surgeon ergonomics, it has also been reported to cause discomfort and physical symptoms in up to 56.1% of surgeons, mostly involving the fingers and neck. Physical symptoms were less common for surgeons who expressed confidence in the ergonomic settings of their console.[29]

Postoperative Complications

Often the major benefit of a minimally invasive technique is short-term wound morbidity. A systematic review of 63 studies showed that compared with open anterior component separation technique (CST), endoscopic CST carried a significantly lower risk of wound morbidity including superficial infections (3.5 vs 8.9%), skin dehiscence (5.3 vs 8.2%), necrosis (2.1 vs 6.8%), hematoma/seroma formation (4.6 vs 7.4%), and fistula tract formation (0.4 vs 1.0%).[34] This difference in wound morbidity is logical in the setting of an anterior CST but is less obvious for a posterior CST, which does not create large subcutaneous flaps. One study comparing 76 open TAR to 38 rTAR reported one seroma in the robotic group versus 9 (11.8%) in the open arm. Additionally, the rate of systemic complications was significantly lower in the robotic group (0% vs 17.1%, $P = .026$).[23] Multiple retrospective studies have noted similar decrease in wound complications between robotic-hybrid TAR compared with open TAR.[35–37] In an effort to control for selection bias, Carbonell and colleagues published a 2:1 propensity score matched cohort study of robotic and open retromuscular ventral hernia repairs from the ACHQC. This data demonstrated a significantly higher surgical site occurrences (SSO) incidence in the robotic group (32% vs 14%, $P < .001$), which was driven by a higher rate of seromas not requiring intervention (28/111 vs 9/222, $P < .001$).[35] This higher seroma rate in robotic repairs may be driven by residual hernia sac, which can be easily excised in an open approach. This assumption is supported by another propensity-matched analysis of open TAR versus hybrid robot-assisted TAR, which demonstrated lower SSO rates in the hybrid robotic group (5% vs 15%, $P = .015$), with no difference in SSI, SSOPI, or SSO subtypes including seroma.[38] A recent meta-analysis of robotic vs open TAR demonstrated that robotic TAR was associated with lower risk of complications rate (9.3 vs 20.7%, OR 0.358, 95% CI 0.218–0.589, $P < .001$) and lower risk of developing SSO (5.3 vs 11.5%, OR 0.669, 95% CI 0.307–1.458, $P = .02$).[39] There is an ongoing randomized controlled trial to evaluate the difference in composite complications at 30 days between robotic and open AWR for ventral hernias 7 to 15 cm (NCT03007758).

Length of Stay

Although open AWR with TAR has been shown to be a durable option for repair, the technique is associated with high rates of short-term complications and long hospitalizations.[40,41] One of the most cited benefits to robotic AWR is decreased length of stay, and there have been multiple retrospective studies supporting this. Martin-del-Campo previously reported a mean length of stay of 1.3 days for robotic TAR compared with 6 days for open TAR ($P < .001$) but the significance of this result is clouded by more comorbid patients (ASA class III: 47% vs 74%, $P = .01$) and recurrent hernias in the open TAR group (29% vs 65%, $P = .001$).[23] Similarly, Bittner and colleagues reported significant reduction in length of stay for robotic TAR compared with open TAR (6.7 ± 4.3 vs 3.5 ± 0.9 days, $P < .01$) but the open cohort included more patients undergoing concomitant procedures (16/76 vs 0/26, $P < .01$).[25] Both studies demonstrated a reduction in length of stay; however, they were highly biased. A 2:1 propensity-score matched cohort of 333 patients (222 open, 111 robotic) showed a significant reduction in length of hospital stay from 3 days to 2 days for patients undergoing robotic AWR ($P < .001$).[35] This was further supported by a systematic review, which concluded that there was consistent, moderate evidence supporting a reduction in length of hospital stay.[42]

Cost

Cost is widely thought to be a disadvantage of the robotic platform, although the existing literature is mixed and difficult to interpret. Most of the prospective literature describing costs of robotic ventral hernia repair does not include AWR but much of the principles can be extrapolated. The capital costs are high for robotic surgery. For example, the cost of purchasing and maintaining the robotic platforms has been estimated at US$1700 per procedure.[8] Another driver of higher costs in the robotic platform compared with traditional laparoscopy is the use of disposable instrumentation. For example, the "Robotic Inguinal vs Transabdominal Laparoscopic Inguinal Hernia Repair: The RIVAL Randomized Clinical Trial" comparing robotic and laparoscopic inguinal hernia repairs reported increased median costs associated with disposable instruments (US$1784 vs US$623, $P < .01$) and total costs (US$3258 vs US$1421, $P < .001$).[43] Olavarria and colleagues similarly reported increased adjusted absolute costs of US$2767 in their randomized controlled trial comparing robotic IPOM to laparoscopic IPOM.[28]

In contrast, the PROVE-IT trial demonstrated no difference in the cost of disposable/reusable instruments, likely secondary to the use of suture fixation of the mesh in the robotic group compared with mechanical fixation using a tacking device in the laparoscopic arm. The robotic IPOM group did demonstrate significantly longer median operative time than laparoscopic IPOM (146 vs 94 minutes; $P < .001$), which translated to higher operating room time–cost ratios (1.25 vs 0.85, $P < .001$).[27]

In a retrospective analysis of costs incurred for open compared with laparoscopic and robotic AWR, Belyansky and colleagues reported higher operating room supply costs associated with minimally invasive surgical (MIS) repairs (US$4893 vs US$3189, $P = .15$) but lower total hospital costs (US$12,295 vs US$20,924, $P < .001$),[44] which were driven by a reduction in length of stay (1.4 vs 5.3 days, $P < .001$). Interpretation of these cost savings for the robotic platform is limited by the retrospective nature of the review and by the inclusion of only 9 robotic cases. Comprehensive costs analysis of 10 open and 16 robotic-assisted AWR with TAR in an Austrian hospital similarly revealed 2.7-fold higher procedure-related costs for robotic repairs but 60% lower total cost of the inpatient stay.[45]

The majority of evidence supports the robotic platform presents higher direct cost than laparoscopic approaches to ventral hernia repair. However, the difference that difference may be offset by the reduction in length of stay.

Hernia Recurrence

Long-term outcomes of robotic AWR compared with open AWR are not well understood. Most retrospective reviews have a follow-up of 180 days or less,[6,23,25,26,37,46] although other cohorts have reported follow-up of an average of 319 days without hernia recurrence.[47] An ACHQC review of robotic and open retromuscular hernia repairs reported no difference in hernia recurrence at 1-year (24% vs 20%, $P = .54$) as well as equivalent improvements in hernia-related quality of life as measured by the change in HerQLes score from baseline (29 vs 34, $P = .66$).[48] Similar hernia recurrence rates (5.6% vs 5.1%, $P > .9$) between robotic and open TAR were also reported in a cohort study with a mean follow up of 19 months in the robotic TAR group and 43 months in the open TAR group.[22] Based on current evidence, there does not seem to be a significant difference in hernia recurrence or quality of life for the robotic versus open AWR. Future prospective clinical trials focusing on long-term follow-up are needed to evaluate hernia recurrence, quality of life, and long-term mesh-related morbidities.

SUMMARY

There is clearly a role for robotics in AWR surgery. Early trials have demonstrated longer operating times, higher direct hospital costs, and decreased length of stay. Other outcomes seem to be similar to open AWR techniques. Robotic AWR is an exciting technique to offer patients with complex ventral hernias.

CLINICS CARE POINTS

- Robotic abdominal wall reconstruction is an young and evolving field with some retrospective data to support its current use.
- There is a need for high-quality randomized trials to support clinical benefit to the patient when applying this technology in the clinical setting.
- A robotic hernia repair may confer a reduced length of stay and decreased wound complications, yet this remians unanswered.

DISCLOSURE

L. Beffa has received honorarium from Intuitive Surgical.

REFERENCES

1. Sheetz KH, Claflin J, Dimick JB. Trends in the Adoption of Robotic Surgery for Common Surgical Procedures. JAMA Netw Open 2020;3(1):e1918911.
2. Holihan JL, Nguyen DH, Nguyen MT, et al. Mesh Location in Open Ventral Hernia Repair: A Systematic Review and Network Meta-analysis. World J Surg 2016; 40(1):89–99.
3. Appleton ND, Anderson KD, Hancock K, et al. Initial UK experience with transversus abdominis muscle release for posterior components separation in abdominal wall reconstruction of large or complex ventral hernias: a combined approach by general and plastic surgeons. Ann R Coll Surg Engl 2017;99(4):265–70.
4. Madion M, Goldblatt MI, Gould JC, et al. Ten-year trends in minimally invasive hernia repair: a NSQIP database review. Surg Endosc 2021;35(12):7200–8.
5. Kelley WE. The evolution of laparoscopy and the revolution in surgery in the decade of the 1990s. J Soc Laparoendosc Surg 2008;12(4):351–7.
6. Warren JA, Cobb WS, Ewing JA, et al. Standard laparoscopic versus robotic retromuscular ventral hernia repair. Surg Endosc 2017;31(1):324–32.
7. Köckerling F, Hoffmann H, Mayer F, et al. What are the trends in incisional hernia repair? Real-world data over 10 years from the Herniamed registry. Hernia 2021; 25(2):255–65.
8. Childers CP, Maggard-Gibbons M. Estimation of the Acquisition and Operating Costs for Robotic Surgery. JAMA 2018;320(8):835–6.
9. Jayne D, Pigazzi A, Marshall H, et al. Effect of Robotic-Assisted vs Conventional Laparoscopic Surgery on Risk of Conversion to Open Laparotomy Among Patients Undergoing Resection for Rectal Cancer: The ROLARR Randomized Clinical Trial. JAMA 2017;318(16):1569–80.

10. Jeong IG, Khandwala YS, Kim JH, et al. Association of Robotic-Assisted vs Laparoscopic Radical Nephrectomy With Perioperative Outcomes and Health Care Costs, 2003 to 2015. JAMA 2017;318(16):1561–8.
11. Wright JD, Ananth CV, Lewin SN, et al. Robotically assisted vs laparoscopic hysterectomy among women with benign gynecologic disease. JAMA 2013;309(7): 689–98.
12. Huger WE. The anatomic rationale for abdominal lipectomy. Am Surg 1979;45(9): 612–7.
13. Sauerland S, Korenkov M, Kleinen T, et al. Obesity is a risk factor for recurrence after incisional hernia repair. Hernia 2004;8(1):42–6.
14. Liu JK, Purdy AC, Moazzez A, et al. Defining a Body Mass Index Threshold for Preventing Recurrence in Ventral Hernia Repairs. Am Surg 2022;88(10):2514–8.
15. Petro CC, Prabhu AS. Preoperative Planning and Patient Optimization. Surg Clin 2018;98(3):483–97.
16. Bernardi K, Olavarria OA, Dhanani NH, et al. Two-year Outcomes of Prehabilitation Among Obese Patients With Ventral Hernias: A Randomized Controlled Trial (NCT02365194). Ann Surg 2022;275(2):288–94.
17. Liang MK, Holihan JL, Itani K, et al. Ventral Hernia Management: Expert Consensus Guided by Systematic Review. Ann Surg 2017;265(1):80–9.
18. Al-Mansour MR, Vargas M, Olson MA, et al. 144 lack of association between glycated hemoglobin and adverse outcomes in diabetic patients undergoing ventral hernia repair: an ACHQC study. Surg Endosc 2022. https://doi.org/10.1007/s00464-022-09479-1. Published online August 15.
19. DeLancey JO, Blay E, Hewitt DB, et al. The effect of smoking on 30-day outcomes in elective hernia repair. Am J Surg 2018;216(3):471–4.
20. Borad NP, Merchant AM. The effect of smoking on surgical outcomes in ventral hernia repair: a propensity score matched analysis of the National Surgical Quality Improvement Program data. Hernia 2017;21(6):855–67.
21. Petro CC, Haskins IN, Tastaldi L, et al. Does active smoking really matter before ventral hernia repair? An AHSQC analysis. Surgery 2019;165(2):406–11.
22. Dewulf M, Hiekkaranta JM, Mäkäräinen E, et al. Open versus robotic-assisted laparoscopic posterior component separation in complex abdominal wall repair. BJS Open 2022;6(3):zrac057.
23. Martin-Del-Campo LA, Weltz AS, Belyansky I, et al. Comparative analysis of perioperative outcomes of robotic versus open transversus abdominis release. Surg Endosc 2018;32(2):840–5.
24. Belyansky I, Reza Zahiri H, Sanford Z, et al. Early operative outcomes of endoscopic (eTEP access) robotic-assisted retromuscular abdominal wall hernia repair. Hernia 2018;22(5):837–47.
25. Bittner JG, Alrefai S, Vy M, et al. Comparative analysis of open and robotic transversus abdominis release for ventral hernia repair. Surg Endosc 2018;32(2): 727–34.
26. Halpern DK, Howell RS, Boinpally H, et al. Ascending the Learning Curve of Robotic Abdominal Wall Reconstruction. J Soc Laparoendosc Surg 2019;23(1): e2018, 00084.
27. Petro CC, Zolin S, Krpata D, et al. Patient-Reported Outcomes of Robotic vs Laparoscopic Ventral Hernia Repair With Intraperitoneal Mesh: The PROVE-IT Randomized Clinical Trial. JAMA Surg 2021;156(1):22–9.
28. Olavarria OA, Bernardi K, Shah SK, et al. Robotic versus laparoscopic ventral hernia repair: multicenter, blinded randomized controlled trial. BMJ 2020;370: m2457.

29. Lee GI, Lee MR, Green I, et al. Surgeons' physical discomfort and symptoms during robotic surgery: a comprehensive ergonomic survey study. Surg Endosc 2017;31(4):1697–706.

30. Moore LJ, Wilson MR, Waine E, et al. Robotic technology results in faster and more robust surgical skill acquisition than traditional laparoscopy. J Robotic Surg 2015;9(1):67–73.

31. van der Schatte Olivier RH, van't Hullenaar CDP, Ruurda JP, Broeders IAMJ. Ergonomics, user comfort, and performance in standard and robot-assisted laparoscopic surgery. Surg Endosc 2009;23(6):1365–71.

32. Berguer R, Smith W. An Ergonomic Comparison of Robotic and Laparoscopic Technique: The Influence of Surgeon Experience and Task Complexity. J Surg Res 2006;134(1):87–92.

33. Park A, Lee G, Seagull JF, et al. Patients Benefit While Surgeons Suffer: An Impending Epidemic. J Am Coll Surg 2010;210(3):306–13.

34. Switzer NJ, Dykstra MA, Gill RS, et al. Endoscopic versus open component separation: systematic review and meta-analysis. Surg Endosc 2015;29(4):787–95.

35. Carbonell AM, Warren JA, Prabhu AS, et al. Reducing Length of Stay Using a Robotic-assisted Approach for Retromuscular Ventral Hernia Repair: A Comparative Analysis From the Americas Hernia Society Quality Collaborative. Ann Surg 2018;267(2):210–7.

36. Halka JT, Vasyluk A, Demare A, et al. Hybrid robotic-assisted transversus abdominis release versus open transversus abdominis release: a comparison of short-term outcomes. Hernia 2019;23(1):37–42.

37. Halka JT, Vasyluk A, DeMare AM, et al. Robotic and hybrid robotic transversus abdominis release may be performed with low length of stay and wound morbidity. Am J Surg 2018;215(3):462–5.

38. Abdu R, Vasyluk A, Reddy N, et al. Hybrid robotic transversus abdominis release versus open: propensity-matched analysis of 30-day outcomes. Hernia 2021; 25(6):1491–7.

39. Bracale U, Corcione F, Neola D, et al. Transversus abdominis release (TAR) for ventral hernia repair: open or robotic? Short-term outcomes from a systematic review with meta-analysis. Hernia 2021;25(6):1471–80.

40. Zolin SJ, Krpata DM, Petro CC, et al. Long-term Clinical and Patient-Reported Outcomes After Transversus Abdominis Release With Permanent Synthetic Mesh: A Single Center Analysis of 1203 Patients. Ann Surg 2022. https://doi. org/10.1097/SLA.0000000000005443. Publish Ahead of Print.

41. Zolin SJ, Fafaj A, Krpata DM. Transversus abdominis release (TAR): what are the real indications and where is the limit? Hernia 2020;24(2):333–40.

42. Ye L, Childers CP, de Virgilio M, et al. Clinical outcomes and cost of robotic ventral hernia repair: systematic review. BJS Open 2021;5(6):zrab098.

43. Prabhu AS, Carbonell A, Hope W, et al. Robotic Inguinal vs Transabdominal Laparoscopic Inguinal Hernia Repair: The RIVAL Randomized Clinical Trial. JAMA Surg 2020;155(5):380–7.

44. Belyansky I, Weltz AS, Sibia US, et al. The trend toward minimally invasive complex abdominal wall reconstruction: is it worth it? Surg Endosc 2018;32(4): 1701–7.

45. Dauser B, Hartig N, Vedadinejad M, et al. Robotic-assisted repair of complex ventral hernia: can it pay off? J Robot Surg 2021;15(1):45–52.

46. Santos DA, Limmer AR, Gibson HM, et al. The current state of robotic retromuscular repairs—a qualitative review of the literature. Surg Endosc 2021;35(1): 456–66.

47. Kudsi OY, Chang K, Bou-Ayash N, et al. Hybrid Robotic Hernia Repair for Incisional Hernias: Perioperative and Patient-Reported Outcomes. J Laparoendosc Adv Surg Tech 2021;31(5):570–8.
48. Guzman-Pruneda F, Huang LC, Collins C, et al. Abdominal core quality of life after ventral hernia repair: a comparison of open versus robotic-assisted retromuscular techniques. Surg Endosc 2021;35(1):241–8.

Parastomal Hernia Repair

Victoria R. Rendell, MD, Eric M. Pauli, MD*

KEYWORDS

- Parastomal • Hernia • Ostomy • Enterostomy • Stoma • Colostomy • Urostomy
- Ileostomy

KEY POINTS

- Parastomal hernias are common and associated with high rates of recurrence after repair.
- Multiple factors, including patient factors, ostomy site condition, hernia size, hernia contents, prior repair attempts and techniques, and presence of concomitant midline hernia, are important when planning parastomal hernia repair.
- Parastomal hernia repair approaches include open and minimally invasive approaches with primary or mesh-based repair with onlay, sublay, and underlay mesh positions.
- The evidence on best repair method and on mesh choice is limited, and more investigation into parastomal hernia repair techniques is needed.

INTRODUCTION

With over 100,000 stomas created yearly in the United States and greater than 750,000 people living with stomas, stoma-related complications, and associated morbidity are prevalent.[1] Parastomal hernias (PHs) are common after stoma creation. Although reported rates of PHs vary considerably in the literature, they can develop in up to 58% of stomas and can occur with any type of stoma created (end or loop, colostomy, ileostomy, or urostomy).[2–6] Although about 25% of PHs are asymptomatic, the majority negatively affect patient quality of life. Issues range from local effects such as skin breakdown, leakage, difficulty pouching, and discomfort to more serious complications related to bowel obstruction with possibility of incarceration and ischemia.[6–8] Cosmetic and psychological effects of PHs should not be downplayed. Many patients, understandably, have a baseline element of anxiety about the presence of a stoma; even an asymptomatic bulge that is perceived to draw attention to their ostomy can be disconcerting.

Given PH-related symptoms are common, the increasing rate of PH repairs over time is unsurprising.[9] Approaching PH repair presents significant frustration to surgeons

Division of Minimally Invasive and Bariatric Surgery, Department of Surgery, Penn State Health Milton S. Hershey Medical Center, 500 University Drive, Hershey, PA 17033, USA
* Corresponding author. Penn State Hershey Medical Center, 500 University Drive, M.C. H149, Hershey, PA 17033.
E-mail address: epauli@pennstatehealth.psu.edu
Twitter: @EricPauliMD (E.M.P.)

Surg Clin N Am 103 (2023) 993–1010
https://doi.org/10.1016/j.suc.2023.04.008
0039-6109/23/© 2023 Elsevier Inc. All rights reserved.

due to a number of inherent challenges, including the technical difficulty of repairing a hernia that necessitates the continued presence of a fascial defect with bowel intentionally traversing it, the increased complications inherent to higher Center for Disease Control wound classification, the overall high rate of recurrence, the added morbidity of stoma-related complications postoperatively, and the challenge of addressing the common concomitant midline hernias. In addition, the heterogeneity of a wide variety of factors associated with PH presentation and repair presents a challenge for the study of outcomes and has resulted in overall limited data to guide surgical approach for subsets of patients.[2]

EVALUATION
Indications for Repair

Patients present with a variety of complaints related to PHs, which should be carefully considered when discussing repair. Acute symptoms of obstruction, incarceration, or strangulation should be evaluated and treated surgically in an urgent manner. For patients who present for consideration of elective repair, a number of factors related to the patient, their stoma, and their surgical history are essential to evaluate (**Table 1**).[6,8] With the high rate of recurrence after repair and many patients citing tolerable PH-related symptoms, a watchful waiting process is often undertaken; however, there are limited data to guide this practice due to insufficient evidence.[2] Most patients elect to proceed with repair due to worsening PH-related symptoms over time. As surgeons consider the timing and approach of repair, it is essential to consider eligibility for stoma reversal as the first approach as this results in the lowest recurrence rate. Unfortunately, only about 25% of PHs are associated with stomas eligible for reversal.[10]

Classification and Evaluation of Imaging

Although the sensitivity of diagnosing a PH with physical examination alone is high, it is virtually impossible to determine the size of the fascial defect in a PH patient in clinic. Cross-sectional imaging offers details related to the stoma, the hernia, and the

Table 1	
Factors to consider when evaluating a patient for parastomal hernia repair	
Patient factors	Obesity
	Age
	Immunosuppressed status
	Active smoking
	Diagnosis of inflammatory bowel disease
	Cardio-pulmonary comorbidities
Stoma factors/symptoms	Leakage/difficulty with pouching (*How frequently are bag changes required?*)
	Skin irritation/infections
	Prolapse
	Size of bulge
	Cosmesis
	Pain/discomfort
	Symptoms of obstruction
Surgical history/details	Type of ostomy (loop vs end, colostomy vs ileostomy vs urostomy)
	Indication for creation (urgent vs elective)
	Eligibility for reversal
	History of prior repair attempts
	History of prior ostomy relocation
	Presence of previously placed mesh

abdominal wall that help considerably with surgical planning.[2,11,12] The following items should be evaluated when reviewing a computed tomography (CT) scan to help determine the approach for repair: (1) the type of ostomy and the path of the mesentery, (2) the size of the PH defect, (3) the location of the defect in relation to the ostomy and to the midline, (4) the location of the trephine through the abdominal wall relative to the semilunar line, and (5) the contents of the hernia sac and amount of bowel involvement. In addition, it is important to note the presence and characteristics of any concomitant midline hernia(s). If the hernia has been repaired previously, it is important to note the location of any residual mesh. Identification of mesh is best performed after review of previous operative notes that contain critical information about mesh type and plane of implant.

Several classification systems have been developed to help characterize PHs, and the most frequently used system is the European Hernia Society (EHS) classification.[13] This classification centers on the size of the defect (> or ≤ 5 cm), the presence of a concomitant midline hernia defect (yes/no), and the status of the hernia as primary or recurrent (**Fig. 1**). Although intended as an intraoperative method, EHS classification is commonly applied to preoperative imaging studies of PHs. Although such a classification system is helpful to structure reporting of outcomes in the study of PH

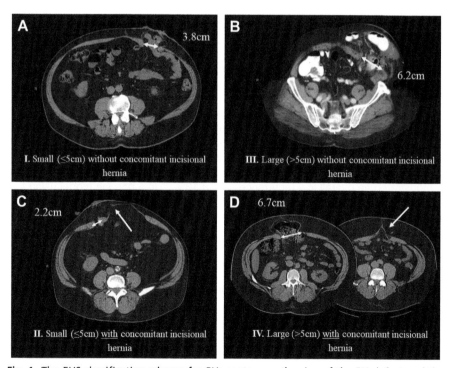

Fig. 1. The EHS classification scheme for PHs centers on the size of the PH defect and the presence of a concomitant incisional hernia. Types I (*A*) and II (*C*) are small hernias (≤5 cm) with and without additional midline incisional hernias. Types III (*B*) and IV (*D*) are large hernias (>5 cm) with and without midline incisional hernias. Of note a "P" and an "R" are added to the types to signify whether the PH is a primary or recurrent hernia.[13] Double-ended arrows represent the transverse width of the PH component, and the single-ended arrows denote the midline hernia component.

repairs, there is no system that directs surgeons to the most appropriate repair by type of classification.

SURGICAL TECHNIQUES

Many techniques for PH have been described. The options for repair currently center on the following variations in approaches: primary repair versus mesh-based repair, open versus minimally invasive technique, mesh position with respect to the abdominal layers, mesh configuration surrounding the stoma site, and whether the stoma is left in situ, revised or resited. **Table 2** provides an overview of PH repair approaches.

Primary Fascial Repair

Open primary repairs involve a midline or lateral approach to the stoma or mucocutaneous junction take down and revision of the stoma at the same site.[14,15] In this repair, the hernia content is reduced, the sac is removed, and the fascial defect is closed with suture. If the hernia is approached directly, extensive adhesiolysis of the peritoneal cavity can be avoided. In addition, no foreign body is used, which makes this a preferred option in some urgent cases where there is significant contamination, in cases where a repeat operation is planned, or in patients who are not candidates for extensive surgery. The main downside to primary fascial repair is the very high recurrence rates demonstrated up to 48% to 66%.[16] In repairs done from the midline, complete sac removal can be challenging, especially if the parastomal defect is smaller. Sutured closure from a posterior approach is also challenging as the following all must be accomplished: obtain robust bites of anterior fascia, avoid large muscular bites, avoid injury to the stoma, and avoid taking bites of posterior fascia alone.

Mesh Suture Repair

As an alternative to primary suture repair, Dumanian and colleagues developed a primary closure technique using mesh strips (**Fig. 2**).[17] These self-made 2 cm strips of lightweight microporous polypropylene mesh were used to approximate the fascial defect around the stoma in 1 cm interrupted bites. Although there are limited data on this technique, a case series of 48 patients with median follow-up of 11.8 months demonstrated an overall low recurrence rate of 13%.[17] In a porcine model using the now commercially available mesh suture option, mesh suture had a lower rate of hernia formation compared with monofilament suture and had good tissue incorporation.[18] Further evaluation is needed to assess long-term recurrence and other complication rates.

Mesh-Based Repair

Mesh-based PH repairs were first described in 1977, as a response to the high recurrence rate associated with primary repairs.[19] Mesh reinforcement can occur with placement of mesh in an onlay, sublay (retromuscular or preperitoneal space), or underlay (intraperitoneal space) fashion. A wide array of mesh configurations around the ostomy have been described, but three main variations dominate the literature. The slit or keyhole configuration involves cutting one side of the mesh toward the center to enable wrapping the mesh around the stoma (**Fig. 3**). Many surgeons remove a circle from the center of the mesh to accommodate the bowel. The slit is then reapproximated with permanent material (sutures or tacks). A cruciate configuration necessitates the stoma be taken down as this involves making a central incision within the mesh and passing the stoma through this opening to prevent dividing a side of the mesh. Some surgeons simply cut a central hole in the mesh rather than creating a

Table 2
Surgical techniques in parastomal hernia repair

Type of Repair	Stoma Management	Mesh Position and Configuration	Approach	Citation Describing Repair
Suture repair (primary)	In situ	n/a	Open	Thorlakson et al,[14] 1965
	Revise/resite			Prian et al,[15] 1975
Mesh suture repair	In situ	Mesh strips used as suture material in fascia	Open	Dumanian et al,[17] 2018
	Revise/resite			
Mesh-based repair	In situ	Onlay mesh: slit/keyhole	Open	Kald et al,[44] 2001; Rosin & Bonardi,[19] 1977
		Underlay: Sugarbaker or slit/keyhole	Open	Sugarbaker,[21] 1985
			MIS	Ayuso et al,[25] 2021
		Sublay: slit/keyhole	Open	Hofstetter et al,[24] 1998
			MIS	Maciel et al,[45] 2019
		Sublay: Sugarbaker PPHR	Open	Pauli et al,[32] 2016
			MIS	Lambrecht,[33] 2021
	Revise/resite	Onlay: slit/keyhole or cruciate	Open	Rosin & Bonardi,[19] 1977
		Underlay: slit/keyhole, Sugarbaker, or cruciate	Open	Raigani et al,[29] 2014
			MIS	DeAsis et al,[26] 2015
		Sublay: cruciate mesh or STORRM	Open	Majumder et al,[31] 2018; Rosen et al,[30] 2010
		Sublay: Sugarbaker PPHR	Open	Pauli et al,[32] 2016

Abbreviations: MIS, minimally invasive surgery approach, laparoscopic or robotic; PPHR, Pauli parastomal hernia repair; STORRM, stapled transabdominal ostomy reinforcement with retromuscular mesh.

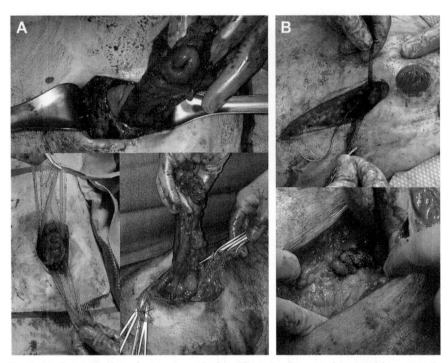

Fig. 2. Mesh strip and mesh suture repairs have been implemented to provide more rein-forcement than a primary suture repair. (*A*) Self-cut 2 cm strips of polypropylene mesh are used in the place of standard sutures to repair the fascial defect around the stoma. (*B*) Newly approved for use in the United States, commercially available mesh suture can be used as an alternative to approximate the fascial defect using mesh rather than standard suture mate-rial. (*Courtesy of* Dr. Gregory Dumanian, Chicago, IL.)

cruciate. Finally, repairs that position an intact piece of mesh underneath the bowel to lateralize the trajectory of the bowel as it exits the peritoneal cavity are termed a Sug-arbaker configuration, which is described in more detail below.

Technical Considerations of Mesh-Based Repairs

This section provides a detailed overview of each type of mesh-based PH repair.

Open Repair with Onlay Mesh: The onlay mesh placement relies on creating a sub-cutaneous space above the fascia surrounding the stoma location for placement of the mesh and affixing the mesh to the anterior rectus and external oblique fascial layers. Originally described by Rosin and Bonardi, this repair involved reducing the hernia sac, narrowing the fascial defect used for the trephine with sutures and then placing the stoma through an opening created in a polyethylene mesh. The mesh was then sutured to the surrounding fascia.[19] Since then, variations of this repair have been described. The stoma can be approached with a lateral peristomal incision, through a midline incision, or by taking down the mucocutaneous junction of the stoma to reach the subcutaneous space. The mesh can be configured in a keyhole fashion around the stoma, or if the stoma is taken down, it can be passed through a cruciate opening in the mesh (see **Fig. 3**). The mesh can be secured with sutures (absorbable or nonabsorbable), staples, and/or with fibrin sealants to the surrounding fascia. Another modification described includes the "stove pipe

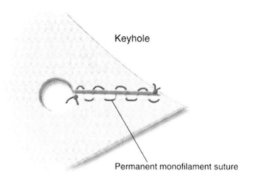

Keyhole

Permanent monofilament suture

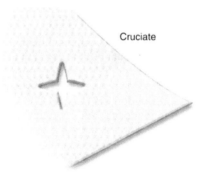

Cruciate

OPTIONS FOR STOMA APERTURES IN MESH

Fig. 3. Mesh configurations around a stoma involving an aperture for the stoma can be fashioned in keyhole or cruciate fashion. The keyhole method involves a slit along one side of the mesh to enable encircling the stoma. Generally, the slit is then reapproximated with suture. The cruciate involves no lateral slit or weakness in the mesh but requires that the stoma is revised/resited for placement. (*From* Winder JS, Pauli EM. Open parastomal hernia repair. In: Rosen MJ, editor. Atlas of abdominal wall reconstruction. 2nd edition. Philadelphia: Elsevier; 2017. p. 124–49; with permission.)

hat" technique in which a second piece of mesh is affixed to the stoma circumferentially as it travels toward the skin.[20] Although not always used, drains can be left in the subcutaneous pocket to help with seroma formation and surgical site infections (SSIs). As with any onlay repair, it is critical to assure that the mesh is positioned on the fascia and not on a layer of subcutaneous fat and that adequate overlap of the defect is achieved.

Open Repair with Underlay Mesh: Between 1980 and 1985, Paul Sugarbaker described a new technique for mesh placement in the underlay space that did not involve dividing the mesh.[21,22] Instead, the mesh was circumferentially secured to the parastomal fascial edges after all the hernia contents were reduced. The stoma bowel exited the peritoneal cavity at an unsecured lateral edge of the mesh and then traversed the fascia to reach the skin. Subsequent iterations of this method would increase the overlap of the mesh in all directions around the fascial defect. Laterally, this created a tunnel that allows the stoma bowl to course between the mesh and the peritoneum until it enters the trephine. A second technique for intraperitoneal mesh reinforcement is the keyhole or slit method.[23,24] This involves cutting the side of the mesh to allow it to surround the stoma, reapproximating the cut edge after placement.

With this technique, there is no lateralization of the stoma as the loop of bowel enters the peritoneal cavity directly through the mesh underneath its fascial opening.

Minimally Invasive Repair with Underlay Mesh: With the advent of minimally invasive techniques, laparoscopic and robotic versions of the intraperitoneal mesh placement have been introduced and are increasingly used.[20,25,26] With these approaches, three to four lateral ports are placed opposite to the stoma side for abdominal access. Adhesions are lysed to free the stoma bowel loop and associated mesentery. Generally, sutures are placed to reestablish a normal sized fascial defect for the stoma. This step is facilitated by use of the robotic approach.[25] The mesh is introduced into the abdomen and either draped across the stoma for lateralization in Sugarbaker fashion or the mesh is applied as a keyhole (**Fig. 4**). It is then sutured (intraperitoneally or with trans-fascial sutures) or tacked to the abdominal wall. Another modification that has been described is a "sandwich" technique involving the placement of two meshes in the underlay space allowing an intact edge of mesh to be sandwiched over the keyhole lateral slit of the first mesh laterally with the keyhole portion of the second mesh extending medially.[27]

Open Repair with Sublay Mesh: The existing approaches to PH repair were inadequate to apply in the not uncommon scenario of a concomitant midline hernia with a PH. Description of sublay repair involving the formation of myofascial flaps can be found as far back as 1993, but these repairs commonly involved division of the neurovascular bundles entering the rectus abdominis muscle at its lateral boundary.[28] Between 2010 and 2014, Rosen and colleagues reported a more contemporary retromuscular PH repair method.[29,30] After a midline laparotomy and adhesiolysis, the stoma was taken down and mobilized for planned resiting at a new location. A sublay space was then formed by entering the retrorectus plane bilaterally and extending laterally with a transversus abdominis release (TAR) (**Fig. 5**). The posterior sheath was reapproximated in the midline and an opening created to allow the stoma bowel to exit the peritoneal cavity underneath the planned new stoma site. The mesh was then placed to fill the retromuscular pocket, generally with a cruciate defect to allow the stoma bowel to traverse. The mesh was secured with transfascial fixation sutures and the plane widely drained. The bowel was brought through a new trephine in the

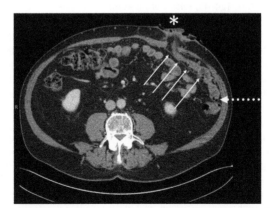

Fig. 4. A postoperative CT scan after a minimally invasive Sugarbaker repair demonstrates the position of the mesh in the underlay space. The mesh (*solid arrows*) drapes underneath the bowel segment descending from the stoma (marked with *asterisk*) toward the lateral abdominal wall, where the bowel then enters the peritoneal cavity at the lateral most edge of the mesh (*dotted arrow*).

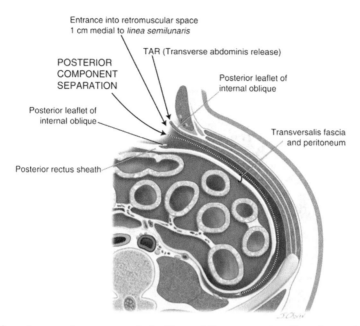

Entrance into retromuscular space
1 cm medial to *linea semilunaris*

TAR (Transverse abdominis release)

POSTERIOR
COMPONENT
SEPARATION

Posterior leaflet of
internal oblique

Posterior leaflet of
internal oblique

Transversalis fascia
and peritoneum

Posterior rectus sheath

Fig. 5. The retromuscular space created with a midline retrorectus dissection and TAR enables a sublay space for mesh placement during PH repair. After opening the midline and entering the posterior rectus sheath, the posterior leaflet of the internal oblique is incised medial to the linea semilunaris, and the underlying transversus abdominis muscle is transected to enter the pre-transversalis/preperitoneal space that extends laterally to the retroperitoneum and psoas muscle. (*From* Winder JS, Pauli EM. Open parastomal hernia repair. In: Rosen MJ, editor. Atlas of abdominal wall reconstruction. 2nd edition. Philadelphia: Elsevier; 2017. p. 124–49; with permission.)

subcutaneous tissue and rectus muscle to the skin where it was matured following midline closure.

A modification of this approach was described by Majumder and colleagues to address the difficulty of aligning all of the independent layers of this repair as well as to alleviate concerns of erosion of mesh related to scissoring within the retromuscular plane.[31] This approach, termed Stapled Transabdominal Ostomy Reinforcement with Retromuscular Mesh (STORRM) also facilitated the vertical alignment of the stomal conduit as it passes through the various layers, which was a particularly challenging aspect of the prior approach (**Fig. 6**). In this technique, the abdominal access, takedown of the stoma, dissection of the retromuscular plane and TAR, closure of the posterior layer, and creation of an opening for the stoma bowel are accomplished similarly. In the STORRM modification, the planned path of the stoma through the mesh and abdominal wall is marked. The anvil of a circular end-to-end anastomosis (EEA) stapler is then passed through the mesh. The stapler is passed through the new stoma site through the abdominal wall and coupled with the anvil. The stapler is then fired. This creates a staple-reinforced opening through the mesh and the abdominal wall for stoma maturation.

An alternative approach was introduced by Pauli and colleagues, which allowed lateralization of the stoma within the retromuscular space as well as the option to leave the stoma in situ.[32] This approach, the Pauli PH repair (PPHR), involves placing a mesh in the retromuscular space in a Sugarbaker configuration with respect to the stoma

(**Fig. 7**). A midline approach with adhesiolysis is performed. The stoma bowel is freed intraperitoneally of adhesions but is not taken down. The retrorectus space is then entered, and the portion of the stoma above the posterior sheath is circumferentially freed. A TAR is performed medial to the linea semilunaris as is typically performed and extended laterally behind the stoma bowel loop, connecting the preperitoneal plane laterally around the stoma. At this point, based on the path of the mesentery of the stoma bowel, a lateralized path is determined, and a posterior layer opening is created along this planned path (**Fig. 8**). The posterior layer is then reapproximated medially, which lateralizes the exit site of the stoma bowel loop from the peritoneal cavity. A large mesh is placed within this space and positioned above the posterior

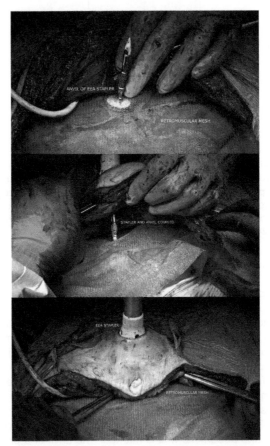

Fig. 6. The STORRM approach involves using an EEA stapler to assist with more precise alignment of the stoma's path through the mesh and the abdominal wall. The planned path for the bowel from the defect in the posterior sheath to the chosen skin site is marked and then created using a fire of an EEA stapler that is passed down through the stoma site and coupled with the anvil that is placed through the chosen site for the mesh defect. (*From* Majumder A, Orenstein SB, Miller HJ, Novitsky YW. Stapled Transabdominal Ostomy Reinforcement with retromuscular mesh (STORRM): Technical details and early outcomes of a novel approach for retromuscular repair of parastomal hernias. Am J Surg. 2018;215(1):82-87. https://doi.org/10.1016/j.amjsurg.2017.07.030; with permission.)

layer and below the bowel in a Sugarbaker configuration. Operative photos of an open PPHR are displayed in **Fig. 9**.

Minimally Invasive Repair with Sublay Mesh: The PPHR repair has been recently adapted for a minimally invasive approach with laparoscopy and the robotic platform.[33] The same principles of the open approach are followed with a retrorectus dissection and TAR extending around the intact stoma (**Fig. 10**). The bowel is lateralized through an incision in the posterior layer and then sutured medially. The mesh is placed in similar fashion. In patients with a midline hernia as well as the PH, contralateral access can be obtained for contralateral retromuscular dissection and TAR.

COMPLICATIONS/CONCERNS

Regardless of the approach, the complications of PH repair include the standard complications known for all hernia repairs. However, the inherent nature of an operation involving a stoma adds additional concerns.[10,34] A stoma can become ischemic as a result of a tight closure of the fascial opening during repair combined with postoperative edema related to intraoperative bowel manipulation. Injury to the stoma or its blood supply can happen as a result of content reduction, stoma mobilization, and fascial closure. The risk of ileus with the operation increases with more invasive approaches involving extensive bowel manipulation. The tight closure of parastomal fascia can also be responsible for stoma-level obstruction. Surgical site occurrences (SSOs) and SSIs are a concern with any hernia repair, particularly when mesh is used. With PH repairs, the operation is clean-contaminated or contaminated by default, which increases infection risk. In addition, for all mesh-based repairs, the mesh is placed in proximity to bowel, which introduces the risk of adhesion formation, mesh erosion, and entero-prosthetic fistula formation. Finally, the recurrence risk is substantially higher for PHs than for other abdominal wall hernias.[34]

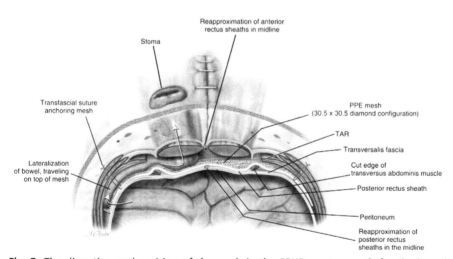

Fig. 7. The dissection and position of the mesh in the PPHR create a path for the bowel within the retromuscular space with mesh reinforcement. The technique avoids a cruciate or keyhole area of weakness in the mesh and separates the inner posterior layer defect in the abdominal wall from the anterior opening in the rectus muscle. (With permission from Joe Chovan.)

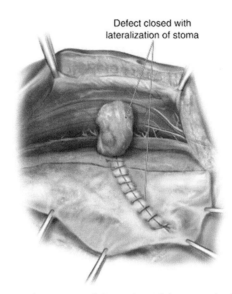

Defect closed with
lateralization of stoma

Fig. 8. In the PPHR approach, a purposeful opening of the posterior layer allows lateralization of the stoma. A path is selected for the stoma based on the most natural lie of the mesentery to the stoma. Once lateralized, the medial portion of the posterior layer is reapproximated in preparation for a Sugarbaker positioning of the mesh in the retromuscular space. (*From* Winder JS, Pauli EM. Open parastomal hernia repair. In: Rosen MJ, editor. Atlas of abdominal wall reconstruction. 2nd edition. Philadelphia: Elsevier; 2017. p. 124–49; with permission.)

CURRENT EVIDENCE
Outcomes for Parastomal Hernia Repair Techniques

A central challenge for PH repairs is the overall lack of high-quality data to drive decision-making. The 2018 EHS guidelines highlighted this challenge as they could not offer a recommendation for six of the nine key questions due to insufficient evidence.[2] Indeed, the only question addressed with strong evidence was that suture repair for elective PH repair should not be done because of higher recurrence rates. Suture repair had a significantly increased recurrence rate compared with all other techniques (69.4% vs 2.1–34.6% for the remainder of the techniques, $P < .0001$) in a systematic review.[20] Other techniques had similar recurrence with the exception of the laparoscopic Sugarbaker technique, which had a lower recurrence rate compared with the keyhole technique (OR 2.3, 95% CI 1.2–4.6; $P = 0.016$). A more recent national cohort study from Finland involving 235 repairs at nine hospitals tracked recurrence with a median follow-up of 39 months. Their findings mirrored the earlier results with keyhole technique having a higher recurrence rate than the Sugarbaker (35.9% vs 21.5%). Recently, a systematic review and meta-analysis again found Sugarbaker configuration mesh repairs to have significantly less recurrence when compared with keyhole repairs (OR 0.38; CI 0.18–0.78; $P = .008$).[35] Interestingly, in a subgroup analysis of studies performed more recently (2015–2021), this difference disappeared. There are no randomized controlled trials or systematic reviews comparing original techniques with the newer sublay techniques. A recent multicenter randomized controlled trial of mesh choice involving 253 Center for Disease Control (CDC) Class II and III retromuscular hernia repairs included 108 PH patients.[36] A

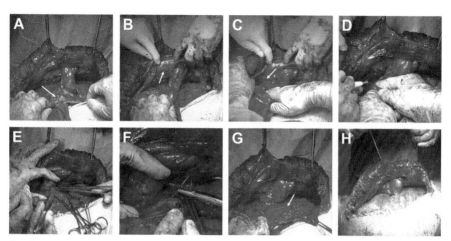

Fig. 9. Open PPHR repair lateralizes the stoma bowel within the retromuscular space to enable Sugarbaker configuration of the mesh. (*A*) The posterior layer (noted with *white arrow*) is dissected free from the stoma bowel and associated mesentery, and a lateral TAR has been performed. (*B*) The posterior layer (*white arrow*) is lifted here to demonstrate the intraperitoneal path of the stoma bowel. The mesentery and bowel naturally lay along a right inferior direction noted in (*C*) with a white arrow, and the posterior layer is then opened along this line (*D*). (*E*) The defect in the posterior layer is then closed from the stoma bowel side toward the medial edge (*F*), resulting in lateralization of the bowel within the retromuscular space, demonstrated in (*G*) (*white arrow* marks the closed posterior layer defect). (*H*) The mesh is then positioned within the retromuscular space in a Sugarbaker configuration with respect to the stoma bowel.

subgroup analysis of the PH patients found an overall recurrence rate of 27.8% at 2 years.[37] Recurrence rate was 10.7% for patients who underwent PPHR, and 30.4% for patients who underwent repairs with a keyhole or cruciate configuration mesh. While clinically relevant, this difference was not statistically significant ($P = .07$), likely because the study was powered to detect differences in outcomes based on mesh type (biologic or synthetic) and not powered to detect differences in recurrent PHs based on mesh configuration. The investigators of this trial are actively completing a single-center prospective randomized trial to directly address the issue of retromuscular mesh configuration and PH recurrence rates.[38]

For other outcomes, including SSO/SSI rates, mesh erosion, mesh infection, and postoperative morbidity, the data are limited, but no particular technique or approach stands out as clearly superior for any of these outcomes.[2,20] For retromuscular PH repairs, mesh erosion seems to be more related to mesh configuration (higher rates with cruciate/keyhole vs Sugarbaker) than to mesh choice (no difference between macroporous polypropylene or acellular dermal matrix).[37] The heterogeneity of the techniques, patient characteristics, hernia characteristics, and mesh choices present significant challenges for the ability to have reliable direct comparisons of the various techniques. In addition, there is noted lack of research involving patient-reported outcomes for PH repairs.[39]

Choice of Mesh for Repair

An important recurring question for PH repair involves the use of mesh and which type is the best to use to achieve the lowest recurrence rate as well as the lowest

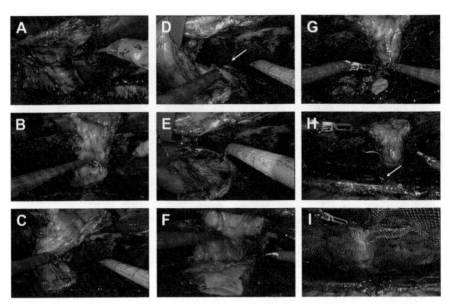

Fig. 10. Minimally invasive PPHR accomplishes the same mesh configuration within the retromuscular repair as the open PPHR. The posterior rectus sheath is taken down and the TAR performed by incising medial to the semilunar line. The TAR is extended laterally beyond the bowel stoma by working cranial and caudal to the stoma and connecting the planes laterally (*A–C*). The posterior layer lateral to the stoma bowel entry site is then incised along the planned trajectory (*D, white arrow*) so that the bowel with its mesentery can be lateralized (*E–F*). The posterior layer defect created is then closed medial to the stoma, which is now lateralized (*G–H*). The white arrow in (*H*) denotes the closure line of the posterior layer. The mesh is then positioned in the retromuscular space and secured with interrupted sutures to hold its Sugarbaker configuration in place (*I*).

complication rate. All types of mesh, including synthetic meshes such as polypropylene, expanded polytetrafluroethylene (ePTFE), and polyester as well as biologic, bioabsorbable, and composite meshes, have been used for PH repair. The concern for higher rates of mesh infection with permanent synthetic mesh in the contaminated field of a PH repair led to increased use of biologic mesh once this became available. However, in the subsequent study of biologic versus synthetic mesh for PH repair, there has been no support for the use of biologic mesh providing any advantage over synthetic mesh.[40,41] Most recently, a multicenter randomized controlled trial of biologic versus synthetic mesh for contaminated ventral hernia repairs released a post hoc analysis for PH repairs and found no difference in recurrence rates (28.9% for biologic vs 25.5% for synthetic mesh, $P = .77$) or reoperation rates with mesh erosions present in 3.5% and 3.9% of cases for each mesh type.[37] Importantly, biologic mesh presents over 200 times the expense of synthetic mesh.[36] Other than the need for a coated surface mesh or an inert mesh (ePTFE) to face the intraperitoneal space during an intraperitoneal underlay repair, there are no clear guidelines to drive the selection of a specific type of mesh over another for most repairs.[2]

DISCUSSION

PHs present a challenge for surgeons as they are associated with significant morbidity for patients and are likely to recur after repair. Many factors are important to consider related to the patient, the hernia, the stoma, and the situation, when planning for a surgical repair. We have outlined the many techniques that are available for PH repair. All repairs have higher than desired recurrence rates. With real gaps in the data available to drive decision-making in PH repair, it generally falls on the surgeon and their comfort level with various techniques to determine a plan for repair while considering the many important patient, hernia, and stoma characteristics that factor into the decision-making process. Continued efforts to design and implement high-quality studies comparing outcomes for the various techniques and approaches should be encouraged.

Emerging literature suggests that the centralization of PH repairs to dedicated centers results in improved outcomes.[42] In 2010, Denmark preferentially filtered PH repairs to five dedicated centers, which resulted in more total elective repairs being performed on patients with more overall comorbidities without any change in the rates of readmission, reoperation, or death. For emergency repairs, reoperation rates (from 44.9% to 23%) and mortality (from 10.3% to 2%) were significantly reduced post-centralization.

Centralization in a country with a nationalized health care system represents a best-case scenario; even still it took 7 years to achieve 95% of case volume performed at a regional hernia center. Such a process in the United States would be challenging, especially as new current procedural terminology (CPT) coding for PHs (repair of PH, any approach, initial or recurrent; 49,621—reducible and 49,622—incarcerated/strangulated) increases the financial incentive for these repairs to be managed surgically. However, given the improved PH repair outcomes from Denmark as well as other successful centralization processes in the United States (eg, esophageal cancer surgery[43]), this process bears discussing and surgeons should consider transferring PH patients to centers with experience, interest, and resources to successfully manage these patients.

SUMMARY

PHs are a common complication associated with stoma creation. Surgical repair is challenging due to the many individual factors that are relevant when considering the approach to repair and the inherent inability to completely close the fascial defect. Although many options for repair have been developed, all have a higher than desired recurrence rate. Continued study of repairs and innovation is needed to tackle PHs.

CLINICS CARE POINTS

- The evaluation of PH for repair must include consideration of patient factors, stoma site condition and associated symptoms, hernia size, hernia contents, the presence of concomitant midline hernia defects, and the urgency of presentation.

- Consideration of ostomy reversal should always be the first approach to a PH repair as this will be associated with the lowest recurrence rate.

- The main categories of surgical approaches to PH repairs are primary versus mesh-based repairs and open versus minimally invasive approaches. For mesh-based repairs, mesh can be placed in the onlay, sublay, or underlay positions in a variety of configurations.

- Open primary repairs are associated with unacceptably high recurrence rates and should be reserved for nonelective cases.

- The evidence on the best overall approach to PH repair is limited by the lack of quality evidence.

- There is no clear guideline on the most appropriate mesh to use for PH repair; however, there are no data to support using biologic mesh over synthetic mesh.
- Sugarbaker configuration mesh (whether performed as an underlay or a sublay operation) seems to be preferable to cruciate or keyhole repairs in terms of hernia recurrence rates and mesh erosions.
- PH repairs should be performed at higher volume centers with experience in a wide array of repair methods and the resources to manage this complex patient population.

DISCLOSURE

Dr V.R. Rendell has nothing to disclose. Dr E.M. Pauli has the following disclosures: Consulting: Actuated Medical, Allergan, Becton-Dickinson, Boston Scientific, Cook Biotech, ERBE, Medtronic, Integra, Intuitive Surgical, Neptune Medical, Noah Medical, Steris, Surgimatix. Royalties: UpToDate (Wolters Kluwer), Springer. Financial Interests: Actuated Medical, Contamination Source Identification, Cranial Devices, Inc.

REFERENCES

1. Advocate Tools. United Ostomy Associations of America, Inc (UOAA). Available at: https://www.ostomy.org/wp-content/uploads/2021/09/AAH_Ostomy_White-Paper _20210827.pdf. Accessed January 16, 2023.
2. Antoniou SA, Agresta F, Garcia Alamino JM, et al. European Hernia Society guidelines on prevention and treatment of parastomal hernias. Hernia 2018; 22(1):183–98.
3. Carne PWG, Robertson GM, Frizelle FA. Parastomal hernia. Br J Surg 2003;90(7): 784–93.
4. Feng D, Wang Z, Yang Y, et al. Incidence and risk factors of parastomal hernia after radical cystectomy and ileal conduit diversion: a systematic review and meta-analysis. Transl Cancer Res 2021;10(3):1389–98.
5. Liu L, Zheng L, Zhang M, et al. Incidence and risk factors for parastomal hernia with a permanent colostomy. J Surg Oncol 2022;126(3):535–43.
6. Malik T, Lee M, Harikrishnan A. The incidence of stoma related morbidity – a systematic review of randomised controlled trials. Ann R Coll Surg Engl 2018;100(7): 501–8.
7. Correa Marinez A, Bock D, Carlsson E, et al. Stoma-related complications: a report from the Stoma-Const randomized controlled trial. Colorectal Dis 2021; 23(5):1091–101.
8. Krishnamurty D, Blatnik J, Mutch M. Stoma Complications. Clin Colon Rectal Surg 2017;30(03):193–200.
9. Gavigan T, Rozario N, Matthews B, et al. Trends in parastomal hernia repair in the United States: a 14-y review. J Surg Res 2017;218:78–85.
10. Gavigan T, Stewart T, Matthews B, et al. Patients Undergoing Parastomal Hernia Repair Using the Americas Hernia Society Quality Collaborative: A Prospective Cohort Study. J Am Coll Surg 2018;227(4):393.
11. de Smet GHJ, Lambrichts DPV, van den Hoek S, et al. Comparison of different modalities for the diagnosis of parastomal hernia: a systematic review. Int J Colorectal Dis 2020;35(2):199–212.
12. Lambrecht JR. Diagnostic methods in parastomal hernia; research and clinical relevance. Hernia 2021;25(3):817–20.

13. Śmietański M, Szczepkowski M, Alexandre JA, et al. European Hernia Society classification of parastomal hernias. Hernia 2014;18(1):1–6.
14. Thorlakson RH. Technique of Repair of Herniations Associated with Colonic Stomas. Surg Gynecol Obstet 1965;120:347–50.
15. Prian GW, Sawyer RB, Sawyer KC. Repair of peristomal colostomy hernias. Am J Surg 1975;130(6):694–6.
16. Al Shakarchi J, Williams JG. Systematic review of open techniques for parastomal hernia repair. Tech Coloproctology 2014;18(5):427–32.
17. Dumanian GA, Lanier ST, Souza JM, et al. Mesh sutured repairs of contaminated incisional hernias. Am J Surg 2018;216(2):267–73.
18. Dumanian GA. Suturable Mesh Demonstrates Improved Outcomes over Standard Suture in a Porcine Laparotomy Closure Model. Plast Reconstr Surg Glob Open 2021;9(10):e3879.
19. Rosin JD, Bonardi RA. Paracolostomy hernia repair with Marlex mesh: A new technique. Dis Colon Rectum 1977;20(4):299–302.
20. Hansson BME, Slater NJ, van der Velden AS, et al. Surgical Techniques for Parastomal Hernia Repair: A Systematic Review of the Literature. Ann Surg 2012; 255(4):685–95.
21. Sugarbaker PH. Peritoneal Approach to Prosthetic Mesh Repair of Paraostomy Hernias. Ann Surg 1985;201(3):344.
22. Sugarbaker PH. Prosthetic mesh repair of large hernias at the site of colonic stomas. Surg Gynecol Obstet 1980;150(4):576–8.
23. Byers JM. Repair of Parastomal Hernias Using Polypropylene Mesh. Arch Surg 1992;127(10):1246.
24. Hofstetter WL, Vukasin P, Ortega AE, et al. New technique for mesh repair of paracolostomy hernias. Dis Colon Rectum 1998;41(8):1054–5.
25. Ayuso SA, Shao JM, Deerenberg EB, et al. Robotic Sugarbaker parastomal hernia repair: technique and outcomes. Hernia 2021;25(3):809–15.
26. DeAsis FJ, Lapin B, Gitelis ME, et al. Current state of laparoscopic parastomal hernia repair: A meta-analysis. World J Gastroenterol 2015;21(28):8670–7.
27. Berger D, Bientzle M. Laparoscopic Repair of Parastomal Hernias: A Single Surgeon's Experience in 66 Patients. Dis Colon Rectum 2007;50(10):1668–73.
28. Alexandre JH, Bouillot JL. Paracolostomal hernia: Repair with use of a Dacron prosthesis. World J Surg 1993;17(5):680–2.
29. Raigani S, Criss CN, Petro CC, et al. Single-Center Experience With Parastomal Hernia Repair Using Retromuscular Mesh Placement. J Gastrointest Surg 2014; 18(9):1673–7.
30. Rosen MJ, Reynolds HL, Champagne B, et al. A novel approach for the simultaneous repair of large midline incisional and parastomal hernias with biological mesh and retrorectus reconstruction. Am J Surg 2010;199(3):416–21.
31. Majumder A, Orenstein SB, Miller HJ, et al. Stapled Transabdominal Ostomy Reinforcement with retromuscular mesh (STORRM): Technical details and early outcomes of a novel approach for retromuscular repair of parastomal hernias. Am J Surg 2018;215(1):82–7.
32. Pauli EM, Juza RM, Winder JS. How I do it: novel parastomal herniorrhaphy utilizing transversus abdominis release. Hernia 2016;20(4):547–52.
33. Lambrecht JR. Endoscopic preperitoneal parastomal hernia repair (ePauli repair) : an observational study. Surg Endosc 2021;35(4):1903–7.
34. Harries RL, Daniels IR, Smart NJ. Outcomes of surgically managed recurrent parastomal hernia: the Sisyphean challenge of the hernia world. Hernia 2021;25(1): 133–40.

35. Fleming AM, Phillips AL, Drake JA, et al. Sugarbaker Versus Keyhole Repair for Parastomal Hernia: a Systematic Review and Meta-analysis of Comparative Studies. J Gastrointest Surg 2022. https://doi.org/10.1007/s11605-022-05412-y.

36. Rosen MJ, Krpata DM, Petro CC, et al. Biologic vs Synthetic Mesh for Single-stage Repair of Contaminated Ventral Hernias: A Randomized Clinical Trial. JAMA Surg 2022;157(4):293–301.

37. Miller BT, Krpata DM, Petro CC, et al. Biologic vs Synthetic Mesh for Parastomal Hernia Repair: Post Hoc Analysis of a Multicenter Randomized Controlled Trial. J Am Coll Surg 2022;235(3):401.

38. Miller BT, Thomas JD, Tu C, et al. Comparing Sugarbaker versus keyhole mesh technique for open retromuscular parastomal hernia repair: study protocol for a registry-based randomized controlled trial. Trials 2022;23:251.

39. Sandø A, Rosen MJ, Heniford BT, et al. Long-term patient-reported outcomes and quality of the evidence in ventral hernia mesh repair: a systematic review. Hernia 2020;24(4):695–705.

40. Carbonell AM, Criss CN, Cobb WS, et al. Outcomes of synthetic mesh in contaminated ventral hernia repairs. J Am Coll Surg 2013;217(6):991–8.

41. Slater NJ, Hansson BME, Buyne OR, et al. Repair of Parastomal Hernias with Biologic Grafts: A Systematic Review. J Gastrointest Surg 2011;15(7):1252–8.

42. Helgstrand F, Henriksen NA. on behalf of the Danish Hernia Database. Outcomes of parastomal hernia repair after national centralization. Br J Surg 2023; 110(1):60–6.

43. Schlottmann F, Strassle PD, Charles AG, et al. Esophageal Cancer Surgery: Spontaneous Centralization in the US Contributed to Reduce Mortality Without Causing Health Disparities. Ann Surg Oncol 2018;25(6):1580–7.

44. Kald A, Landin S, Masreliez C, et al. Mesh repair of parastomal hernias: new aspects of the Onlay technique. Tech Coloproctology 2001;5(3):169–71.

45. Maciel V, Mata W, Arevalo G, et al. Robotic retro-rectus repair of parastomal hernias. J Robot Surg 2019;13(3):483–9.

Devices in Hernia Surgery

Ajita S. Prabhu, MD

KEYWORDS

- Medical device regulation • Hernia mesh devices • Ventral hernia • Hernia mesh
- Premarket notification

KEY POINTS

- Although mesh is commonly utilized in hernia repair, further exploration is needed to identify populations who may benefit from primary repair.
- It is difficult to remain current regarding mesh types, however further emphasis of educational concepts on mesh types should be prioritized in surgical training.
- Regulation of mesh devices continues to evolve; coordinated registry networks and unique device identifiers are ostensibly innovative approaches to achieving higher level device regulation without stifling innovation of technology.

If we could artificially produce tissues of the density and toughness of fascia and tendon, the secret of the radical cure of hernias would be discovered.
—Theodore Bilroth, 1878

Hernia surgery is a unique field in terms of its heavy dependence on mesh and biomaterials. Given that the frequency of ventral hernia repairs alone has almost doubled from 2006 to 2022 in the United States to 611,000 per year,[1] the national and potentially global implications of devices in hernia repair are sweeping. Nonetheless, considerable controversy remains regarding the indications and even the need for mesh in ventral hernia repair. Here, we attempt to frame some of the contemporary arguments about mesh and biomaterials in hernia repair and shed light on the complexities of the mesh industry and its relationship with surgeons.

DO ALL HERNIA REPAIRS NEED MESH?

Although Theodore Bilroth made a prescient statement about mesh almost 150 years ago, the debate about appropriate candidates for mesh placement remains active to date. Likely, one of the main drivers of surgeon adoption of mesh was the publication by Luijendijk and colleagues published in 2000 in the New England Journal of Medicine.[2] The authors compared polypropylene mesh placement with continuous polypropylene suture closure for primary or first-time incisional hernia defects 6 cm or lesser in length or width. The authors concluded that mesh was indicated for all midline

Cleveland Clinic Lerner College of Medicine, 9500 Euclid Avenue, Crile A-100, Cleveland, OH 44195, USA
E-mail address: prabhua@ccf.org

Surg Clin N Am 103 (2023) 1011–1017
https://doi.org/10.1016/j.suc.2023.04.009
surgical.theclinics.com

incisional hernias, regardless of size. Surgeons rapidly adopted mesh into their practices, perhaps due to the wide exposure received by the article, and soon enough the use of mesh was extrapolated to many incisional hernias as well as primary umbilical and epigastric hernias. To date, this article remains one of the most impactful and practice-changing in general surgery. Nonetheless, it is unclear whether extrapolation of the findings from Luijendijk is reasonable and/or appropriate today. Although it remained the highest level of evidence surgeons could use to determine care for hernia patients until that point, the Luijendijk study did not account for multiply recurrent hernias, presence of contamination, larger hernia defects, or underlying patient comorbidities. Since that time, although, great progress has been made in recognizing the importance of tailoring operative techniques to specific patient scenarios.

There are some technical aspects of the Luijendijk trial, which would likely be considered differently today. Notably, the Luijendijk study utilized 1.0 polypropylene suture with estimated 1-cm bites in the suture arm of the trial, which brings to question the accuracy of technique used as well as whether the so-called small bites technique popularized by Deerenberg[3] and Fortelny[4] utilizing 2.0 slow-absorbing suture for laparotomy closure could also have a place in suture repair of ventral hernia today. (Small bites technique has not been formally studied in ventral hernia repair yet, however recruitment for a mesh vs suture trial for ventral hernia repair utilizing small bites technique is currently ongoing [Clinicaltrials.gov Identifier: NCT05599750]). Additionally, where the mesh arm was expected to achieve exclusion of the viscera by suturing omentum or peritoneum closed versus bridging the intra-abdominal elements with Vicryl mesh, the authors also state that some patients (the number is not reported) had bridging of the anterior fascia when tension was present, calling into question whether this technique is a true evaluation of a mesh repair as we consider it today. A more contemporary consideration for a mesh repair would reflect the current emphasis on achieving reapproximation of the linea alba, often through a retromuscular dissection and broad (3–5 cm) overlap of the defect.

Furthermore, more emphasis has been called to increasingly specific scenarios such as mesh utilization or mesh type in contaminated fields,[5,6] staging of hernia repairs in contaminated situations,[7] and patient-specific factors such as obesity and other modifiable comorbidities[8,9] which may affect wound morbidity in the short-term and, ostensibly, hernia recurrence in the long-term.

Finally, little attention was previously paid to potential long-term consequences of mesh usage. Recent high-quality literature suggests that while the incidence of mesh-related reoperation is only about 5% for all patients receiving mesh,[10] the nature of the complications including mesh infections, erosions, fistulae, and hernia recurrence can be devastating for patients.

Overall, the practice of ventral hernia repair has heavily shifted toward the use of mesh devices, and the consequences of that shift are overall unclear. However, given the rare but catastrophic potential for mesh-related reoperation and the progression of operative techniques particularly for open surgery, including retromuscular mesh placement and a potentially advantageous suturing strategy, the authors note that a more current exploration regarding the need for mesh in all hernia repair utilizing updated techniques is warranted and may indeed identify a population of patients who could benefit from mesh avoidance.

WHICH MESH FOR WHICH PATIENT?

A key factor in ventral hernia repair is the type of mesh material used for patients undergoing repair with mesh. Ideal characteristics of mesh have been described throughout surgical literature for decades: they are chemically inert, cause minimal foreign body reaction, are not physically modified in vivo, do not produce allergy or hypersensitivity, are noncarcinogenic, are resistant to mechanical strains, can be shaped to the form required, and can be sterilized. Still, no mesh is perfect for every case or every patient, and determining appropriate applications of the hundreds of mesh brands and materials on today's market is further stymied by the lack of high-level evidence to support or refute the use of each device. Further complicating the situation is the significant heterogeneity in reporting of clinical outcomes of hernia repair (variable definitions and terminology) and lack of emphasis placed on patient-reported outcomes.[11] Head-to-head trials comparing meshes to each other are understandably rare because small comparative trials are impractical for making broad generalizations about mesh materials, and larger scale trials are costly and cumbersome to execute. Thus, prospective clinical trials are likely not a pragmatic step forward in the path toward determining best uses for specific mesh devices. Moreover, little in the way of governmental funding is earmarked toward investigating concepts related to hernia repair because it is not viewed as a national health priority, and device industry stands to benefit very little from nonessential investment in device trials where there is a so-called winner and a loser.

Additionally, although surgical education seems to appropriately emphasize hernia repair as a topic that residents should be familiar with, education around mesh and biomaterials varies significantly from program to program[12]; this likely, in part, depends on the increasing trend toward hospitals purchasing and stocking mesh portfolios recommended by group purchasing organizations. In that case, determinations of mesh purchases are largely driven by contracts, and the combined lack of high-level clinical evidence to support the use of one device over another further serves to result in the stocking of meshes being driven by finance as opposed to clinical context. This may limit the device brands to 1 or 2 per hospital, thereby limiting the exposure of trainees to different mesh brands and materials. Surgeon preferences may further complicate this, and the increasing trend toward referring complex hernias to tertiary and quaternary centers may also limit resident exposure to the full spectrum of hernia disease. Finally, surgeons must be aware that contemporary literature regarding specific mesh devices may suffer the unintended consequences of the opaque relationships between surgeon investigators and the mesh device industry. Although most surgeons have an altruistic interest in best serving their patients, and those surgeons authoring articles regarding the performance of mesh devices expectedly use the high volumes of those devices about which they publish, conflict-of-interest reporting is notoriously inaccurate, and unconscious bias may occur in those publications.[13,14]

Due to the seemingly insurmountable quest for "the perfect mesh," the hernia market has continued to expand unabated, with each new iteration of mesh devices purporting to resolve mesh-related issues and/or overcome undesirable clinical scenarios and patient-related conditions. To date, the 4 major categories of mesh and biomaterials in hernia repair include permanent synthetic, absorbable synthetic, absorbable biosynthetic, and biologic. Each of these broad categories can contain hundreds of variations on the main, or building block, material. For the most part, permanent synthetic materials remain based on polypropylene, polyester, and expanded polytetrafluoroethylene (ePTFE). Still, within those categories, there is further variation based on filament size, pore size, presence or absence of a barrier coating, and other technical specifications. Although a comprehensive review of each available mesh and biomaterial on today's market is outside the scope of this article, this example serves to illustrate not only the sheer volume of information surgeons must familiarize themselves with regarding mesh and biomaterials but also the impractical expectation that clinically busy surgeons are able to keep abreast of the rapidly changing mesh landscape. Still, arguably, the surgeon must bear some responsibility for the long-term performance of implantable devices and the associated effects on their patients given the inherent but often-unacknowledged conflict of the surgeon: the need to operate to support one's livelihood.

Likely, some broad generalizations can be made regarding "best mesh type" to use for various common clinical scenarios, such as using a barrier-coated synthetic mesh for laparoscopic ventral hernia repair. Additional complexities of the cases, such as contamination related to a permanent stoma, underlying patient comorbidities, the surgeon's training and technical skillset, or the surgeon's judgment regarding patient candidacy and operative technique, however, can result in varying clinical outcomes for patients and can quickly complicate the discussion. Improvement of educational concepts through professional societies and surgical training as well as intentional efforts by surgeons to stay current on hernia literature are the most practical approaches to gain basic understanding of device selection and utilization.

HOW ARE MESH DEVICES REGULATED?

One of the perhaps most important yet rarely discussed concepts regarding mesh devices is the regulatory process by which new devices are vetted to come to market. Because this topic is seldom discussed in surgical training, most practicing surgeons are not familiar with the US Food and Drug Administration (FDA) processes or terminology associated with the status of devices that are on the market.[15] Thus, the terms "cleared" and "approved" are often used interchangeably; however, they have markedly different regulatory implications and levels of scientific scrutiny. Although a full and detailed discussion regarding FDA regulatory processes is outside of the scope of this article, the specific application of FDA clearance for meshes will be described here.

Briefly, the FDA's Center for Devices and Radiological Health is responsible for premarket and postmarket device surveillance and regulation. Within the regulatory framework, there are 3 classes of medical devices based on the level of control considered necessary to assure the safety and effectiveness of the device as well as the perceived risk associated with the device, where Class I is the least stringent/risky and Class III is the most rigorous/risky. Mesh devices are categorized as Class II, which requires a premarket approval application (also known as PMA/510K process) to be submitted before marketing the device.[16] Class II devices and specifically meshes are considered "cleared" through the Premarket Notification process for marketing if they demonstrate "substantial equivalence" to a legally marketed device, known as a "predicate device," before 1976, when the Medical Device Amendment Act was enacted in the United States. Although there is some requirement above and beyond general controls for Class II devices, which may include postmarket surveillance, labeling requirements, registry data, and accepted testing standards, the level of regulation for these devices is essentially intermediate, and premarket clinical testing is not required.[15] Practically speaking, this results in newer or more contemporary mesh devices being cleared based on predicate devices that never underwent testing to ensure their safety. Thus, so-called "descendant devices" may inadvertently continue to propagate unidentified design flaws or safety issues from predicate devices, which may have already been recalled for device failure.[17]

FDA regulatory practices are not included in the curriculum of surgical trainees. Thus, with little to no knowledge of the device classification system and how devices were evaluated before market, surgeons may maintain a false sense of security and therefore assume that most or all devices (meshes) on the market must be "safe." Further complicating this notion is the rapid and continual expansion of the mesh market, driven by the perpetual search for the "perfect mesh," as mentioned previously. Although the Class II classification was intended to balance the competing agendas of innovation and device regulation, the sheer volume of surgical innovations hinders close surveillance of each device throughout its life cycle after entering the market. Although the FDA has an existing Manufacturer and User Device Experience database expressly designed to capture adverse events from postmarket implant/device performance, the quality of the data is compromised by reliance on end user reporting, lack of a denominator of total devices implanted, and missing, duplicated, or nonstandardized entries.[18]

More recent initiatives for device surveillance include the addition of a unique device identifier (UDI) system and coordinated registry networks (CRNs). UDIs are specific types of labels, which allow devices to remain identifiable from manufacturing to distribution to patient use.[19] CRNs are currently in evolution and will leverage UDI, electronic health records, and real-world evidence gathered from patient registries to provide a more robust regulatory system throughout device life cycles, which can ostensibly serve a role in postmarket surveillance with benefit to all stakeholders—patients, surgeons, and the medical device industry.[20] Given the relatively recent initiation of UDIs and CRNs, it will understandably take time to leverage them into a robust and reproducible system for device surveillance. The interest in leveraging large disease-specific patient registries may also result in more early identification of device signals when device-related complications occur, due to the ability to efficiently accrue large volumes of patient-level data where devices are also identifiable.[21]

SUMMARY

Although the field of hernia repair has made exponential advancements regarding improved understanding of operative techniques, disease-related algorithms, and the application of minimally invasive technology, mesh devices remain one of the most important yet least well understood contributors to clinical and patient-reported outcomes from ventral (and all other) hernia repairs. Although hernia disease occupies a notable share of the medical device marketplace, little high-quality evidence is available to help guide the decision-making of surgeons selecting devices, and the lack of prioritizing investigation of hernia disease in the government and industry sectors only serves to propagate what is already a challenging field to navigate.[22] Moving forward, the American Board of Surgery and professional societies such as the American College of Surgeons should be encouraged to play a larger role in emphasizing the importance of education regarding the concepts of device regulation, hernia repair techniques, and technical specifications of mesh types, if only at a broad level. Finally, despite the challenge in maintaining current knowledge of all contemporary mesh types, general surgeons should be urged to take responsibility for having at minimum a basic understanding of mesh and biomaterials given the high volume of these operations that they will continue to perform throughout their careers.

CLINICS CARE POINTS

- Although mesh technology has outstripped the scope of surgical training, more emphasis should be placed on the basic technical specifications of mesh and biomaterials.

- Further, surgeons should have a basic understanding of the regulatory processes associated with mesh devices.
- Some patients may benefit from primary hernia repair, and further work will help delineate those populations.

REFERENCES

1. Schlosser KA, Renshaw SM, Tamer RM, et al. Ventral hernia repair: an increasing burden affecting abdominal core health. Hernia 2022. https://doi.org/10.1007/S10029-022-02707-6.
2. Luijendijk RW, Hop WCJ, van den Tol MP, et al. A Comparison of Suture Repair with Mesh Repair for Incisional Hernia. N Engl J Med 2000;343(6). https://doi.org/10.1056/nejm200008103430603.
3. Deerenberg EB, Harlaar JJ, Steyerberg EW, et al. Small bites versus large bites for closure of abdominal midline incisions (STITCH): a double-blind, multicentre, randomised controlled trial. Lancet (London, England) 2015;386(10000): 1254–60.
4. Fortelny RH, Andrade D, Schirren M, et al. Effects of the short stitch technique for midline abdominal closure on incisional hernia (ESTOIH): randomized clinical trial. Br J Surg 2022;109(9):839–45.
5. Carbonell AM, Cobb WS. Safety of prosthetic mesh hernia repair in contaminated fields. Surg Clin North Am 2013;93(5):1227–39.
6. Rosen MJ, Krpata DM, Petro CC, et al. Biologic vs Synthetic Mesh for Single-stage Repair of Contaminated Ventral Hernias: A Randomized Clinical Trial. JAMA Surg 2022;157(4):293–301.
7. Petro CC, Rosen MJ. Fight or flight: The role of staged approaches to complex abdominal wall reconstruction. Plast Reconstr Surg 2018;142(3S):38S–44S.
8. Tastaldi L, Krpata DM, Prabhu AS, et al. The effect of increasing body mass index on wound complications in open ventral hernia repair with mesh. Am J Surg 2019; 218(3). https://doi.org/10.1016/j.amjsurg.2019.01.022.
9. Alkhatib H, Tastaldi L, Krpata DM, et al. Impact of modifiable comorbidities on 30-day wound morbidity after open incisional hernia repair. Surgery 2019;166(1): 94–101.
10. Kokotovic D, Bisgaard T, Helgstrand F. Long-term recurrence and complications associated with elective incisional hernia repair. JAMA 2016;316(15):1575–82.
11. Harji D, Thomas C, Antoniou SA, et al. A systematic review of outcome reporting in incisional hernia surgery. BJS Open 2021;5(2). https://doi.org/10.1093/BJSOPEN/ZRAB006.
12. Hope WW, O'Dwyer B, Adams A, et al. An evaluation of hernia education in surgical residency programs. Hernia 2014;18(4):535–42.
13. Olavarria OA, Shah P, Bernardi K, et al. Lack of Regulations and Conflict of Interest Transparency of New Hernia Surgery Technologies. J Surg Res 2019;9:1–8.
14. Sekigami Y, Tian T, Char S, et al. Conflicts of Interest in Studies Related to Mesh Use in Ventral Hernia Repair and Abdominal Wall Reconstruction. Ann Surg 2022; 276(5):E571–6.
15. Buch B. FDA Medical Device Approval: Things You Didn't Learn in Medical School or Residency. Am J Orthop 2007;36(8):407–12.
16. Classify Your Medical Device | FDA. Available at: https://www.fda.gov/medical-devices/overview-device-regulation/classify-your-medical-device. Accessed March 7, 2023.

17. Zargar N, Carr A. The regulatory ancestral network of surgical meshes. PLoS One 2018;13(6). https://doi.org/10.1371/JOURNAL.PONE.0197883.
18. Sandberg JM, Gray I, Pearlman A, et al. An evaluation of the Manufacturer And User Facility Device Experience database that inspired the United States Food and Drug Administration's Reclassification of transvaginal mesh. Investig Clin Urol 2018;59(2):126–32.
19. UDI basics | FDA. Available at: https://www.fda.gov/medical-devices/unique-device-identification-system-udi-system/udi-basics. Accessed March 7, 2023.
20. Sedrakyan A, Campbell B, Graves S, et al. Surgical registries for advancing quality and device surveillance. Lancet 2016. https://doi.org/10.1016/s0140-6736(16)31402-7.
21. Prabhu AS, Poulose BK, Rosen MJ. Harnessing the power of collaboration for postmarket surveillance of hernia mesh devices. Ann Surg 2020;271(2):221–2.
22. Poulose BK, Shelton J, Phillips S, et al. Epidemiology and cost of ventral hernia repair: Making the case for hernia research. Hernia 2012;16(2):179–83.

Mesh Selection in Abdominal Wall Reconstruction

An Update on Biomaterials

Ryan Ellis, MD, Benjamin T. Miller, MD*

KEYWORDS

- Abdominal wall reconstruction • Ventral hernia repair • Synthetic mesh
- Biologic mesh • Biosynthetic mesh • Absorbable mesh

KEY POINTS

- The ideal mesh for abdominal wall reconstruction is inert, resists degradation, allows for host tissue ingrowth, is able to clear an infection, and escapes patient detection.
- Permanent synthetic mesh material, pore size, and density are characteristics that affect the optimal position of mesh placement and mesh durability. Surgeons must be familiar with the properties of the prosthetics they are placing in patients.
- For clean retromuscular abdominal wall reconstruction, we prefer to use heavy weight permanent synthetic mesh.
- For clean-contaminated or contaminated retromuscular abdominal wall reconstruction cases, we prefer medium weight permanent synthetic mesh. Biologic mesh has been shown to have acceptable wound event and hernia recurrence rates when used in contaminated abdominal wall reconstruction cases.
- For hernias repaired in a "staged" fashion under contaminated or suboptimal conditions, we use short-term absorbable mesh as an inlay repair. Biologic or biosynthetic mesh may also be used in these situations.

If we could artificially produce tissue of the density and toughness of fascia and tendon, the secret of the radical cure of the hernia repair would be discovered.[1]
— *Theodore Billroth, 1857.*

INTRODUCTION

Mesh reinforcement has become the standard of care for repair of large or complex incisional hernias because it reduces hernia recurrences.[2] However, understanding

Department of Surgery, Cleveland Clinic Center for Abdominal Core Health, Cleveland Clinic Foundation, 9500 Euclid Avenue, Cleveland, OH 44195, USA
* Corresponding author.
E-mail address: millerb35@ccf.org

Surg Clin N Am 103 (2023) 1019–1028
https://doi.org/10.1016/j.suc.2023.04.010
0039-6109/23/© 2023 Elsevier Inc. All rights reserved.

surgical.theclinics.com

Table 1
Permanent synthetic and short-term absorbable synthetic mesh options

Mesh (Manufacturer)	Material	Pore Size (mm)	Mesh Density (g/m²)	Absorption
Prolene (Ethicon)	Polypropylene	0.9	76	Permanent
Physiomesh (Ethicon)	Monocryl/PDS/Prolene	2.4	30	Permanent
Vicryl (Ethicon)	92% PGA; 8% PLLA	-	-	2–3 mo
Parietex (Medtronic)	Polyester/collagen film	1.29	90	Film—20 d Polyester—permanent
Parietene (Medtronic)	Polypropylene	2.4	46	Permanent
Symbotex (Medtronic)	Polyester	3.3	64	Permanent

Abbreviations: P4HB, poly-4-hydroxybutyric acid; PDS, polydioxanone; PGA, polyglycolic acid; PLA, polylactic acid; PLLA, poly-L-lactic acid; TMC, trimethylene carbonate.

which mesh to use and when can be challenging. Hernia size and complexity, case contamination, surgeon experience, and available resources all factor into mesh choice considerations. Furthermore, new mesh varieties are frequently added to the market, and no standardized hernia mesh curriculum exists. It can also be difficult to understand mesh characteristics because they are often not listed on the packaging or the manufacturer's website. Faced with these obstacles, mesh selection in abdominal wall reconstruction can quickly become overwhelming. It is no wonder, then, that surgeons typically use mesh they are most familiar with and can be reluctant to change their practice when new mesh or evidence become available.

In our practice, abdominal wall reconstruction is performed with posterior components separation, often with the addition of a transversus abdominis release (TAR) procedure.[3] We do not perform anterior component separations, so this article will likely be biased toward mesh selection for retromuscular ventral hernia repairs. The ideal mesh for these hernia repairs has several key features. It is well incorporated into the native tissues of the abdominal wall; it resists degradation and fracture; it does not elicit a host foreign body reaction; the host immune response is able to clear an infection from it; and it escapes patient detection. Many meshes have been engineered in the last half century to achieve these goals, with varying degrees of success. The goal of this article is to simplify mesh selection in abdominal wall reconstruction. Common mesh types—permanent synthetic, short-term absorbable, long-term absorbable, and biologic—and their unique characteristics will be discussed. Recent evidence supporting certain mesh features in clean and contaminated ventral hernia repairs will be reviewed. Finally, we will give our recommendations for mesh use in abdominal wall reconstruction using posterior components separation.

MESH CHARACTERISTICS AND CLASSIFICATIONS
Permanent Synthetic Mesh

Mesh material and pore size
An implanted mesh faces 2 possible fates. It is either incorporated into the patient's tissues or it is degraded by the host immune response. Mesh is often broadly classified according to these 2 outcomes: permanent or absorbable. Permanent mesh, as the name suggests, is incorporated into the host's tissues and resists degradation by the host immune response. Permanent mesh can be further classified by the material it is made from, which is typically 1 of 3 materials: polypropylene, polyester, or

polytetrafluorethylene (PTFE). Polypropylene and polyester are carbon polymers and PTFE is a fluoropolymer.[4] These materials imbue each permanent mesh type with certain properties (**Table 1**).

One of these characteristics is mesh pore size. Mesh with a pore diameter greater than 100 μm is considered macroporous mesh and mesh with a pore diameter less than 75 μm is microporous mesh.[5] Polypropylene and polyester can be made into macroporous mesh, whereas PTFE is often made into microporous mesh.[4] Macroporous mesh is thought to have 2 advantages over microporous mesh in abdominal wall reconstruction. Pores larger than 75 μm permit the passage of host immune cells and blood vessels, allowing the body to clear a bacterial infection from the mesh.[5] Moreover, larger pores allow migration of host fibroblasts through the mesh, encouraging collagen deposition and mesh incorporation into the surrounding tissues.[6] Microporous mesh, however, does not allow tissue ingrowth. Instead, it is encapsulated by surrounding tissues.[7] This feature of microporous mesh can have advantages in some instances. Because microporous products, such as PTFE mesh, inhibit tissue ingrowth, it can be placed against the viscera, whereas bare polypropylene or polyester meshes have been known to erode into the bowel.[8]

Mesh "Weight"

Mesh pore size is linked to another mesh feature—mesh density, or "weight." Larger mesh pores often result in lighter mesh and smaller pores in heavier mesh. Synthetic mesh weights fall into 1 of 3 categories: lightweight, medium weight, or heavyweight. Lightweight mesh has a density less than 40 g/m^2.[4] Lighter, more flexible meshes were thought to generate less host inflammation and therefore decrease the patient-perceived mesh sensation and chronic pain.[9] However, this flexibility comes at a cost. Lightweight mesh has been associated with central mesh fractures and subsequent hernia repair failure.[10] These mesh fractures are likely caused by a combination of mesh degradation in host tissues and fatigue under the repeated forces generated by the abdominal wall.

Medium weight mesh density falls somewhere between 40 and 60 g/m^2. Medium weight mesh was purported to leverage the advantages of both lightweight and heavyweight mesh. Compared with heavyweight mesh, it has larger pores, which may allow it to clear an infection more easily. It is also denser than lightweight mesh, perhaps making it less likely to fracture. However, we have recently questioned the durability of medium weight mesh in abdominal wall reconstruction. In a retrospective review of medium weight mesh, Maskal and colleagues found the central mesh fracture rate to be 4.1%.[11] Central mesh fracture rates were particularly high among patients who underwent a bridged repair (30%). Although 4.1% may not seem like a significant fracture rate, we perform some 400 abdominal wall reconstructions annually, making the number of central mesh fractures—and therefore hernia recurrences—on the order of 16 per year. We interpret this number as unacceptably high because these patients are often subjected to redo posterior components separation with TAR, which carries high morbidity.[12]

Heavyweight mesh has a density of at least 75 g/m^2. Its higher density makes it less vulnerable to fracture under the physiologic stress of the abdominal wall. This durability was thought to have a downside as reports surfaced of patients experiencing mesh sensations after implantation of heavyweight mesh. Early studies found that heavyweight mesh was associated with more chronic pain than lightweight mesh.[13] However, Krpata and colleagues, in a randomized controlled trial (RCT) comparing medium weight to heavyweight mesh in open, clean retromuscular ventral hernia repairs, found that pain scores at 30 days and 1 year were identical in both groups.[14] Quality of life between the 2 study arms was also similar at 1 year. Given the similar patient-reported outcomes between heavyweight and medium weight mesh and the lower long-term durability of medium weight mesh, we prefer to use permanent heavyweight mesh in clean abdominal wall reconstruction cases. We do not know if permanent heavyweight mesh is safe to use in contaminated cases.

Composite Mesh

One additional permanent synthetic mesh deserves to be discussed—composite mesh. Composite mesh comprises at least 2 materials and is designed to be placed in the peritoneal cavity. One side of the mesh is permanent material, often polypropylene, which reinforces the hernia repair. The other side is a resorbable collagen barrier that inhibits visceral adhesions.[4] The collagen coating also prevents tissue ingrowth, making them unattractive for abdominal wall reconstruction. We use composite mesh for laparoscopic or robotic intraperitoneal onlay mesh repairs; we do not use composite mesh for retromuscular abdominal wall reconstruction.

Short-Term Absorbable Mesh

Mesh that is replaced by the host's tissues is absorbable mesh. Absorbable mesh is further classified either as short-term or long-term absorbable mesh. Short-term absorbable mesh types include Dexon (Covidien, Mansfield, MA), a polyglycolic acid mesh, and Vicryl (Ethicon, Inc., Somerville, NJ), a polyglactin 910 mesh. These meshes are completely resorbed in 60 to 90 days[15] and, because they are absorbed, can be placed directly on the bowel.[16] Short-term absorbable mesh plays important roles in abdominal wall reconstruction.

Staged Hernia Repairs

One way these fast-absorbing meshes can be used is in "staged" situations. Incisional hernias are often encountered in "less-than-ideal" circumstances, including emergent hernia repairs, stoma takedowns, infected mesh excisions, and enterocutaneous fistula closures. The decision to proceed with abdominal wall reconstruction in these instances is not straightforward. When faced with this situation, several factors should be considered.

- Will the patient likely need additional abdominal operations?
- Can the circumstances (eg, level of contamination, patient hemodynamics, or patient comorbidities) be improved to optimize the outcome for the patient?
- Am I comfortable performing abdominal wall reconstruction given the hernia size and setting?

If the answer is yes to the first 2 questions and no to the third, we recommend consideration of a "staged" approach to abdominal wall reconstruction.[16] This staged approach involves either closing the hernia primarily, or, if it is too wide, closing the hernia with an absorbable mesh inlay. In these situations, we prefer to use fast-absorbing mesh, such as Vicryl mesh, for 2 reasons. Earlier studies support low fistula rates (5%) when it is used in under these circumstances and its price is lower than biologic or biosynthetic mesh.[17] A biologic or long-term absorbable synthetic (biosynthetic) mesh may also be used as a mesh inlay, and prospective studies have also shown low rates of fistula formation (5%) when these meshes are used.[18] If the hernia recurs after placement of an absorbable mesh bridge, definitive abdominal wall reconstruction can be performed when the patient and operating conditions are optimized.

Short-term absorbable mesh has a second important use in abdominal wall reconstruction. It can be used to bridge the posterior fascial elements when they cannot be closed without tension. This situation may occur during the repair of large lateral or loss of domain hernias. Short-term absorbable mesh may also be used to close fenestrations in the peritoneum of the posterior fascia. These fenestrations must be closed to prevent intraparietal hernia formation.[19] Short-term absorbable mesh, such as polyglactin 910 mesh, is thought to be replaced with peritoneum; however, high-quality studies in the space are lacking.[20] We advise against bridging the posterior fascia with composite mesh to avoid a synthetic mesh-on-synthetic mesh situation that would limit mesh incorporation into the retromuscular space.

LONG-TERM ABSORBABLE MESH
Biosynthetic Mesh

A dreaded complication of permanent synthetic mesh use in hernia repair is mesh infection. For decades, permanent mesh has been thought to be particularly susceptible to infection when used in a contaminated case. Many complex hernia repairs, however, involve some level of contamination. Concomitant gastrointestinal procedures may be performed or chronic abdominal wounds may be encountered. Parastomal hernia repairs also involve some level of contamination. Given the purported risks associated with permanent synthetic mesh use in contaminated fields, long-term absorbable meshes, or biosynthetic meshes were engineered. Biosynthetic mesh provides hernia repair reinforcement while ultimately becoming replaced by native tissue over time, possible making them less likely to harbor chronic infections than permanent synthetic mesh.[14] One biosynthetic mesh has been prospectively evaluated in contaminated ventral hernia repairs—GORE BIO-A Tissue Reinforcement (W.L. Gore & Associates, Inc., Newark, DE).

The COBRA study prospectively evaluated GORE BIO-A in the single-stage repair of contaminated ventral hernias across 9 sites in the United States and the Netherlands.[21] GORE BIO-A is a polyglycolide-trimethylene carbonate copolymer that is resorbed by about 6 months.[22] A total of 104 patients were included in the study with a mean hernia width of 9 cm. Study participants underwent open ventral hernia repair with Centers for Disease Control (CDC) class II (23%) and III (77%) wounds. At 2 years postoperatively, 28% had experienced a wound event but no complete mesh excisions were required. The hernia recurrence rate was 14% at 2 years postoperatively, and patient quality of life improved from baseline. Overall, this single-arm, prospective study found that GORE-BIO mesh had adequate durability with high wound event rates in the single-stage repair of contaminated ventral hernias.

A second biosynthetic mesh, Phasix Mesh (BD, Franklin Lakes, NJ), was recently studied in CDC class I ventral hernia repairs. Phasix mesh is a poly-4-hydroxybutyrate (P4HB) polymer that is resorbed between 12 and 18 months.[14] A recent study of 5-year outcomes after open abdominal wall reconstruction with Phasix mesh showed mixed results.[23] A total of 121 patients were enrolled with a mean hernia width of 8.6 cm. At 30 days postoperatively, the surgical site infections (SSIs) rate was 10.1% and no mesh excisions were required. The overall hernia recurrence rate was 22.0% at 5 years, although the recurrence rate in retromuscular repairs was only 11.4%. These results should be interpreted with caution, however, because just 44.6% of patients were available for follow-up at 5 years. The authors deserve to be commended for the 5-year follow-up in this study, which showed acceptable wound event and hernia recurrence rates (**Table 2**).

Biologic Mesh

Biologic meshes are acellular collagen matrices derived from human or animal tissue and tend to be classified according to their tissue source—dermal, pericardial, or

Table 2
Biosynthetic mesh options

Mesh (Manufacturer)	Material	Pore Size (mm)	Mesh Density (g/m²)	Absorption
Phasix (Bard-Davol)	P4HB	0.26	182	12–18 mo
TIGR Matrix (Novus)	1. Primary matrix—PLA:TMC	-	-	Partial after 4 mo, complete after 3 y
	2. Secondary matrix—PGA:TMC			
BIO-A (GORE)	67% PGA; 33% TMC	-	-	6 mo

Abbreviations: P4HB, poly-4-hydroxybutyric acid; PGA, polyglycolic acid; PLA, polylactic acid; TMC, trimethylene carbonate.

submucosal. Because biologic mesh undergoes neovascularization and host immune cell infiltration, it was initially considered to be a safer alternative to permanent synthetic mesh.[24,25] Early studies also indicated that biologic mesh was safe in contaminated hernia repairs, although only 2 meshes have been prospectively studied in this setting—Strattice Reconstructive Tissue Matrix (LifeCell Corporation, Branchburg, NJ) and OviTex Reinforced Tissue Matrix (TELA Bio Inc., Malvern, PA) (**Table 3**).

The RICH study, a prospective, single-arm trial, evaluated Strattice mesh, a porcine dermal matrix, in the single-stage repair of contaminated ventral hernias across 12 United States sites.[26] This study included 85 patients with large hernias (mean hernia width was 16 cm) with CDC wound classes II (49%), III (49%), and IV (2%). At 2 years postoperatively, the majority of patients (66%) had experienced a wound event but no complete mesh excisions were required. The hernia recurrence rate for repairs with complete fascial closure was 23% at 2 years. In general, Strattice mesh allowed for successful, single-stage abdominal wall reconstruction in contaminated cases for greater than 70% of patients but the wound event rate was high.

The BRAVO study, a prospective, single-arm, multicenter study evaluated OviTex 1S mesh in ventral hernia repair. OviTex 1S mesh is an ovine rumen matrix with a permanent or absorbable synthetic polymer embroidered into the mesh.[27] A total of 92 patients underwent both open and minimally invasive repairs with OviTex mesh. Study participants had a mean hernia width of 8.11 cm, and the trial included mostly CDC class I cases (80.4%), with some class II (15.2%) and III (4.4%) cases. At 2 years postoperatively, wound events were seen in 38% of patients, and 3 patients underwent partial or complete mesh removal. The hernia recurrence rate was 4.5% at 2 years but the authors did not describe how they determined hernia recurrence. Global and hernia-specific quality of life improved from baseline for study participants.

Table 3
Biologic mesh options

Mesh (Manufacturer)	Material	Mesh Density (g/m²)	Absorption
Alloderm (AbbVie)	Human cadaveric matrix	Variable	Permanent
Strattice (AbbVie)	Porcine dermal matrix	Variable	Permanent
Flex HD (MTF Biologics)	Human cadaveric matrix	Variable	Permanent
OviTex (TELA Bio)	PGA; sheep rumen	12–15 g/m²	Permanent

Abbreviation: PGA, polyglycolic acid.

Overall, this trial of mostly clean ventral hernia repairs, found that OviTex mesh was a viable option but the wound event rate was high.

These prospective, single-arm studies have shown that biologic and biosynthetic meshes perform adequately in contaminated ventral hernia repairs. An additional consideration, however, is the cost of these meshes. Biologic and biosynthetic mesh cost more than synthetic mesh. Some biologic meshes are 200 times more expensive than their synthetic counterparts.[28] Biologic and biosynthetic mesh should therefore outperform synthetic mesh in contaminated ventral hernia repair to justify their cost. However, early hopes that biologic mesh would outperform synthetic mesh have not been borne out in the data.

Synthetic or Biologic Mesh in Contaminated Hernia Repair

No prospective, head-to-head studies have yet compared biosynthetic with synthetic mesh for contaminated ventral hernia repairs; however, 3 RCTs have compared biologic with synthetic mesh in the single-stage repair of contaminated ventral hernias. Olivarria and colleagues compared biologic mesh (porcine acellular dermal matrix) with synthetic mesh (medium weight, macroporous polypropylene) in open retromuscular ventral hernia repair.[29] Most cases (68%) were CDC class II to IV, and median hernia width was 6 cm. A total of 87 patients were included (44 biologic and 43 synthetic mesh). At 1 year postoperatively, the rate of major complications (a composite of mesh infection, hernia recurrence, and reoperation) was higher in the biologic than synthetic group, although this was not statistically significant (42.4% vs 21.6%, respectively; $P = .071$).

The second RCT performed by Harris and colleagues found similar results.[30] They compared Strattice with synthetic (Ventralight ST or Soft Mesh, CR Bard, Murray Hill, NJ) mesh in ventral hernia repair. Some contaminated cases (CDC class II to IV) were included (31%). They found that SSIs rates were similar between the 2 groups (biologic 39% vs synthetic 34%, $P = .227$). However, the use of synthetic mesh was associated with lower hernia recurrence rates than biologic mesh at 2 years (22% vs 40%, respectively, $P = .035$).

The third RCT, by Rosen and colleagues, compared Strattice mesh with medium weight, macroporous polypropylene mesh (Bard Soft Mesh, CR Bard, Murray Hill, NJ) in CDC class II and III retromuscular ventral hernia repairs.[28] Synthetic mesh outperformed biologic mesh with respect to hernia recurrence at 2 years (5.6% vs 20.5%, respectively), with an absolute risk reduction of 14.9% with synthetic mesh (95% CI, −23.8 to −6.1; $P = .001$). Mesh safety, defined as surgical site occurrences requiring procedural intervention, was similar between the 2 groups up to 2 years postoperatively (odds ratio, 1.22; 95% CI, 0.60–2.44; $P = .58$). Quality of life was also similar between the 2 groups at 2 years postoperatively.

A meta-analysis of studies comparing synthetic to biologic mesh, published in 2023, found that hernia recurrence rates were higher for biologic compared with synthetic mesh (OR 2.75; 95% CI 1.76–4.31; $P < .00001$).[31] SSIs were higher in the biologic versus the synthetic group (OR 1.53; 95% CI 1.02–2.29; $P = .04$). Rates of hematomas, seromas, and mesh excision were similar between the 2 groups.

Although these recent studies support the safety and durability of synthetic mesh for contaminated ventral hernia repairs, a more nuanced understanding of these results is important. These studies were performed by surgeons with advanced training in abdominal wall reconstruction, so these results may not be generalizable to surgeons or institutions that perform these operations at low volumes. Furthermore, some of the cases included in these studies could have been staged and the subsequent operation performed under clean conditions. For example, 57% of the patients in the study by Rosen and colleagues, essentially all those who did not have a parastomal hernia repair, could have undergone a staged hernia repair with definitive abdominal wall reconstruction and permanent mesh placement at a later date.

Authors' Mesh Choice for Abdominal Wall Reconstruction

The mesh characteristics discussed all play a role in mesh selection for abdominal wall reconstruction. For complex hernia repair, we perform posterior components separation, often with a TAR procedure. This is essentially a wide preperitoneal dissection, which creates a large retromuscular pocket outside the peritoneal cavity. This space is the ideal location for bare, permanent synthetic mesh for a few reasons. The retromuscular space is well vascularized, which optimizes tissue ingrowth into the macroporous permanent mesh while excluding it from the peritoneal cavity. The retromuscular space can also be matured widely, allowing placement of a large piece of mesh for sufficient overlap of the hernia defect.

For clean abdominal wall reconstruction cases, we prefer to use heavyweight mesh in clean cases because it is more durable than medium weight mesh and is not associated with increased pain or a patient-perceived mesh sensation. For clean-contaminated and contaminated abdominal wall reconstruction cases, we feel the data justify the use of medium weight polypropylene mesh. It should be noted, however, that no mesh—synthetic, biologic, or biosynthetic—is US Food and Drug Administration—approved for use in CDC class II, III, or IV cases. The use of heavyweight mesh under contaminated circumstances has not been rigorously studies, and we therefore cannot recommend its use in these settings.

SUMMARY

A wide variety of mesh choices is available for abdominal wall reconstruction. Each mesh has unique characteristics that give it certain advantages and disadvantages, depending on the position of its placement in the abdominal wall and the circumstances under which it is used. If the prosthetic is permanent, surgeons should be familiar with the features of the mesh they are placing in the patient, including mesh material, pore size, and density. If hernia repair circumstances are suboptimal, a staged approach to abdominal wall reconstruction is probably the safest approach.

CLINICS CARE POINTS

- Evidence supports the use of heavy weight over medium weight permanent synthetic mesh in clean retromuscular abdominal wall reconstruction cases.
- For clean-contaminated or contaminated retromuscular abdominal wall reconstruction cases, evidence supports medium weight permanent synthetic mesh over biologic mesh.
- For hernias repaired in a "staged" fashion under contaminated or suboptimal conditions when the fascia cannot be closed primarily, evidence supports the use of short-term absorbable mesh, biologic, or biosynthetic mesh as an inlay repair.

DISCLOSURE

The authors have nothing to disclose.

REFERENCES

1. Read R. Milestones in the history of hernia surgery: prosthetic repair. Hernia 2004;8:8–14.
2. Luijendijk RW, Hop WC, van den Tol MP, et al. A comparison of suture repair with mesh repair for incisional hernia. N Engl J Med 2000;343(6):392–8.
3. Krpata DM, Blatnik JA, Novitsky YW, et al. Posterior and open anterior components separations: a comparative analysis. Am J Surg 2012;203(3):318–22.
4. Bilsel Y, Abci I. The search for ideal hernia repair; mesh materials and types. Int J Surg 2012;10(6):317–21.
5. Sanders D, Lambie J, Bond P, et al. An in vitro study assessing the effect of mesh morphology and suture fixation on bacterial adherence. Hernia 2013;17(6): 779–89.
6. Greca FH, de Paula JB, Biondo-Simões ML, et al. The influence of differing pore sizes on the biocompatibility of two polypropylene meshes in the repair of abdominal defects: experimental study in dogs. Hernia 2001;5(2):59–64.
7. Orenstein SB, Saberski ER, Kreutzer DL, et al. Comparative analysis of histopathologic effects of synthetic meshes based on material, weight, and pore size in mice. J Surg Res 2012;176(2):423–9.
8. Aldridge AJ, Simson JN. Erosion and perforation of colon by synthetic mesh in a recurrent paracolostomy hernia. Hernia 2001;5(2):110–2.
9. Cobb WS, Kercher KW, Heniford BT. The argument for lightweight polypropylene mesh in hernia repair. Surg Innov 2005;12(1):63–9.
10. Petro CC, Nahabet EH, Criss CN, et al. Central failures of lightweight monofilament polyester mesh causing hernia recurrence: a cautionary note. Hernia 2015;19:155–9.
11. Maskal S, Miller B, Ellis R, et al. Mediumweight polypropylene mesh fractures after open retromuscular ventral hernia repair: incidence and associated risk factors, *Surg Endosc*, 2023. doi: 10.1007/s00464-023-10039-4. Online ahead of print.
12. Montelione KC, Zolin SJ, Fafaj A, et al. Outcomes of redo-transversus abdominis release for abdominal wall reconstruction. Hernia 2021;25(6):1581–92.
13. DeLong CG, Doble JA, Schilling AL, et al. Delineating the burden of chronic postoperative pain in patients undergoing open repair of complex ventral hernias. Am J Surg 2018;215(4):610–7.
14. Deeken CR, Matthews BD. Characterization of the mechanical strength, resorption properties, and histologic characteristics of a fully absorbable material (poly-4-hydroxybutyrate-PHASIX mesh) in a porcine model of hernia repair. ISRN Surg 2013;2013:238067.
15. Krpata DM, Petro CC, Prabhu AS, et al. Effect of hernia mesh weights on postoperative patient-related and clinical outcomes after open ventral hernia repair. JAMA Surg 2021;156(12):1085–92.
16. Petro CC, Rosen MJ. Fight or Flight: The Role of Staged Approaches to Complex Abdominal Wall Reconstruction. Plast Reconstr Surg 2018 Sep;142:38S–44S.
17. Fabian TC, Croce MA, Pritchard FE, et al. Planned ventral hernia. Staged management for acute abdominal wall defects. Ann Surg 1994;219(6):643–53.
18. De Vries FEE, Claessen JJM, Arterna JJ, et al. Immediate closure of abdominal cavity with biologic mesh versus temporary abdominal closure of open abdomen in non-trauma emergency patients (CLOSE-UP study). Surg Inf 2020;21(8): 694–703.
19. Carbonell AM. Interparietal hernias after open retromuscular hernia repair. Hernia 2008;12(6):663–6.

20. Liu L, Petro C, Majumder A, et al. The use of Vicryl mesh in a porcine model to assess its safety as an adjunct to posterior fascial closure during retromuscular mesh placement. Hernia 2016;20(2):289–95.

21. Rosen MJ, Bauer JJ, Harmaty M, et al. Multicenter, Prospective, Longitudinal Study of the Recurrence, Surgical Site Infection, and Quality of Life After Contaminated Ventral Hernia Repair Using Biosynthetic Absorbable Mesh: The COBRA Study. Ann Surg 2017;265(1):205–11.

22. Katz AR, Mukherjee DP, Kaganov AL, et al. A new synthetic monofilament absorbable suture made from polytrimethylene carbonate. Surg Gynecol Obstet 1985; 161:213–22.

23. Roth JS, Anthone GJ, Selzer DJ, et al. Long-term, prospective, multicenter study of poly-4-hydroxybutyrate mesh (Phasix mesh) for hernia repair in cohort at for complication: 60-month follow-up. J Am Coll Surg 2022;235(6):894–904.

24. Sandor M, Xu H, Connor J, et al. Host response to implanted porcine-derived biologic materials in a primate model of abdominal wall repair. Tissue Eng Part A 2008;14:2012–31.

25. Burns NK, Jaffari MV, Rios CN, et al. Non-cross-linked porcine acellular dermal matrices for abdominal wall reconstruction. Plast Reconstr Surg 2010;125: 167–76.

26. Itani KMF, Rosen MJ, Vargo D, et al. Prospective study of single-stage repair of contaminated hernias using a biologic porcine tissue matrix: the RICH study. Surgery 2012;152(3):498–505.

27. DeNoto G III, Ceppa EP, Pacella SJ, et al. 24-month results of the BRAVO study: A prospective, multi-center study evaluating the clinical outcomes of a ventral hernia cohort treated with OviTex® 1S permanent reinforced tissue matrix. Ann Med Surg 2022;83:104745.

28. Rosen MJ, Krpata DM, Petro CC, et al. Biologic vs synthetic mesh for single-stage repair of contaminated ventral hernias: a randomized clinical trial. JAMA Surgery 2022 1;157(4):293–301.

29. Olavarria OA, Bernardi K, Dhanani NH, et al. Synthetic versus biologic mesh for complex open ventral hernia repair: A pilot randomized controlled trial. Surg Infect 2021;22(5):496–503.

30. Harris HW, Primus F, Young C, et al. Preventing recurrence in clean and contaminated hernias using biologic versus synthetic mesh in ventral hernia repair: the PRICE randomized controlled trial. Ann Surg 2021;273(4):648–55.

31. Mazzola Poli de Figueiredo S, Tastaldi L, Mao RD, et al. Biologic versus synthetic mesh in open ventral hernia repair: A systematic review and meta-analysis of randomized controlled trials [published online ahead of print, 2023 Jan 7]. Surgery 2023;173(4):1001–7.

Hernia Mesh Complications

Management of Mesh Infections and Enteroprosthetic Fistula

Kathryn A. Schlosser, MD[a], Jeremy A. Warren, MD[b,*]

KEYWORDS

- Prosthetic mesh infection • Ventral hernia repair • Mesh salvage
- Abdominal wall reconstruction • Enteroprosthetic fistula

KEY POINTS

- Mesh infection is a potentially devastating complication, which can lead to chronic morbidity, significant cost, and multiple reinterventions after elective hernia repair.
- There is little high-quality data to guide the management of mesh infection.
- The risk of mesh infection is minimized through preoperative patient optimization, perioperative strategies to prevent contamination, choice of operative approach, mesh selection, and placement.
- Mesh characteristics and location in the abdominal wall are key factors to successful salvage. Macroporous, monofilament mesh in an extraperitoneal position is salvageable in most cases.

INTRODUCTION
Significance of Mesh Infection

Prosthetic mesh infection (PMI) is a potentially devastating complication of ventral hernia repair (VHR). Although the risk of PMI after VHR is relatively low, with an average of 610,000 VHR performed annually in the United States, the prevalence of this complication warrants a clear understanding of patient and surgical risk factors for PMI and optimal treatment strategies.[1] PMI may result in significant cost, multiple additional procedures, patient disability, and negative impact on quality of life. However, due to low quality of evidence in the literature, limited postmarket surveillance, and significant heterogeneity in the technical aspects of VHR, surgeons are often left with only

a Department of Surgery, Prisma Health, 701 Grove Road, Support Tower 3, Greenville, SC 29605, USA; b Department of Surgery, Division of Minimal Access Surgery, University of South Carolina School of Medicine Greenville, Prisma Health, 701 Grove Road, Support Tower 3, Greenville, SC 29605, USA
* Corresponding author.
E-mail address: Jeremy.warren@prismahealth.org
Twitter: @KT_Schlosser (K.A.S.)

Surg Clin N Am 103 (2023) 1029–1042
https://doi.org/10.1016/j.suc.2023.04.011
0039-6109/23/© 2023 Elsevier Inc. All rights reserved.

surgical.theclinics.com

personal experience and expert opinion to guide the prevention and management of PMI. Herein, we outline strategies for the prevention, diagnosis, and treatment of PMI.

Definition

There is a lack of standardized reporting of PMI. Diagnostic criteria for PMI include positive culture of periprosthetic fluid collection, mesh exposure, poor mesh incorporation, and/or signs of infection such as wound breakdown, necrosis, enteric fistula or purulence, and clinical suspicion.[2] Large databases such as the American College of Surgeons National Surgical Quality Improvement Program, National Inpatient Survey, and National Ambulatory Surgical Sample capture surgical site infections (SSI) but lack a distinct category for PMI.[3] The Abdominal Core Health Quality Collaborative (ACHQC) is the only national registry that specifically captures PMI but is a voluntary database with a relatively small sample of participating surgeons across the country.[4]

Incidence and risk factors

Understanding the risk of PMI and management options is critical to avoid the "vicious cycle" of PMI; mesh explantation, hernia recurrence, and subsequent repair of a more complex recurrent hernia.[5] Due to nonstandardized reporting, the incidence of PMI varies widely in the literature and is often extrapolated based on reported rates of surgical site occurrence (SSO), SSI, SSO/SSI requiring procedural intervention (SSOPI), or subsequent operations for mesh explantation.[6] Incidence of PMI after open VHR ranges from 1% to 10.1%. This is lower after minimally invasive repair (MIS) 1% to 3%.[7–12] However, with multiple techniques used for VHR and numerous mesh materials available, PMI risk factors and prevention strategies are difficult to generalize.[13–16] The indolent nature of PMI further obscures the true incidence of mesh infections, which often presents months to years after index VHR, well outside of standard follow-up duration.[17]

Recognition of modifiable risk factors for SSI, technical factors that may increase the risk of PMI, and mesh characteristics that affect both risk and management of PMI are all critical for successful management. Patient factors that may increase the risk of PMI include immunosuppression, methicillin-resistant *Staphylococcus aureus* (MRSA) colonization, uncontrolled diabetes mellitus, smoking, and obesity. Operative factors such as intraoperative contamination, duration of surgery, and repair of recurrent hernias also increase this risk, as does development of postoperative SSO or SSI.[14,18–21] The impact of operative approach, surgical technique, and mesh selection on the risk and management of PMI are discussed below.

Microbiology

Initial bacterial inoculation most often occurs intraoperatively from skin flora, which is the most common source, or enteric contamination but may also derive from hematogenous spread with oral, enteric, or other flora. Bacteria at this stage have a free-floating "planktonic" phenotype, are metabolically active, and are more susceptible to antibiotics. Once bacteria adhere to tissue or prosthetic, they enter a proliferation and accumulation phase. Presentation at this stage is likely a periprosthetic fluid collection or purulent drainage. Bacteria may also progress to secrete a protein-polysaccharide matrix known as a biofilm. As biofilm matures, bacteria enter a quiescent state, making them less susceptible to antibiotic therapy.[20] Biofilm creates an environment that promotes antibiotic resistance through mechanical shielding, protection from immunoglobulins and host phagocytes, and increasing antimicrobial resistance through lateral gene transfer.[22,23] Diagnosis of PMI is more difficult if biofilm forms because bacteria often fail to grow using standard culture methods. Advanced microscopic or fluorescence in situ hybridization techniques are capable of capturing quiescent bacteria in biofilm but are not commonly used.[16] When explanted mesh is and examined using these techniques, even in the absence of clinical infection, biofilm formation with one or more microbes is often identified.[24] Clinically, this state is associated with a low-grade inflammatory response but rarely suppuration.

S aureus is the dominant organism associated with PMI (70%–80%), and up to half are MRSA.[2,13,20] MRSA produces a particularly pernicious biofilm, making eradication and mesh salvage with antibiotics or local wound care alone nearly impossible. Other infectious organisms include skin flora such as *Staphylococcus epidermidis*, enteric flora such as *Escherichia coli* and *Enterococcus faecalis*, or oral and dental flora due to poor dentition and associated bacteremia. Presence of enteric organisms should raise the suspicion of enteroprosthetic fistula, particularly with delayed presentation. However, in the absence of a fistula, these bacteria are more often associated with successful salvage in our experience.

Technique and Textiles

Physiomechanical properties and biocompatibility of mesh play a major role in bacterial penetrance, adhesion, and propagation of biofilm. In particular, the porosity and interfilament distance largely determines bacterial adhesion, with smaller pore size and interfilament distance increasing the risk of adherence.[10,25] Interfilament distance also impacts scar plate formation, which is associated with mesh contraction, encapsulation, and changes in permeability.[20,23] The effective porosity of a mesh may be further decreased by antiadhesive barrier coatings and host foreign body reaction (**Fig. 1**).[26] Decreasing the effective porosity inhibits host immune response and tissue integration and enhances bacterial adhesion, decreasing the likelihood of mesh salvage.[23]

Recent studies provide insight into mesh characteristics and operative technique that are optimal for prevention and clearance of PMI.[27–29] Microporous and multifilament mesh may promote bacterial adherence while impairing host immune response and antibiotic penetration.[20,27] In contrast, macroporous monofilament mesh is associated with greater tissue ingrowth, lower bacterial adherence, and decreased biofilm formation, which clinically translates into greater mesh salvage.[30] Barrier coatings designed to prevent adhesions may also play a role in PMI and impact mesh salvage. These materials are most often placed in an intraperitoneal position (IPOM) where PMI is least salvageable. When placed in a retromuscular position, they seem to increase the risk of SSO compared with noncoated mesh.[31]

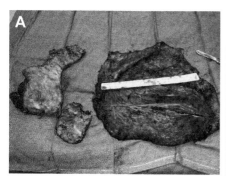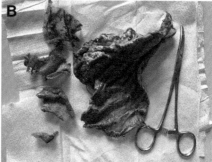

Fig. 1. (*A*) Fibrous encapsulation of an intraperitoneal composite mesh of PTFE + PP. (*B*) Contraction and deformation of an intraperitoneal PTFE mesh (*right*) and separate microporous barrier-coated PP.

The interplay of mesh characteristics and position in the abdominal wall further affects the incidence and outcome of PMI. Mesh onlay has a higher rate of SSI and SSO than sublay mesh placement.[32] Retromuscular repair places mesh in a well-vascularized compartment that promotes tissue ingrowth, decreases the risk of SSI, and improves the likelihood of salvage should PMI develop.[29,33] The combination of retromuscular repair with a noncoated, macroporous, monofilament polypropylene (PP) seems to be ideal for minimizing the risk of PMI and mesh explantation,[16] and in fact demonstrates safety and efficacy even in the setting of clean-contaminated and contaminated cases.[34,35] MIS repair consistently demonstrates the lowest risk of PMI. However, standard laparoscopic ventral hernia repair (LVHR) involves mesh placed in the IPOM,[36,37] making salvage difficult. Up to 25% of patients will require a subsequent abdominal operation (SAO) after VHR, and a significant proportion are clean-contaminated or contaminated cases, posing a significant risk for secondary PMI with intraperitoneal mesh (**Fig. 2**).[38] Thus, the impact of mesh selection and position at the time of index VHR is significant, and the short-term outcomes are not the only consideration for long-term success. The introduction of robotic VHR greatly facilitates MIS placement of extraperitoneal mesh, although the long-term impact of this development remains unclear.[39,40]

Biologic and absorbable synthetic meshes theoretically provide a scaffold for tissue ingrowth while decreasing or eliminating the risk of SSI and PMI. Unfortunately, this purported advantage has not been confirmed in the literature, and behavior in vivo can vary widely based tissue source, processing, polymers, and as yet uncharacterized host tissue interactions.[41] Clinically these products have similar rates of SSO and SSI and higher rates of hernia recurrence.[39,41,42] In the only randomized control trial to date, Rosen and colleagues demonstrate superiority of macroporous PP over porcine acellular dermis for open retromuscular VHR in clean-contaminated and contaminated cases for hernia recurrence, with no difference in the risk of SSO, SSI, SSOPI, or mesh explantation.[43] It should be noted that no mesh is currently approved by the Federal Drug Administration for placement in clean-contaminated, contaminated, or dirty cases.

PATIENT EVALUATION AND TREATMENT

PMI often presents with new or persistent pain, cellulitis, exposed mesh, or purulent drainage (**Fig. 3**). Delayed presentation is common, and in our experience occurs a

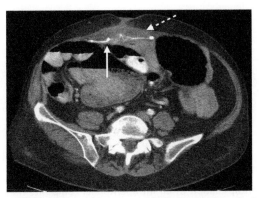

Fig. 2. Secondary infection of PTFE mesh after exploration for bowel obstruction requiring resection. Solid arrow—PTFE mesh; dashed arrow—periprosthetic fluid collection.

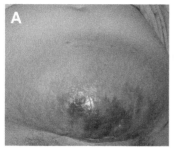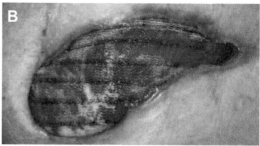

Fig. 3. (*A*) Patient presenting with new abdominal wall cellulitis and distant history of LVHR with IPOM. (*B*) Exposed PP mesh after onlay repair complicated by superficial SSI. Ultimately salvaged with the use of NPWT.

mean of 19.9 months after repair.[38] A history of SSI, seroma, or hematoma is common.[20,21,44] Patients with an SAO after index VHR, particularly if contaminated, should raise the index of suspicion for secondary PMI. If drainage or an open wound is present, a culture should be obtained and empiric antibiotics initiated, with or without wound opening. Computed tomography (CT) imaging is useful in confirming the diagnosis and defining the extent of infection. Periprosthetic fluid collection, inflammatory changes, adherent adjacent viscera, extraluminal air, or enteric contrast extravasation suggest PMI or enteroprosthetic fistula. Culture of periprosthetic fluid should guide antibiotic therapy and drainage may aid in clearance of infection.

Patient expectations and goals of treatment affect the management strategy of PMI. Operative debridement and mesh excision, coupled with a likely inevitable hernia recurrence is an arduous undertaking. Some patients may prefer long-term antibiotic suppression with local wound management as needed, which may in fact provide a better quality of life. Treatment must be tailored for each patient depending on their clinical presentation, and conditions may evolve that necessitate alterations in that management plan over time. When surgical intervention is needed, preoperative optimization is recommended, whenever feasible, to improve the outcomes of mesh explantation. This includes weight loss, smoking cessation, glycemic control, and nutritional support. The inflammatory state induced by PMI will itself exacerbate hyperglycemia, however, and will limit the ability to lower glycosylated hemoglobin (HbA1c). Delaying treatment in such cases is unnecessary, and the removal of the infectious source will likely improve HbA1c. Our algorithm outlining workup and management of PMI is shown in **Fig. 4** and elaborated upon in the following sections.

Mesh Salvage

Antibiotic therapy
In the absence of enteroprosthetic fistula or severe systemic infection, attempts at mesh salvage is reasonable and begins with local wound care and antibiotic therapy. Empiric antibiotics should reflect local antibiograms and target skin flora, particularly MRSA. Cultures should guide antibiotics whenever possible. Local wound care with wet to dry dressings and/or negative pressure wound therapy (NPWT) is indicated for any wound breakdown, with or without mesh exposure. In cases with favorable mesh characteristics and position, particularly macroporous monofilament PP placed in an extraperitoneal plane, these measures are often adequate for mesh salvage.[17,36,45–47] Antibiotic therapy should be continued while there are signs of active soft tissue or systemic infection, until mesh removal is performed, or in rare

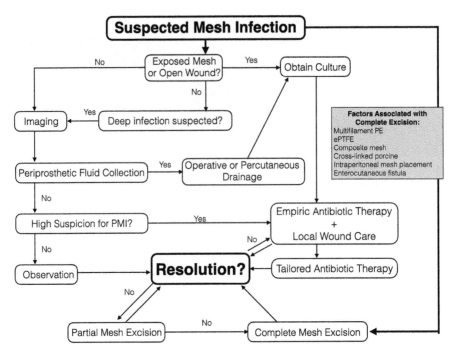

Fig. 4. Algorithm for the evaluation and management of PMI.

cases for chronic suppression in patients not suitable for surgical explantation. For patients with exposed mesh with planned mesh salvage, antibiotics are typically not required throughout the duration of wound care as long is it remains well drained without surrounding soft tissue infection.

Negative pressure wound therapy
Treatment with NPWT promotes fibroblast migration to aid in granulation tissue formation, clears proteinaceous exudate, stimulates neovascularization, and is useful in the treatment of PMI (see **Fig. 3**B). Successful mesh salvage with NPWT is almost exclusively confined to extraperitoneal (sublay, onlay), macroporous, monofilament mesh. Infected PTFE or multifilament polyester mesh resists the formation of granulation tissue even with NPWT,[33,38] and mesh explantation is required.

Drainage and lavage
Antibiotic lavage via percutaneous drains can also successfully salvage PMI in select cases.[48,49] Similarly, some NPWT therapy systems allow continuous irrigation of exposed mesh with antibiotic solution. Both of these methods may improve salvage but also impose a significant wound care burden on the patient and care team.[50]

Partial mesh excision
When conservative measures fail, partial or complete mesh excision (CME) is required. Partial mesh excision (PME) with debridement of unincorporated mesh and surrounding nonviable tissue, with continued local wound therapy may be adequate for salvage. Success is typically limited to materials favoring bacterial clearance, and microporous, multifilament, and intraperitoneal meshes are typically not salvaged with PME. Comparison consistently demonstrates a lower rate of postoperative wound complications, reoperation, and recurrent infection with CME (25.5%–29%)

versus PME (35%–100%).[17,51–54] However, studies are limited by sample size, and mesh properties and position are frequently underreported. Generalizable recommendations for PMI management based only on these studies, without specifically considering mesh type and location, may deter attempts at mesh salvage and subject patients to unnecessary reoperations.

Complete Mesh Excision

In cases of persistent PMI, unfavorable mesh characteristics, intraperitoneal mesh, and confirmed or suspected enteroprosthetic fistula, CME is warranted. Laminar PTFE and multifilament polyester mesh rarely clear infection and require complete excision.[18,55] Similarly, microporous mesh is more likely to require complete excision, and successful salvage of intraperitoneal mesh is rare. For PMI of intraperitoneal mesh in the absence of fistula, laparoscopic or robotic mesh excision will minimize the risk of early morbidity and improve patient recovery. It is imperative to ensure that all mesh and permanent fixation material be removed to minimize persistent or recurrent infection. For PTFE mesh, this is typically easy to do; for multifilament or microporous mesh, fibers often fray and require a more tedious dissection to guarantee complete removal.

Enteroprosthetic Fistula

Fistulization of bowel to a previously placed mesh is a unique subset of PMI (**Fig. 5**). This occurs almost exclusively with intraperitoneal mesh. Patients may present with drainage of enteric contents but often simply present with delayed onset of PMI well after index repair or SAO. In our experience, enteroprosthetic fistula presents a mean of 48.1 months after VHR, thus there should be a high index of suspicion for any PMI remote from VHR.[38] Imaging will often demonstrate extraluminal air, periprosthetic fluid, and sometimes contrast extravasation. When enteroprosthetic fistula is suspected but not confirmed on CT, a fistulogram may aid in diagnosis. However, advanced imaging is not required, given that CME is indicated in most cases of intraperitoneal PMI, particularly when fistula is suspected. Surgical management involves resection of the affected bowel and complete removal of intraperitoneal mesh. For fistulas occurring through a well-incorporated extraperitoneal mesh, PME of only the unincorporated and grossly involved mesh may be adequate. Management of the abdominal wall, discussed in more detail below, is typically limited to primary closure with staged definitive abdominal wall reconstruction (AWR).

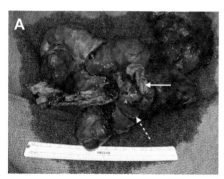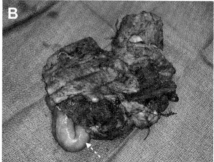

Fig. 5. (*A*) Enteroprosthetic fistula with intraluminal PTFE mesh (*solid arrow; dashed arrow—small bowel*). (*B*) Enteroprosthetic fistula of composite PTFE + PP mesh to the small bowel.

Chronic enteroprosthetic fistula resulting from erosion of the prosthetic into the viscera is a distinctly different pathologic condition than early enterocutaneous fistula resulting from bowel injury or anastomotic leak. For patients who develop PMI after extraperitoneal VHR, native tissue is interposed between the viscera and the mesh, and many early fistulae will close spontaneously. In such cases, standard treatment with control of sepsis, wound care, and nutritional optimization is appropriate, with delayed surgical resection for persistent fistulae (**Fig. 6**).

ABDOMINAL WALL MANAGEMENT

Management of any remaining abdominal wall defects after partial or CME is an important consideration, posing significant risk of recurrent infection with immediate definitive repair or the near certainty of recurrent hernia with primary closure. Up to 30% of patients will develop recurrent PMI after mesh explantation with a single-stage VHR with synthetic mesh placement.[6] Single-stage repair may be feasible when infection is sufficiently suppressed with antibiotic therapy, limited to a local area, and a new separate plane for mesh placement is available with good-quality tissue. A single-stage approach has even been described in the setting of enterocutaneous or enteroprosthetic fistula with acceptable results.[34,46,47,56] A "delayed-immediate" approach, in which mesh resection or fistula takedown with primary closure is performed initially, followed by a short course of antibiotics and definitive AWR later during the same hospitalization,[57] is also feasible. Often, however, chronic infection or fistula renders the surrounding tissue unsuitable for mobilization and closure and a staged approach is indicated. Biologic or absorbable synthetic mesh may be considered for single-stage or delayed-immediate AWR but available data do not clearly support this practice, and no mesh is currently approved for placement in a contaminated field.[34,58,59] For the majority of patients who undergo staged AWR, any operative approach is acceptable but consideration should be given for the risk of SSI and SAO.

NEW DEVELOPMENTS AND FUTURE IMPLICATIONS

Intraoperative measures, including glove change, redraping, minimizing operating room traffic, minimizing implant handling, wound irrigation, and antimicrobial

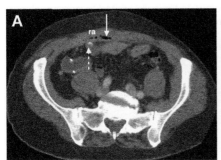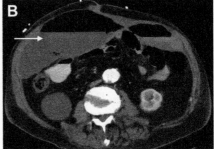

Fig. 6. (*A*) Chronic enterocutaneous fistula through a macroporous PP mesh in the retromuscular space. Ultimately required small bowel resection and PME for persistent low-output fistula. Solid arrow—air and fluid in retromuscular space; dashed arrow—staple line adherent to posterior sheath; ra—rectus abdominis. (*B*). Large infected retromuscular hematoma ultimately found to be an enterocutaneous fistula. Closed spontaneously after percutaneous drainage only, and is now 3-year postop. Solid arrow—large retromuscular abscess with air-fluid level.

dressings, have been shown to reduce prosthetic infections in orthopedic and plastic surgery.[60–63] However, data specific to PMI prevention are limited. Presoaking or intraoperative mesh irrigation with antibiotic solution does affect subsequent bacterial adhesion and biofilm formation, although this depends on mesh type and clinical evidence is limited.[30,64]

Integration of antimicrobial substances with prosthetic implants is an intriguing option for preventing PMI. Silver ion, titanium, chlorhexidine, and various antibiotics have been applied to mesh in order to reduce bacterial adhesion and infection. For example, Dualmesh Plus (W.L. Gore & Associates, Inc, Newark, DE), a laminar PTFE mesh coated with silver chlorhexidine, demonstrated lower adherence of *S aureus* compared with PP or PTFE. To date, there is no large-scale clinical evidence for any of these augmented products to support their routine use, and the complex interaction of mesh construct, tissue ingrowth, and host immunity play a larger role than the materials' antimicrobial properties alone.[65]

The best treatment of PMI remains prevention. As outlined above, mesh selection and choice of operative approach significantly affects the incidence and management of PMI.[10,12] Optimization of patient comorbidities such as glycemic control, weight loss, smoking cessation, decrease or cessation of immunosuppression, and MRSA decolonization all impact the overall risk of SSO/SSI after VHR.[11,66,67] With an estimated 610,000 VHR performed annually in the United States with an estimated cost of US$9.7 billion, any reduction in PMI has significant financial implications.[1] In 2016, Cox and colleagues estimated that preventable patient comorbidities increased hospital cost significantly after VHR, even in the absence of postoperative complications.[68] The added cost of PMI increases this calculation exponentially due to prolonged antibiotic therapy, local wound care, rehospitalization, and an average of 2 to 4 reoperations for mesh excision and recurrent VHR.[69] This does not include the impact on a patients' time, well-being, disability, or quality of life.[70]

This reality should stimulate a greater focus on understanding the risk of PMI, the technical and textile factors at play, and the optimal management, all of which are impeded by poor postmarket surveillance and the vast array of mesh products and surgical techniques in use. Comparative research is difficult due to lack of funding, heterogenous surgical techniques, the sheer number of available mesh options, and lack of detailed information on mesh properties. Most studies are retrospective, lack adequate data to derive a true incidence of PMI, and do not provide generalizable and actionable information to surgeons. The ACHQC has the potential to provide clarity to this issue but unfortunately captures only a small proportion of cases performed and is not yet scalable to the entire breadth of VHR.[4] Until long-term surveillance mechanisms for reporting mesh implantation and complications is standardized and mandated, VHR and management of PMI will at the discretion of individual surgeons guided by personal experience and expert opinion alone.

SUMMARY

Optimal management of PMI after VHR is based on limited low-quality evidence due to the heterogeneity of patient comorbidities, hernia morphology, surgical technique, mesh selection, lack of standardized reporting, poor postmarket surveillance, and shortage of high-quality long-term data. However, available evidence does provide valuable insight into the mesh characteristics and surgical techniques that can minimize the incidence of PMI and afford the best opportunity for mesh salvage. Macroporous, monofilament mesh placed in an extraperitoneal position, particularly when placed with a minimally invasive approach, seems to be ideal for decreasing the risk of PMI and promoting mesh salvage. In contrast, Intraperitoneal, microporous, multifilament, and barrier-coated meshes are least amenable to mesh salvage, typically requiring CME and staged AWR.

CLINICS CARE POINTS

- PMI is diagnosed by positive culture of periprosthetic fluid, mesh exposure, enteroprosthetic fistula, or purulence. Skin flora, particularly *S aureus* and MRSA, are the most common organisms. Biofilm formation creates a significant obstacle to diagnosis and clearance of infection.

- Presentation of PMI can be delayed by months or years after hernia repair. Delayed presentation, particularly with intraperitoneal mesh and the absence of an SAO, should raise suspicion for enteroprosthetic fistula.

- Risk factors for PMI mirror the risk factors for SSI but also include mesh characteristics, mesh location, and surgical technique used.

- PMI of macroporous PP mesh in an extraperitoneal can be salvaged in most cases with drainage, local wound care, and antibiotic therapy.

- PMI of microporous, multifilament, barrier coated, or intraperitoneal mesh will require CME in most cases. Whenever possible, we recommend MIS approach for mesh removal.

- Management of the abdominal wall after mesh excision should most often be done in a staged fashion. In select cases with limited area of infection, minimal tissue inflammation, and a new clean plane for mesh placement, a single-stage approach can be performed.

- Biologic and absorbable synthetic meshes lack sufficient evidence to recommend their routine use for either prevention of PMI or single-stage AWR after mesh excision.

DISCLOSURE

J. Warren: Intuitive Surgical, honoraria, consulting; Absolutions, nonpaid consultant; ACHQC board.

REFERENCES

1. Schlosser KA, Renshaw SM, Tamer RM, et al. Ventral hernia repair: an increasing burden affecting abdominal core health. Hernia 2022. https://doi.org/10.1007/s10029-022-02707-6.
2. Bueno-Lledó J, Ceno M, Perez-Alonso C, et al. Biosynthetic Resorbable Prosthesis is Useful in Single-Stage Management of Chronic Mesh Infection After Abdominal Wall Hernia Repair. World J Surg 2021;45:443–50.
3. NIS. National Inpatient Sample. Healthcare Cost and Utilization Project (HCUP). Available at: https://hcup-us.ahrq.gov/databases.jsp. Accessed January 2023.
4. Poulose BK, Roll S, Murphy JW, et al. Design and implementation of the Americas Hernia Society Quality Collaborative (AHSQC): improving value in hernia care. Hernia 2016;20:177–89.
5. Warren JA, Ewing JA, Carbonell AM, et al. Ventral Hernia Repair in Contaminated Field: Additional Comparative Analysis of Risks of Recurrence and Infection: In Reply to Liang and colleagues. J Am Coll Surg 2020;230:1125–6.
6. Dipp Ramos R, O'Brien WJ, Gupta K, et al. Events, care, and outcomes after hernia mesh explantation for infection. Am J Surg 2022;224:174–6.
7. Olavarria OA, Bernardi K, Shah SK, et al. Robotic versus laparoscopic ventral hernia repair: multicenter, blinded randomized controlled trial. BMJ 2020;370.

8. Mohan R, Yeow M, Wong JYS, et al. Robotic versus laparoscopic ventral hernia repair: a systematic review and meta-analysis of randomised controlled trials and propensity score matched studies. Hernia 2021;25:1565–72.

9. Pierce RA, Spitler JA, Frisella MM, et al. Pooled data analysis of laparoscopic vs. open ventral hernia repair: 14 years of patient data accrual. Surg Endosc 2007; 21:378–86.

10. Pérez-Köhler B, Bayon Y, Bellón JM. Mesh Infection and Hernia Repair: A Review. Surg Infect 2016;17:124–37.

11. Sanchez VM, Abi-Haidar YE, Itani KMF. Mesh infection in ventral incisional hernia repair: incidence, contributing factors, and treatment. Surg Infect 2011;12: 205–10.

12. Engelsman AF, van der Mei HC, Ploeg RJ, et al. The phenomenon of infection with abdominal wall reconstruction. Biomaterials 2007;28:2314–27.

13. Cobb WS, Carbonell AM, Kalbaugh CL, et al. Infection risk of open placement of intraperitoneal composite mesh. Am Surg 2009;75:762–8.

14. Hawn MT, Gray SH, Snyder CW, et al. Predictors of mesh explantation after incisional hernia repair. Am J Surg 2011;202:28–33.

15. Dipp Ramos R, O'Brien WJ, Gupta K, et al. Incidence and Risk Factors for Long-Term Mesh Explantation Due to Infection in More than 100,000 Hernia Operation Patients. J Am Coll Surg 2021;232:872–80.e2.

16. Quiroga-Centeno AC, Quiroga-Centeno CA, Guerrero-Macías S, et al. Systematic review and meta-analysis of risk factors for Mesh infection following Abdominal Wall Hernia Repair Surgery. Am J Surg 2022;224:239–46.

17. Levy S, Moszkowicz D, Poghosyan T, et al. Comparison of complete versus partial mesh removal for the treatment of chronic mesh infection after abdominal wall hernia repair. Hernia 2018;22:773–9.

18. Kao AM, Arnold MR, Augenstein VA, et al. Prevention and Treatment Strategies for Mesh Infection in Abdominal Wall Reconstruction. Plast Reconstr Surg 2018;142:149S–55S.

19. Mavros MN, Athanasiou S, Alexiou VG, et al. Risk factors for mesh-related infections after hernia repair surgery: a meta-analysis of cohort studies. World J Surg 2011;35:2389–98.

20. Wilson RB, Farooque Y. Risks and Prevention of Surgical Site Infection After Hernia Mesh Repair and the Predictive Utility of ACS-NSQIP. J Gastrointest Surg 2022;26:950–64.

21. Tolino MJ, Tripoloni DE, Ratto R, et al. Infections associated with prosthetic repairs of abdominal wall hernias: pathology, management and results. Hernia 2009;13:631–7.

22. Katsikogianni M, Missirlis YF, Harris L, et al. Concise review of mechanisms of bacterial adhesion to biomaterials and of techniques used in estimating bacteria-material interactions. Eur Cells Mater 2004;8:37–57.

23. Jacombs ASW, Karatassas A, Klosterhalfen B, et al. Biofilms and effective porosity of hernia mesh: are they silent assassins? Hernia 2020;24:197–204.

24. Kathju S, Nistico L, Melton-Kreft R, et al. Direct demonstration of bacterial biofilms on prosthetic mesh after ventral herniorrhaphy. Surg Infect 2015;16:45–53.

25. Fowler JR, Perkins TA, Buttaro BA, et al. Bacteria Adhere Less to Barbed Monofilament Than Braided Sutures in a Contaminated Wound Model. Clin Orthop Relat Res 2013;471:665–71.

26. Klinge U, Klosterhalfen B. Modified classification of surgical meshes for hernia repair based on the analyses of 1,000 explanted meshes. Hernia Hernia 2012; 16:251–8.

27. Brown GL, Richardson JD, Malangoni MA, et al. Comparison of prosthetic materials for abdominal wall reconstruction in the presence of contamination and infection. Ann Surg 1985;201:705–11.
28. Brown RH, Subramanian A, Hwang CS, et al. Comparison of infectious complications with synthetic mesh in ventral hernia repair. Am J Surg 2013;205:182–7.
29. Cobb WS, Warren JA, Ewing JA, et al. Open Retromuscular Mesh Repair of Complex Incisional Hernia: Predictors of Wound Events and Recurrence. J Am Coll Surg 2014;220:606–13.
30. Sadava EE, Krpata DM, Gao Y, et al. Does presoaking synthetic mesh in antibiotic solution reduce mesh infections? An experimental study. J Gastrointest Surg 2013;17:562–8.
31. Thomas JD, Fafaj A, Zolin SJ, et al. Non-coated versus coated mesh for retrorectus ventral hernia repair: a propensity score-matched analysis of the Americas Hernia Society Quality Collaborative (AHSQC). Hernia 2021;25:665–72.
32. Albino FP, Patel KM, Nahabedian MY, et al. Does mesh location matter in abdominal wall reconstruction? A systematic review of the literature and a summary of recommendations. Plast Reconstr Surg 2013;132:1295–304.
33. Berrevoet F, Vanlander A, Sainz-Barriga M, et al. Infected large pore meshes may be salvaged by topical negative pressure therapy. Hernia 2013;17:67–73.
34. Rosen MJ, Bauer JJ, Harmaty M, et al. Multicenter, Prospective, Longitudinal Study of the Recurrence, Surgical Site Infection, and Quality of Life After Contaminated Ventral Hernia Repair Using Biosynthetic Absorbable Mesh: The COBRA Study. Ann Surg 2017;265:205–11.
35. Carbonell AM, Criss CN, Cobb WS, et al. Outcomes of Synthetic Mesh in Contaminated Ventral Hernia Repairs. J Am Coll Surg 2013;217:991–8.
36. Chelala E, Barake H, Estievenart J, et al. Long-term outcomes of 1326 laparoscopic incisional and ventral hernia repair with the routine suturing concept: a single institution experience. Hernia 2016;20:101–10.
37. Fortelny RH, Hofmann A, May C, et al. Open and Laparo-Endoscopic Repair of Incarcerated Abdominal Wall Hernias by the Use of Biological and Biosynthetic Meshes. Front Surg 2016;3:10.
38. Warren JA, Love M, Cobb WS, et al. Factors affecting salvage rate of infected prosthetic mesh. Am J Surg 2020;220:751–6.
39. Sugiyama G, Chivukula S, Chung PJ, et al. Robot-assisted transabdominal preperitoneal ventral hernia repair. J Soc Laparoendosc Surg 2015;19.
40. Balla A, Alarcón I, Morales-Conde S. Minimally invasive component separation technique for large ventral hernia: which is the best choice? A systematic literature review. Surg Endosc 2020;34:14–30.
41. De Silva GS, Krpata DM, Gao Y, et al. Lack of identifiable biologic behavior in a series of porcine mesh explants. Surgery 2014;156:183–9.
42. Ball CG, Kirkpatrick AW, Stuleanu T, et al. Is the type of biomesh relevant in the prevention of recurrence following abdominal wall reconstruction? A randomized controlled trial. Can J Surg 2022;65:E541–9.
43. Rosen MJ, Krpata DM, Petro CC, et al. Biologic vs Synthetic Mesh for Single-stage Repair of Contaminated Ventral Hernias: A Randomized Clinical Trial. JAMA Surg 2022;157:293–301.
44. Tolino MJ, Tripoloni DE. Late-onset deep mesh infection after inguinal hernia repair. Hernia 2008;12:107 [author reply: 109].
45. Kuo YC, Mondschein JI, Soulen MC, et al. Drainage of collections associated with hernia mesh: is it worthwhile? J Vasc Interv Radiol 2010;21:362–6.

46. Rosen MJ, Krpata DM, Ermlich B, et al. A 5-year clinical experience with single-staged repairs of infected and contaminated abdominal wall defects utilizing biologic mesh. Ann Surg 2013;257:991–6.

47. Krpata DM, Stein SL, Eston M, et al. Outcomes of simultaneous large complex abdominal wall reconstruction and enterocutaneous fistula takedown. Am J Surg 2013;205:354–9.

48. Trunzo JA, Ponsky JL, Jin J, et al. A novel approach for salvaging infected prosthetic mesh after ventral hernia repair. Hernia 2009;13:545–9.

49. Aguilar B, Chapital AB, Madura JA, et al. Conservative management of mesh-site infection in hernia repair. J Laparoendosc Adv Surg Tech A 2010;20:249–52.

50. Hardee I, Wang V, Frank C, et al. Novel use of antibiotic irrigating solution in negative-pressure wound therapy for a chronically infected abdominal wall biologic mesh. Am Surg Southeastern Surgical Congress 2019;85:E596–8.

51. Bueno-Lledó J, Torregrosa-Gallud A, Carreño-Saénz O, et al. Partial versus complete removal of the infected mesh after abdominal wall hernia repair. Am J Surg 2016;214:47–52.

52. Chung L, Tse GH, O'Dwyer PJ. Outcome of patients with chronic mesh infection following abdominal wall hernia repair. Hernia 2014;18:701.

53. Mazzola Poli de Figueiredo S, Tastaldi L, Mao RMD, et al. Biologic versus synthetic mesh in open ventral hernia repair: A systematic review and meta-analysis of randomized controlled trials. Surgery 2023;173(4):1001–7.

54. Kao AM, Arnold MR, Otero J, et al. Comparison of Outcomes After Partial Versus Complete Mesh Excision. Ann Surg 2020;272:177–82.

55. Paton BL, Novitsky YW, Zerey M, et al. Management of infections of polytetrafluoroethylene-based mesh. Surg Infect 2007;8:337–41.

56. Alaedeen DI, Lipman J, Medalie D, et al. The single-staged approach to the surgical management of abdominal wall hernias in contaminated fields. Hernia 2007;11:41–5.

57. Hackenberger PN, Eiferman D, Janis JE. "Delayed-Immediate" Hernia Repairs in Infected Wounds: Clinical and Economic Outcomes. Am Surg 2022. https://doi.org/10.1177/00031348221093804.

58. Petro CC, Rosen MJ. A Current Review of Long-Acting Resorbable Meshes in Abdominal Wall Reconstruction. Plast Reconstr Surg 2018;142:84S–91S.

59. Itani KMF, Rosen M, Vargo D, et al. Prospective study of single-stage repair of contaminated hernias using a biologic porcine tissue matrix: the RICH Study. Surgery 2012;152:498–505.

60. Rivera-Buendía F, Franco-Cendejas R, Román-López CG, et al. Randomized Controlled Trial to Reduce Bacterial Colonization of Surgical Drains with the Use of Chlorhexidine-Coated Dressings After Breast Cancer Surgery. Ann Surg Oncol 2019;26:3883–91.

61. Bejko J, Tarzia V, Carrozzini M, et al. Comparison of Efficacy and Cost of Iodine Impregnated Drape vs. Standard Drape in Cardiac Surgery: Study in 5100 Patients. J Cardiovasc Transl Res 2015;8:431–7.

62. Webster J, Alghamdi A. Use of plastic adhesive drapes during surgery for preventing surgical site infection. Cochrane Database Syst Rev 2015;2015.

63. Ward WG, Cooper JM, Lippert D, et al. Glove and gown effects on intraoperative bacterial contamination. Ann Surg 2014;259:591–7.

64. Fatula LK, Nelson A, Abbad H, et al. Antibiotic Irrigation of the Surgical Site Decreases Incidence of Surgical Site Infection after Open Ventral Hernia Repair. Am Surg 2018;84:1146–51.

65. Mirel S, Pusta A, Moldovan M, et al. Antimicrobial Meshes for Hernia Repair: Current Progress and Perspectives. J Clin Med 2022;11:883.
66. Ventral Hernia Working G, Breuing K, Butler CE, et al. Incisional ventral hernias: review of the literature and recommendations regarding the grading and technique of repair. Surgery 2010;148:544–58.
67. Stremitzer S, Bachleitner-Hofmann T, Gradl B, et al. Mesh graft infection following abdominal hernia repair: risk factor evaluation and strategies of mesh graft preservation. A retrospective analysis of 476 operations. World J Surg 2010;34: 1702–9.
68. Cox TC, Blair LJ, Huntington CR, et al. The cost of preventable comorbidities on wound complications in open ventral hernia repair. J Surg Res 2016;206:214–22.
69. Plymale MA, Davenport DL, Walsh-Blackmore S, et al. Costs and Complications Associated with Infected Mesh for Ventral Hernia Repair. Surg Infect 2020;21: 343–8.
70. Mauch JT, Mellia JA, Heniford BT, et al. End-Stage Hernia Disease: A Conceptual Framework. Plast Reconstr Surg 2021;148:165e–6e.

Moving?

Make sure your subscription moves with you!

To notify us of your new address, find your **Clinics Account Number** (located on your mailing label above your name), and contact customer service at:

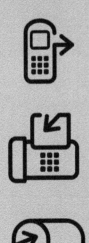

Email: journalscustomerservice-usa@elsevier.com

800-654-2452 (subscribers in the U.S. & Canada)
314-447-8871 (subscribers outside of the U.S. & Canada)

Fax number: 314-447-8029

Elsevier Health Sciences Division
Subscription Customer Service
3251 Riverport Lane
Maryland Heights, MO 63043

Printed and bound by CPI Group (UK) Ltd, Croydon, CR0 4YY

03/10/2024

01040470-0008